An Update on Pediatric Oncology and Hematology

Guest Editors

MAX J. COPPES, MD, PhD, MBA
RUSSELL E. WARE, MD, PhD
JEFFREY S. DOME, MD, PhD

HEMATOLOGY/ONCOLOGY CLINICS OF NORTH AMERICA

www.hemonc.theclinics.com

Consulting Editors
GEORGE P. CANELLOS, MD
NANCY BERLINER, MD

February 2010 • Volume 24 • Number 1

SAUNDERS an imprint of ELSEVIER, Inc.

W.B. SAUNDERS COMPANY
A Division of Elsevier Inc.

1600 John F. Kennedy Blvd. • Suite 1800 • Philadelphia, PA 19103-2899

http://www.theclinics.com

HEMATOLOGY/ONCOLOGY CLINICS OF NORTH AMERICA Volume 24, Number 1
February 2010 ISSN 0889-8588, ISBN 13: 978-1-4377-2202-4

Editor: Kerry Holland

Hematology/Oncology Clinics (ISSN 0889-8588) is published bimonthly by Elsevier Inc., 360 Park Avenue South, New York, NY 10010-1710. Months of issue are February, April, June, August, October, and December. Business and Editorial Offices: 1600 John F. Kennedy Blvd., Ste. 1800, Philadelphia, PA 19103–2899. Customer Service Office: 3251 Riverport Lane, Maryland Heights, MO 63043. Periodicals postage paid at New York, NY and at additional mailing offices. Subscription prices are $306.00 per year (domestic individuals), $483.00 per year (domestic institutions), $152.00 per year (domestic students/residents), $347.00 per year (Canadian individuals), $591.00 per year (Canadian institutions) $413.00 per year (international individuals), $591.00 per year (international institutions), and $206.00 per year (international and Canadian students/residents). International air speed delivery is included in all *Clinics* subscription prices. All prices are subject to change without notice. **POSTMASTER:** Send address changes to *Hematology/Oncology Clinics of North America*, Elsevier Health Sciences Division, Subscription Customer Service, 3251 Riverport Lane, Maryland Heights, MO 63043. Customer Service (orders, claims, online, change of address): Elsevier Health Sciences Division, Subscription Customer Service, 3251 Riverport Lane, Maryland Heights, MO 63043. Tel: 1-800-654-2452 (U.S. and Canada); 314-447-8871(outside U.S. and Canada). Fax: 314-447-8029. E-mail: journalscustomerservice-usa@elsevier.com (for print support); journalsonlinesupport-usa@elsevier.com (for online support).

Reprints. For copies of 100 or more, of articles in this publication, please contact the Commercial Reprints Department, Elsevier Inc., 360 Park Avenue South, New York, New York 10010-1710; Tel.: 212-633-3813, Fax: 212-462-1935, E-mail: reprints@elsevier.com.

Hematology/Oncology Clinics of North America is covered in *MEDLINE/PubMed (Index Medicus), EMBASE/ Excerpta Medica, and BIOSIS.*

Printed and bound in the United Kingdom
Transferred to Digital Print 2011

Contributors

CONSULTING EDITORS

GEORGE P. CANELLOS, MD
William Rosenberg Professor of Medicine, Department of Medical Oncology, Dana-Farber
Cancer Institute, Boston, Massachusetts

NANCY BERLINER, MD
Chief, Division of Hematology, Brigham and Women's Hospital; Professor of Medicine,
Harvard Medical School, Boston, Massachusetts

GUEST EDITORS

MAX J. COPPES, MD, PhD, MBA
Senior Vice President, Center for Cancer and Blood Disorders, Children's National
Medical Center; Director, Center for Cancer and Immunology Research, Children's
Research Institute; Professor of Medicine, Pediatrics and Oncology, Georgetown
University; Clinical Professor of Pediatrics, George Washington University,
Washington, DC

RUSSELL E. WARE, MD, PhD
Lemuel W. Diggs Chair in Hematology, Member, and Chair, Department of Hematology,
St. Jude Children's Research Hospital; and Professor of Pediatrics, University
of Tennessee Health Sciences Center, Memphis, Tennessee

JEFFREY S. DOME, MD, PhD
Chief, Division of Oncology, Center for Cancer and Blood Disorders, Children's National
Medical Center, Washington, DC

AUTHORS

TIMOTHY J. BERNARD, MD
Assistant Professor of Pediatrics, Department of Child Neurology; Co-Director, Pediatric
Stroke Program, University of Colorado and The Children's Hospital; and Mountain States
Regional Hemophilia and Thrombosis Center, Aurora, Colorado

VICTOR BLANCHETTE, FRCP
Chief, Division of Hematology/Oncology, The Hospital for Sick Children; and Department
of Pediatrics, University of Toronto, Toronto, Ontario, Canada

PAULA BOLTON-MAGGS, DM, FRCP
University Department of Hematology, Manchester Royal Infirmary, Manchester,
United Kingdom

HUIB CARON, MD, PhD
Professor of Pediatric Oncology, Department of Pediatric Oncology and Hematology,
Emma Children's Hospital AMC, Amesterdam, the Netherlands

WILLIAM L. CARROLL, MD
Director, Palliative Care Program, Division of Pediatric Hematology/Oncology, New York
University Medical Center, New York, New York

MELODY J. CUNNINGHAM, MD
Director, Palliative Care Program, Le Bonheur Children's Medical Center, Memphis, Tennessee

ANGELIKA EGGERT, MD
Professor of Pediatrics and Head of Pediatric Cancer Research, Department of Hematology/Oncology, University Children's Hospital Essen, Hufelandstr, Essen, Germany

TERRY J. FRY, MD
Chief, Division of Blood/Marrow Transplantation and Immunology, Center for Cancer and Blood Disorders, Children's National Medical Center; and Associate Professor of Pediatrics, George Washington University, Washington, DC

BRENDA GIBSON, MD, Department of Paediatric Haemotology, Royal Hospital for Sick Children, Glasgow, Scotland, United Kingdom

NEIL A. GOLDENBERG, MD
Assistant Professor of Pediatrics and Medicine; Co-Director, Pediatric Stroke Program, University of Colorado and The Children's Hospital; and Associate Director, Mountain States Regional Hemophilia and Thrombosis Center, Aurora, Colorado

MATTHEW M. HEENEY, MD
Instructor of Pediatrics, Department of Pediatrics, Harvard Medical School; and Division of Hematology/Oncology, Children's Hospital Boston, Boston, Massachusetts

JOHANN HITZLER, FRCP(C), FAAP
Assistant Professor, Division of Hematology/Oncology, The Hospital for Sick Children; and Developmental and Stem Cell Biology, The Hospital for Sick Children Research Institute, University of Toronto, Toronto, Ontario, Canada

W. KEITH HOOTS, MD
Professor, Division of Pediatrics, Hematology Section, The University of Texas Health Sciences Center; and Medical Director, Gulf States Hemophilia and Thrombophilia Center, Houston, Texas

LEONTIEN C.M. KREMER, MD, PhD
Department of Pediatric Oncology, Emma Children's Hospital/Academic Medical Center, Amsterdam, the Netherlands

JANET L. KWIATKOWSKI, MD, MSCE
Assistant Professor of Pediatrics, University of Pennsylvania School of Medicine; and Attending Hematologist, Division of Hematology, The Children's Hospital of Philadelphia, Philadelphia, Pennsylvania

ARJAN C. LANKESTER, MD, PhD
Pediatrician and Immunologist, Department of Pediatrics, BMT-Unit, Leiden University Medical Center, Leiden, the Netherlands

TOBEY MacDONALD, MD
Attending Oncologist and Director, Neuro-Oncology Program, Center for Cancer and Blood Disorders; and Center for Cancer Immunology Research, Children's National Medical Center; Associate Professor of Pediatrics, The George Washington University School of Medicine and Health Sciences, Washington, DC

PAUL C. NATHAN, MD, MSc
Division of Hematology/Oncology, Hospital for Sick Children, Toronto, Ontario, Canada

KEVIN C. OEFFINGER, MD
Director, Adult Long-Term Follow-up Program, Departments of Pediatrics and Medicine, Memorial Sloan-Kettering Cancer Center, New York, New York

ROGER J. PACKER, MD
Executive Director, Center for Neuroscience and Behavioral Medicine; Chairman, Division of Neurology; and Director, The Brain Tumor Institute, Children's National Medical Center; Professor of Neurology and Pediatrics, The George Washington University School of Medicine and Health Sciences, Washington, DC

JULIE R. PARK, MD
Associate Professor of Pediatrics, Division of Hematology and Oncology, University of Washington School of Medicine, and Seattle Children's Hospital, Seattle, Washington

ROB PIETERS, MD, MSc, PhD
Head, Department of Pediatric Oncology and Hematology, Erasmus MC-Sophia Children's Hospital, Rotterdam, the Netherlands

DIRK REINHARDT, PD
Ausserplanmassiger Professor, AML-BFM Study Group, Pediatric Hematology/ Oncology, Hannover Medical School, Hannover, Germany

NIDRA I. RODRIGUEZ, MD
Assistant Professor, Division of Pediatrics, Hematology Section, The University of Texas Health Sciences Center; and Assistant Professor, Gulf States Hemophilia and Thrombophilia Center, Houston, Texas

JEFFREY E. RUBNITZ, MD, PhD
Associate Member, Department of Oncology, St. Jude Children's Research Hospital, Memphis, Tennessee

FRANKLIN O. SMITH, MD
Marjory J. Johnson Endowed Chair, Professor of Pediatrics, and Director, Division of Hematology/Oncology, University of Cincinnati College of Medicine, Cincinnati Children's Hospital Medical Center, Cincinnati, Ohio

GILBERT VEZINA, MD
Chief, Division of Neuro-Radiology, Children's National Medical Center; and Professor of Radiology and Pediatrics, The George Washington University School of Medicine and Health Sciences, Washington, DC

PARESH VYAS, FRCPath, DPHil
Reader in Haemato-Oncology, MRC Molecular Haemotology Unit, John Radcliffe Hospital, Weatherall Institute of Molecular Medicine, University of Oxford, Headington, Oxford, United Kingdom

RUSSELL E. WARE, MD, PhD
Lemuel W. Diggs Chair in Hematology, Member, and Chair, Department of Hematology, St. Jude's Children Research Hospital; and Professor of Pediatrics, University of Tennessee Health Sciences Center, Memphis, Tennessee

C. MICHEL ZWAAN, MD, PhD
Department of Pediatric Oncology/Hematology, Erasmus MC-Sophia Children's Hospital, Rotterdam, the Netherlands

Contents

Acute lymphoblastic leukemia (ALL), the most common type of cancer in children, is a heterogeneous disease in which many genetic lesions result in the development of multiple biologic subtypes. Today, with intensive multiagent chemotherapy, most children who have ALL are cured. The many national or institutional ALL therapy protocols in use tend to stratify patients in a multitude of different ways to tailor treatment to the rate of relapse. This article discusses the factors used in risk stratification and the treatment of pediatric ALL.

Children with Down syndrome have an increased risk for developing both acute myeloid as well as lymphoblastic leukemia. These leukemias differ in presenting characteristics and underlying biology when compared with leukemias occurring in non-Down syndrome children. Myeloid leukemia in children with Down syndrome is preceded by a preleukemic clone (transient leukemia or transient myeloproliferative disorder), which may disappear spontaneously, but may also need treatment in case of severe symptoms. Twenty percent of children with transient leukemia subsequently develop myeloid leukemia. This transition offers a unique model to study the stepwise development of leukemia and of gene dosage effects mediated by aneuploidy.

Acute myeloid leukemia (AML) is a heterogeneous group of leukemias that result from clonal transformation of hematopoietic precursors through the acquisition of chromosomal rearrangements and multiple gene mutations. As a result of highly collaborative clinical research by pediatric cooperative cancer groups worldwide, disease-free survival has improved significantly during the past 3 decades. Further improvements in outcomes of children who have AML probably will reflect continued progress in understanding the biology of AML and the concomitant development of new molecularly targeted agents for use in combination with conventional chemotherapy drugs.

> Neuroblastoma, a neoplasm of the sympathetic nervous system, is the second most common extracranial malignant tumor of childhood and the most common solid tumor of infancy. Neuroblastoma is a heterogeneous malignancy with prognosis ranging from near uniform survival to high risk for fatal demise. Neuroblastoma serves as a paradigm for the prognostic utility of biologic and clinical data and the potential to tailor therapy for patient cohorts at low, intermediate, and high risk for recurrence. This article summarizes our understanding of neuroblastoma biology and prognostic features and discusses their impact on current and proposed risk stratification schemas, risk-based therapeutic approaches, and the development of novel therapies for patients at high risk for failure.

> Central nervous system (CNS) tumors comprise 15% to 20% of all malignancies occurring in childhood and adolescence. They may present in a myriad of ways, often delaying diagnosis. Symptoms and signs depend on the growth rate of the tumor, its location in the central nervous system (CNS), and the age of the child. This article describes the presentation, diagnosis, and management of these tumors.

> The past 25 years have seen an increase in our understanding of immunology and further expansion in the clinical use of immunotherapeutic modalities. How immunotherapy will be integrated with chemotherapy, radiation, and surgery remains to be established. Although there have been successes in the field of immunotherapy, they have been inconsistent, and it is hoped that increased understanding of the basic principles of immunology will improve the consistency of beneficial effects. In this article, we briefly provide a general overview of our current understanding of the immune system, with a focus on concepts in tumor immunology, followed by a discussion of how these concepts are being used in the clinic.

> Childhood cancer survivors are at increased risk of serious morbidity, premature mortality, and diminished health status. Proactive and anticipatory risk-based health care of survivors and healthy lifestyles can reduce these risks. In this article, the authors first briefly discuss four common problems of survivors: neurocognitive dysfunction, cardiovascular disease, infertility and gonadal dysfunction, and psychosocial problems. Second, the

authors discuss the concept of risk-based care, promote the use of recently developed evidence-based guidelines, describe current care in the United States, Canada, and the Netherlands, and articulate a model for shared survivor care that aims to optimize life long health of survivors and improve two-way communication between the cancer center and the primary care physician.

Neil A. Goldenberg and Timothy J. Bernard

With improved pediatric survival from serious underlying illnesses, greater use of invasive vascular procedures and devices, and a growing awareness that vascular events occur among the young, venous thromboembolism (VTE) increasingly is recognized as a critical pediatric concern. This review provides background on etiology and epidemiology in this disorder, followed by an indepth discussion of approaches to the clinical characterization, diagnostic evaluation, and management of pediatric VTE. Prognostic indicators and long-term outcomes are considered, with emphasis on available evidence underlying current knowledge and key questions for further investigation.

Timothy J. Bernard and Neil A. Goldenberg

Arterial ischemic stroke (AIS) is a rare disorder in children. Research suggests that risk factors, outcomes, and presentation are different from those of adult stroke. In particular, prothrombotic abnormalities and large vessel arteriopathies that are nonatherosclerotic seem to play a large role in the pathogenesis of childhood AIS. This review examines the epidemiology and etiologies of neonatal and childhood AIS and provides a detailed discussion of approaches to the clinical characterization, diagnostic evaluation, and management. Long-term outcomes of recurrent AIS and neuromotor, speech, cognitive, and behavioral deficits are considered. Emphasis is on evidence underlying current knowledge and key questions for further investigation.

Nidra I. Rodriguez and W. Keith Hoots

This article describes recent clinical and research advances in hemophilia therapy. Different prophylactic regimens for the management of severe hemophilia are described along with the use of adjuvant treatment options to achieve hemostasis. The safety and efficacy of radionuclide synovectomy with phosphorus 32-sulfur colloid to treat existing joint arthropathy also are described. The development of inhibitors to factor VIII or IX remains a challenge for hemophilia care and recent approaches to achieve immune tolerance induction are discussed. Finally, recent advances in hemophilia are mentioned, including the role of iron, inflammation, and angiogenesis in the pathogenesis of hemophilic arthopathy.

RELATED INTEREST

Clinics in Laboratory Medicine, June 2009 (Vol. 29, No. 2)
Hemostasis and Coagulation
Henry M. Rinder, MD, *Guest Editor*

THE CLINICS ARE NOW AVAILABLE ONLINE!

Access your subscription at:
www.theclinics.com

Preface

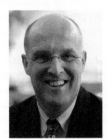 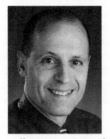 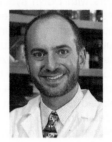

Max J. Coppes, MD, PhD, MBA   Russell E. Ware, MD, PhD   Jeffrey S. Dome, MD, PhD
Guest Editors

The last decade had seen many exciting developments in oncology and hematology. In large part this has been the result of the improved ability to translate laboratory observations to patient care. This is nicely exemplified by the introduction of antibodies targeting tumor-specific antigens, anti-angiogenic compounds, small molecules targeting the genetic lesions that drive cancer cells, and bioactive compounds affecting hematopoiesis or hemostasis. The readers of *Hematology/Oncology Clinics of North America* are probably very familiar with new developments as they pertain to adults. This particular issue highlights some of the exciting developments in pediatric oncology and hematology. The articles were selected from back-to-back issues of the *Pediatric Clinics of North America*, 1 focusing on pediatric oncology and 1 focusing on pediatric hematology. The rationale for the back-to-back issues is that some, mostly large, pediatric hospitals have begun to separate these 2 subspecialties. For many decades, the subspecialties of pediatric hematology and pediatric oncology have been practiced by the same individuals. However, some institutions have come to the realization that the knowledge base and experience to function optimally as a pediatric hematologist or oncologist mandate an operational if not formal separation. The separation of pediatric hematology and oncology disciplines allows specialists to focus on either malignant disorders such as leukemias and lymphomas, solid tumors, and brain tumors or specific nonmalignant hematologic disorders such as sickle cell disease, transfusion medicine, or clotting disorders. We believe that a focused approach is required to further develop these exciting fields of medicine.

With regard to pediatric oncology, this issue includes 3 articles on leukemia, the most common form of pediatric cancer. One article provides an update on acute lymphoblastic leukemia (ALL), with an emphasis on the evolving molecular classification and risk stratification for this disease. A second article focuses on acute myeloid leukemia (AML), highlighting recent improvements in outcome, although much more

Hematol Oncol Clin N Am 24 (2010) xiii–xv
doi:10.1016/j.hoc.2009.12.001
0889-8588/10/$ – see front matter © 2010 Elsevier Inc. All rights reserved.

progress needs to made. A third article is devoted to acute leukemia in patients with Down syndrome, who are at increased risk of developing acute leukemia. AML in patients with Down syndrome is associated with the development of preleukemic clones and transient leukemia; ALL is not associated with an overt preleukemic phase. This issue also includes articles on tumors for which cure remains a challenge: central nervous system (CNS) tumors and neuroblastoma, and an article on advances in cancer immunotherapy. As overall childhood cancer survival rates have improved, the cost of cure is rapidly becoming evident. An article on the challenges experienced by adults who survived a childhood cancer is included. Slowly, guidelines are being developed to ensure that children cured of their cancer have access to health care services tailored to their unique needs. Unlike in adults, the normal (healthy) tissues of children treated for cancer are still in active development and experiencing growth bursts. Consequently, the long-term effects of cancer treatment are not only serious, but, as we have now started to realize, affect a significant proportion of survivors.

Unlike pediatric oncology, for which most treatments are directed or have been established by prospective randomized clinical trials, the management of many primary hematologic conditions in children lacks such guidance. For some conditions, most notably sickle cell disease and, more recently, disorders of hemostasis, the need for prospective clinical trials is currently being addressed, but for other hematologic conditions, some of which are rare, pediatric hematologists need to determine management based on a review of the literature and experience. The articles selected for this issue cover aspects that most hematologists, pediatricians, and pediatric hematologists deal with on a regular basis (eg, sickle cell disease, thalassemia, hemophilia, immune thrombocytopenic purpura [ITP], and thrombosis), but which continue to pose challenges with regard to optimal management. As some authors indicate, we anticipate that the future of pediatric hematology will include a better understanding of the biology that leads to hematologic diseases and multi-institutional trials to further improve life expectancy and/or quality of life of children affected by these disorders.

Many of the contributions in this issue are authored by colleagues from different countries. This reflects that the worlds of pediatric oncology and pediatric hematology are shrinking. This is good as further gains in outcome will require large, occasionally international, clinical trials. We hope that the readers will experience some of the same stimulation and excitement the editors felt as we communicated with the authors.

Max J. Coppes, MD, PhD, MBA
Center for Cancer and Blood Disorders &
Center for Cancer and Immunology Research
Children's National Medical Center
111 Michigan Avenue NW
Washington, DC 20010, USA

Russell E. Ware, MD, PhD
Department of Hematology
St. Jude Children's Research Hospital
262 Danny Thomas Place, MS 355
Memphis, TN 38105, USA

Jeffrey S. Dome, MD, PhD
Division of Oncology, Center for Cancer and Blood Disorders
Children's National Medical Center
111 Michigan Avenue NW
Washington, DC 20010, USA

E-mail addresses:
mcoppes@cnmc.org (M.J. Coppes)
russell.ware@stjude.org (R.E. Ware)
jdome@cnmc.org (J.S. Dome)

Biology and Treatment of Acute Lymphoblastic Leukemia

Rob Pieters, MD, MSc, PhD[a],*, William L. Carroll, MD[b]

KEYWORDS

• Acute lymphoblastic leukemia • Children • Adolescents
• Chemotherapy • Genomics • Targeted therapy

Acute lymphoblastic leukemia (ALL), the most common type of cancer in children, is a heterogeneous disease in which many genetic lesions result in the development of multiple biologic subtypes. The etiology of ALL is characterized by the acquisition of multiple consecutive genetic alterations in the (pre)leukemic cells. In the most common genetic subtypes of ALL, the first hit occurs in utero,[1] as evidenced, for example, by the presence of the *TEL/AML1* gene fusion or hyperdiploidy in neonatal blood spots on Guthrie cards. These first genetic abnormalities are, in fact, initiating preleukemic cells, not leukemic ones, because most children whose neonatal blood spots show a genetic defect typically associated with leukemia never develop leukemia. Also, such preleukemic cells harbor additional genetic abnormalities. T-cell acute lymphoblastic leukemia (T-ALL) is an exception, because the majority of genetic lesions described in T-ALL seem not to occur in the neonatal blood spots.[2]

Today, with intensive multiagent chemotherapy, most children who have ALL are cured. The factors that account for the dramatic improvement in survival during the past 40 years include the identification of effective drugs and combination chemotherapy through large, randomized clinical trials, the recognition of sanctuary sites and the integration of presymptomatic central nervous system (CNS) prophylaxis, intensification of treatment using existing drugs, and risk-based stratification of treatment. The many national or institutional ALL therapy protocols in use tend to stratify patients in a multitude of different ways. Treatment results often are not published for the overall patient group but rather are reported only for selected subsets of patients. This limitation hampers the comparison of outcomes in protocols. In 2000,

A version of this article was previously published in the *Pediatric Clinics of North America*, 55:1.
[a] Department of Pediatric Oncology and Hematology, Erasmus MC-Sophia Children's Hospital, Dr Molewaterplein 60, 3015GJ Rotterdam, The Netherlands
[b] Division of Pediatric Hematology/Oncology, New York University Medical Center, 160 East 32nd Street, 2nd Floor, New York, NY 10016, USA
* Corresponding author.
E-mail address: rob.pieters@erasmusmc.nl (R. Pieters).

the results of ALL trials run in the early 1990s by the major study groups were presented in a uniform way.[3–12] The 5-year event-free survival (EFS) rates seemed not to vary widely, ranging from 71% to 83% (**Table 1**). Overall remission rates usually were 98% or higher.

Risk-based stratification allows the tailoring of treatment according to the predicted risk of relapse. Children who have high-risk features receive aggressive treatment to prevent disease recurrence, and patients who have a good prognosis receive effective therapy but are not exposed to unnecessary treatment with associated short- and long-term side effects. Clinical factors that predict outcome and are used for stratification of patients into treatment arms are age, gender, and white blood cell count at presentation. Biologic factors with prognostic value are the immunophenotype and genotype of the leukemia cells. Another predictive factor is the rapidity of response to early therapy, such as the decrease in peripheral blood blast count in response to a week of prednisone or the decrease in bone marrow blasts after 1 to 3 weeks of multiagent chemotherapy. More recently the determination of minimal residual disease (MRD) in the bone marrow during the first months of therapy using flow cytometry or molecular techniques has been shown to have a high prognostic value and therefore is used for stratification in many contemporary trials. The detection of MRD accurately distinguishes very good responders to therapy from those who will respond poorly to therapy, irrespective of the biologic subtype of ALL and the underlying mechanism of this response.[13] In several protocols, MRD is used to stratify patients for reduction of therapy (ie, patients who are MRD negative especially at early time points) or intensification of therapy (ie, patients who are MRD positive at later time points).

| Table 1 | | | | | |
| **Treatment results from major clinical trials in childhood acute lymphoblastic leukemia conducted in the early 1990s** | | | | | |
Study Group	Years of Study	Patient Number	Overall 5-year Event-free Survival (%)	B-lineage ALL 5-year Event-free Survival (%)	T-lineage ALL 5-year Event-free Survival (%)
DFCI-91-01	1991–1995	377	83	84	79
BFM-90	1990–1995	2178	78	80	61
NOPHO-ALL92	1992–1998	1143	78	79	61
COALL-92	1992–1997	538	77	78	71
SJCRH-13A	1991–1994	167	77	80	61
CCG-1800	1989–1995	5121	75	75	73
DCOG-ALL8	1991–1996	467	73	73	71
EORTC-58881	1989–1998	2065	71	72	64
AIEOP-91	1991–1995	1194	71	75	40
UKALL-XI	1990–1997	2090	63	63	59

Abbreviations: AIEOP, Associazione Italiana Ematologia Oncologia Pediatrica; BMF, Berlin-Frankfurt-Münster; CCG, Children's Cancer Group; COALL, Co-operative Study Group of Childhood Acute Lymphoblastic Leukemia; DCOG, Dutch Childhood Oncology Group; DFCI, Dana Farber Cancer Institute; EORTC-CLG European Organization for the Research and Treatment of Cancer; NOPHO, Nordic Society of Pediatric Haematology and Oncology; SJCHR, St Jude Children's Research Hospital; UKALL United Kingdom Acute Lymphoblastic Leukemia.

AGE AND IMMUNOPHENOTYPE

Over the years, age has remained an independent predictor of outcome (**Table 2**). Children aged 1 to 9 years have the best outcome; children and adolescents aged 10 to 20 years have a slightly worse outcome, which is associated in part with a higher incidence of T-cell leukemia and a lower incidence of favorable genetic abnormalities such as *TEL/AML1* and hyperdiploidy. For adults, survival rates decrease further with increasing age. When results are corrected for differences in immunophenotype, ALL cells from older children and adults are more resistant to multiple antileukemic drugs than are cells from children in the first decade of life.[14,15]

Infants diagnosed at less than 1 year of age have a relatively poor outcome that is associated with a high incidence of the unfavorable very immature proB-ALL phenotype and especially the presence of *MLL* gene rearrangements.[16] The poor outcome has led physicians in the United States, Japan, and the International Interfant collaborative group including European and non-European countries and institutes to develop specific protocols to treat infant ALL.[13,17,18] Biologic characteristics of infant ALL cells are described later in the paragraph discussing the *MLL* gene.

T-cell ALL is detected in approximately 15% of childhood ALL. It is characterized by a relative resistance to different classes of drugs when compared with B-lineage ALL.[14] T-cell ALL cells accumulate less methotrexate polyglutamates and less cytarabine triphosphate than precursor B-ALL cells.[19] With risk-adapted therapy the outcome of T-cell ALL now approaches that of B-lineage ALL in many study groups (see **Table 1**).

Approximately 85% of childhood ALL is of B lineage, mainly common or preB ALL. A very immature subtype characterized by the lack of CD10 expression (proB ALL) is associated with a high incidence of *MLL* gene rearrangements and an unfavorable outcome. Mature B-lineage ALL, defined by the presence of immunoglobulins on the cell surface, has a favorable outcome only when treated with B-non-Hodgkin lymphoma protocols.

GENETICS
Hyperdiploidy

Hyperdiploidy (a DNA index > 1.16 or > 50 chromosomes per leukemia cell) is found in approximately 25% of children who have B-lineage ALL. It is associated with a favorable outcome, especially when extra copies of chromosome 4, 10 or 17 are present.[20] Hyperdiploid ALL cells have an increased tendency to undergo apoptosis, accumulate

---

Table 2
Clinical and biologic factors predicting clinical outcome

Factor	Favorable	Unfavorable
Age at diagnosis	1–9 years	<1 or >9 years
Sex	Female	Male
White blood cell count	Low (eg, <50 or <25 × 10^9/L)	High (eg, >50 or >25 × 10^9/L)
Genotype	Hyperdiploidy (>50 chromosomes) t(12;21) or *TEL/AML1* fusion	Hypodiploidy (<45 chromosomes) t(9;22) or *BCR/ABL* fusion t(4;11) or *MLL/AF4* fusion
Immunophenotype	Common, preB	ProB, T-lineage

high amounts of methotrexate polyglutamates, and are highly sensitive to antimetabolites and L-asparaginase.[21]

TEL/AML1

The *TEL/AML1* fusion, also found in approximately 25% of cases, is mutually exclusive with hyperdiploidy and also is associated with a favorable outcome. It is formed by a fusion of the *TEL* gene on chromosome 12 encoding for a nuclear phosphoprotein of the ETS family of transcription factors and the *AML1* gene on chromosome 21, a transcription factor gene encoding for part of the core-binding factor. The *TEL/AML1* fusion probably inhibits the transcription activity of the normal *AML1* gene involved in proliferation and differentiation of hematopoietic cells. *TEL/AML1* fusion is associated with a high chemosensitivity, especially for L-asparaginase.[22] The mechanism behind this asparaginase sensitivity remains unclear but is not caused by a low asparagines synthetase activity in the leukemic cells.[23,24] *TEL/AML1*-rearranged cells also may be more sensitive to other drugs, especially anthracyclines and etoposide.[25]

Both hyperdiploidy and *TEL/AML1* occur mainly in children younger than 10 years of age with common/preB ALL and are rare above this age and in other ALL immunophenotypes.

MLL

Abnormalities of the mixed lineage leukemia (*MLL*) gene on chromosome 11q23 occur in only approximately 2% of children above the age of 1 year, although it is present in approximately 80% of infants who have ALL. All types of *MLL* gene rearrangements, such as *MLL/AF4* created by t(4;11), *MLL/ENL* created by t(11;19), and *MLL/AF9* created by t(9;11), are associated with a poor outcome in infants who have ALL[17]; in older children this poor outcome may only hold true for the presence of *MLL/AF4*.[26] The *MLL/AF9* rearrangement occurs in older infants and is characterized by a more mature pattern of immunoglobulin gene rearrangements, suggesting another pathogenesis.[17,27]

The precise actions of the fusion products involving *MLL* are not known, but they are associated with abnormal expression of *HOX* genes, which may lead to abnormal growth of hematopoietic stem cells.[28] ALL cells with *MLL* gene abnormalities are highly resistant to glucocorticoids in vitro and in vivo and also to L-asparaginase.[14,17,29] These cells, however, show a marked sensitivity to the nucleoside analogues cytarabine and cladribine.[30] This sensitivity is related to a high expression of the membrane nucleoside transporter ENT1.[31] *MLL*-rearranged ALL cells do not show a defective methotrexate polyglutamation[32] and have no overexpression of multidrug resistance proteins.[33] Methotrexate pharmacokinetics might be different in the youngest infants.[34]

BCR-ABL

The translocation t(9;22) fuses the *BCR* gene on chromosome 22 to the *ABL* gene on chromosome 9 causing an abnormal *ABL* tyrosine kinase activity associated with increased proliferation and decreased apoptosis. The *BCR/ABL* fusion is found mainly in common and preB ALL. The incidence of *BCR/ABL* increases with age: it is seen in approximately 3% of children who have ALL but in approximately 25% of adults who have ALL. The presence of *BCR/ABL* predicts a poor outcome.

Children who have *BCR/ABL*-rearranged ALL or *MLL*-rearranged ALL more often show a poor response to prednisone [29,35] and have high levels of MRD after induction therapy.

Genetics in T-cell Acute Lymphoblastic Leukemia

The prognostic value of genetic abnormalities in T-ALL is less clear.[36] Ectopic expression of *TAL-1* is caused by the translocation t(1;14) in only a few percent of T-ALL cases or, more often, by the *SIL-TAL* fusion transcript. Activation of *HOX11* by the translocations t(10;14) and t(7;10) occur in approximately 10% of T-ALL cases. Two recently described abnormalities occur frequently and exclusively in T-ALL. These are the ectopic expression of *HOX11L2*, mainly caused by the translocation t(5;14), in approximately 25% of T-ALL cases and activating mutations of the *NOTCH1* gene in 50% of T-ALL cases. *NOTCH1* mutations are not associated with a poor outcome and may be associated with a favorable outcome.[37]

Others

Many other recurrent genetic and molecular genetic lesions exist in small subsets of childhood ALL such as the translocation t(1;19) leading to a *E2A-PBX1* fusion detected in less than 5% of precursor B-ALL, mainly preB ALL. Although in the past this translocation had been associated with a poor prognosis, this is not longer true with contemporary treatment protocols. Two percent of precursor B-lineage ALL cases harbor an intrachromosomal amplification of chromosome 21 that is associated with poor survival.[38] Hypodiploidy (<45 chromosomes) is detected in only 1% of children who have ALL and is associated with poor outcome, particularly in the low-hypodiploid (33–39 chromosomes) or near-haploid cases (23–29 chromosomes) as shown in a recent retrospective international study.[39]

A discussion of all other abnormalities is beyond the scope of this article. It should be mentioned that children who have Down syndrome and ALL do not have a better outcome and perhaps even have a worse outcome than other ALL cases because they lack favorable genetic features.[40,41]

THERAPY

The backbone of contemporary multiagent chemotherapeutic regimens is formed by four elements: induction, CNS-directed treatment and consolidation, reinduction, and maintenance.

Induction

The goal of induction therapy is to induce morphologic remission and to restore normal hematopoiesis. Induction therapy contains at least three systemic drugs (ie, a glucocorticoid, vincristine, and L-asparaginase) and intrathecal therapy. The addition of an anthracycline as a fourth drug is matter of debate. In some protocols all patients receive an anthracycline; in other protocols it is reserved for high-risk cases. The induction phase aims to induce complete morphologic remission in 4 to 6 weeks.

Central Nervous System–Directed Treatment and Consolidation

CNS-directed therapy aims to prevent CNS relapses and to reduce the systemic minimal residual leukemia burden. CNS therapy usually is achieved by weekly or biweekly intrathecal therapy along with systemically administered drugs such as high-dose methotrexate (MTX) and 6-mercaptopurine (6-MP). Some groups rely on other drugs (eg, cyclophosphamide, cytarabine) in the consolidation phase to reduce systemic tumor burden further.

Reinduction

Reinduction therapy or delayed (re)intensification most often uses drugs comparable to those used during induction and consolidation therapy and has clearly shown its value by reducing the risk of relapse.

Maintenance

Therapy for ALL is completed by prolonged maintenance therapy for a total treatment duration of 2 years, or even longer in some protocols. Maintenance consists of daily 6-MP and weekly MTX. In some protocols additional pulsed applications of a glucocorticoid and vincristine and intrathecal therapy are administered.

A fifth element, allogeneic stem cell transplantation (SCT), is reserved for only a small number of selected patients in first complete remission. The contribution of specific parts of treatment depends on the total therapy administered to a patient. A few important topics for which new data have been produced recently are discussed in the following sections.

Anthracyclines in Induction?

It is unclear if addition of an anthracycline to a three-drug induction regimen is of benefit. Regimens that do not contain anthracycline are less myelosuppressive. Studies performed by the Children's Cancer Group, however, showed that selected patients younger than 10 years of age did not benefit from the addition of an anthracycline, whereas selected older children did.[42]

Dexamethasone or Prednisone?

Several recent randomized studies have shown that the substitution of prednisone (approximately 40 mg/m^2) by dexamethasone (approximately 6 mg/m^2) significantly decreases the risk of bone marrow and CNS relapses when used in what are thought to be equipotent dosages.[43,44] One Japanese study, however, did not confirm the advantage of using dexamethasone.[45] The benefit of dexamethasone may result from higher free plasma levels and a better CNS penetration or from the fact that the presumed equivalent antileukemic activity for prednisone/dexamethasone is not a 6:1 dose ratio but is higher, as some (but not all) in vitro experiments suggest.[46,47] At this dose ratio dexamethasone also results in more toxicity than prednisone.[43] In vitro, a strong cross-resistance to prednisone and dexamethasone exists in ALL cells.

Which Dose Intensity of Which Asparaginase?

Randomized studies have revealed that at the same dose schedules, the use of L-asparaginase derived from *Escherichia coli* resulted in significant better EFS and overall survival (OS) rates than when asparaginase derived from *Erwinia chrysanthemi* (Erwinase) was used.[48,49] This difference results from differences in the half-lives of the drugs, and the difference presumably would not be found if Erwinase were given in an adequate dose-intensity schedule. The dose-intensity schedule to achieve complete asparagine depletion is 5000 units/m^2 every 3 days for *E coli* asparaginase. Erwinase must be scheduled more frequently than *E coli* asparaginase to achieve the same asparagine depletion. For the pegylated type of *E coli* asparaginase (PEG-asparaginase), 2500 units/m^2 once every 2 weeks leads to the same pharmacodynamic effects. Lower doses of PEG-asparaginase (1000 units/m^2) also lead to complete asparagine depletion in serum but not in the cerebrospinal fluid.[50]

Intensification of asparaginase in induction and reinduction has improved outcomes in different studies.[51–53] Also, asparaginase intolerance was an important factor predicting an inferior outcome.[54,55] Allergic reactions usually are responsible for the discontinuation of asparaginase. Allergic reactions occur mainly when the drug is readministered in reinduction several weeks after first exposure during induction. In addition, the presence of asparaginase antibodies may lead to inactivation of the drug. Consequently, many investigators favor the use of the less immunogenic PEG-asparaginase from therapy outset rather than using it only after allergic reactions have occurred. In the light of these data, pharmacodynamic monitoring of asparaginase administration may prove very important for individual children who have ALL.

Which Central Nervous System–directed Therapy?

To clarify the role of different CNS-directed therapies, a meta-analysis was published in 2003.[56] From this analysis it became clear that long-term intrathecal therapy leads to EFS rates comparable with those of radiotherapy. Radiotherapy seemed to be more effective than high-dose MTX in preventing CNS relapse, but intravenous MTX reduced systemic relapses, resulting in comparable EFS rates for high-dose MTX and radiotherapy. It was concluded that radiotherapy can be replaced by multiple intrathecal doses of chemotherapy and that intravenous MTX reduces systemic relapses. It is still unclear whether intrathecal triple therapy (glucocorticoid, MTX, cytarabine) has any advantage over the use of intrathecal MTX as single drug. A recent Children's Cancer Group study suggested that intrathecal triple therapy prevented CNS relapse but did not improve OS because fewer bone marrow relapses occurred when intrathecal MTX was used as a single agent.[57]

The results of CNS-directed therapy depend on the treatment used. For example, the use of systemic dexamethasone reduces the incidence of CNS relapse. The comparison of different CNS preventive regimens is hampered because results are described for heterogeneous groups of patients. In several protocols, radiotherapy is still given to selected groups of high-risk patients such as those who have T-ALL with high white cell counts and children who have CNS involvement at diagnosis. Cranial radiotherapy is specifically toxic for very young children because of its detrimental effect on cognitive function.

What Type of Reinduction/Intensification and Maintenance?

Maintenance therapy consists of daily oral 6-MP and weekly intravenous or oral MTX. The intravenous administration of MTX may overcome compliance problems, but there is no evidence that it is more effective than oral MTX. Several randomized studies have shown that the use of thioguanine offers no advantage over 6-MP in maintenance therapy.[58,59] For unknown reasons, 6-MP is more effective when administered in the evening than in the morning. Continuous adaptations of the doses of MTX and 6-MP based on peripheral blood counts are necessary to reduce the risk of relapse, on the one hand, and the risk of infections, on the other.[60,61] There are large interindividual differences in the doses that are tolerated or needed to reduce cell counts. This variability reflects pharmacogenetic differences, for instance in the status of thiopurine methyltransferase, a key enzyme that inactivates thiopurines.[60,62a] Also, large intraindividual differences in doses occur (eg, because of concurrent viral infections). Recently, the major ALL study groups reached consensus on how to adjust the doses of 6-MP and MTX during maintenance so that the white blood cell count remains between 1.5 and 3.0 $\times$ 10^9/L.[62b] Routine measurements of liver function are not necessary in patients who do not have symptoms of liver dysfunction.

A meta-analysis of 42 trials showed that both longer maintenance (3 years versus 2 years) and the use of pulses of vincristine and a glucocorticoid during maintenance result in lower relapse rates but increased death rates.[63] The most important factor that has helped reduce relapses and improve survival is the use of an intensive reinduction course at the start of maintenance therapy. Several randomized studies proved the value of reinduction therapy for childhood ALL.[64,65] Attempts to omit reinduction led to a significant increase in relapse rate.[66] More than 50% of patients who were treated without reinduction did not relapse, however, illustrating that not all patients really need this intensification element. The question, of course, is how to identify these patients early on. When an intensive reinduction course is given, neither longer maintenance nor the use of vincristine/glucocorticoid pulses may contribute significantly to a better OS.[63]

The results of the meta-analysis do not exclude the possibility that subgroups of patients may benefit from a longer duration of maintenance. Several study groups use longer maintenance therapy for boys than for girls. Reduction of the duration of maintenance below 2 years in a Japanese study led to an increased risk of relapse.[67] This study, however, also demonstrates that not all patients need 2 years of maintenance therapy. Again, the important question is how to identify these patients. It might be that a long maintenance therapy is less effective in high-risk leukemias with a very aggressive behavior, such as *MLL* gene–rearranged ALL, *bcr-abl*–positive ALL, and T-ALL, in which relapses occur relatively early; the more smoldering types of ALL, such as hyperdiploid and *TEL/AML1*-gene rearranged ALL, might benefit more from maintenance therapy.

A recent large, randomized study did not show a benefit for the use of pulses with vincristine and a glucocorticoid in a selected group of patients treated on a Berlin/Frankfurt/Münster regimen.[68] The benefit of these pulses therefore may be found only in studies that use no or a less intensive reinduction course, such as in the Dutch Childhood Leukemia Study Group-6 study[69] or in studies in which the upfront therapy is relatively mild.

Who Should (not) be Transplanted?

Autologous SCT is not effective in childhood ALL and therefore should not be performed. A collaborative study of several large study groups has shown that *BCR/ABL*-positive ALL benefits from allogeneic SCT from a matched related donor both in terms of EFS and OS.[12] For other types of donor this benefit was not proven. A comparable analysis for children who had t(4;11) could not detect a beneficial effect of SCT from any type of donor.[26] Recently, a comparison was performed between children who had very high-risk ALL in first remission who were assigned by the availability of a compatible related donor to receive SCT or to receive chemotherapy when no donor was available.[70] "Very high risk" was defined in this study by the presence of one or more of the following criteria: failure to achieve complete remission after 5 weeks' therapy, t(9;22) or t(4;11) positivity, a poor prednisone response associated with T-cell phenotype, or a white blood cell count higher than $100 \times 10^{e}9/L$. The 5-year disease-free survival rate was better for the patients who received SCT from a matched related donor than for those who received chemotherapy. Only one in six of these high-risk patients had a suitable family donor, however. SCT from alternative donors resulted in an inferior outcome. Therefore the role of allogeneic SCT in first complete remission is limited in these very high-risk patients. Another recent study failed to prove a benefit for allogeneic SCT in very high-risk cases,[71] whereas the Berlin/Frankfurt/Münster study group showed that high-risk T-cell ALL cases may benefit from SCT.[72]

Treatment of Adolescents

Four recent reports from four different countries show that outcome for adolescents who have ALL is better when these patients are treated on a pediatric rather than an adult protocol.[73–76] The 5-year EFS of patients aged 15 to 21 years was approximately 30% higher when they were treated according to a pediatric protocol (**Table 3**). This result could not be explained by differences in immunophenotype and genetic abnormalities, but there seemed to be large differences in the dose intensity used during treatment. The pediatric protocols contained more glucocorticoids, vincristine, L-asparaginase, MTX, and 6-MP. In addition, it is conceivable that the longer delays between different parts of treatment noted in adolescents treated according to the adult protocols might have played a role. It is possible that hematologists have a different approach in managing toxicities because they generally treat older patients who do not tolerate intensive therapy well. Also, the toxicity caused by SCT usually is accepted as part of therapy, whereas adult hematologists have less experience with glucocorticoid- and asparaginase-induced toxicities. In the Dutch study, use of the adult ALL treatment protocol resulted in both a higher relapse rate and in a higher toxic death rate for adolescents.[74]

Side Effects

Nearly all chemotherapy side effects seen in children treated for ALL are temporary. The single most important cause of toxic death is infections: 0.5% to 1.5% of patients die from infections during induction therapy, and between 1% and 3% die from infections while in complete remission.[77] Many toxicities result from using a combination of drugs; some, however, are drug specific. Drug-specific toxicities include neuropathy and constipation caused by vincristine, mucositis caused by MTX, diabetes, behavior disturbances, Cushingoid appearance, osteoporosis, and avascular necrosis of bone caused by glucocorticoids, and allergic reactions and thrombosis caused by asparaginase.[78]

Toxicity increases with patient age. For example, children older than 10 years have a higher incidence of side effects to glucocorticoids such as avascular necrosis of bone and hyperglycemia, and pancreatitis and thromboembolic complications caused by L-asparaginase.[55] About 5% to 15% of children older than 10 years of age and adolescents experience one or more of these side effects. It has been shown that short pulses of glucocorticoids (5 days) lead to fewer side effects than more continuous schedules with the same cumulative doses of glucocorticoids.

Table 3
Outcome of adolescents treated on a pediatric or adult acute lymphoblastic leukemia protocol

Study Group [Reference]	Patient Number	Age Category (in Years)	5-year Event-free Survival (%)
United Sates: pediatric[75]	196	16–21	64
United States: adult[75]	103	16–21	38
Dutch: pediatric[74]	47	15–18	69
Dutch: adult[74]	44	15–18	34
French: pediatric[73]	77	15–20	67
French: adult[73]	100	15–20	41
United Kingdom: pediatric[72]	61	15–17	65
United Kingdom: adult[72]	67	15–17	49

PERSPECTIVES
New Genomic Techniques

The recent sequencing of the human genome and technical advances in high through-put analysis of DNA copy number and mRNA expression now allow a "molecular portrait" of leukemia. Gene-expression profiling can be helpful in classifying ALL patients, in revealing new insights into the pathways involved in different genetic subtypes of ALL, and in identifying new pathways involved in therapy resistance and new therapeutic targets.[79]

The first studies using gene-expression profiling showed that known morphologic, immunophenotypic, and genetic subclasses of ALL had specific gene-expression profiles.[28,80,81] Gene-expression profiling may be even more suitable for classifying ALL cases because it takes into consideration the biologic state and genetic progres-sion. Gene-expression patterns have been revealed that are related to in vitro resistance to several classes of individual agents, to clinical outcome, and to cross-resistance to multiple antileukemic drugs.[82,83] These studies, for example, have shown that *MCL-1* overexpression is involved in glucocorticoid resistance in ALL. Modulation of *MCL-1* expression sensitizes ALL cells to glucocorticoids.[84]

Bhojwani and colleagues [85] revealed that gene-expression profiles of early relapsed ALL samples were characterized by the overexpression of genes involved in cell-cycle regulation; this finding might identify attractive new targets for therapy. Armstrong [86] and Stam[87] showed high levels of wild-type *FLT3* in *MLL*-rearranged ALL. High levels of *FLT3* are related to a poor outcome,[88] and inhibition of this tyrosine kinase is very effective in *MLL*-rearranged ALL cells in vitro [87] as well as in an in vivo mouse model.[86] This finding has led to the design of two different phase I/II studies of these inhibitors in *MLL*-rearranged ALL.

Genome-wide techniques to screen for mutations and amplifications and for single-nucleotide polymorphisms (SNPs) recently have revealed many recurrent genetic alter-ations that are important for the development of ALL[89–92] and for the sensitivity to chemotherapy. For example, polymorphisms in folate-related genes are related to the MTX sensitivity of ALL cells.[93] Mulligan and colleagues[89] used SNP arrays to reveal that childhood ALL samples show recurrent gene deletions and amplifications including somatic *PAX5* deletion, which is present in about one third of all ALL cases.[89] Overall deletions were more common than amplification, specifically deletions of genes involved in B-cell differentiation, indicating that arrested development is a key feature of leukemia transformation. In the forthcoming years, large-scale studies will analyze the profile of microRNAs in ALL subtypes[94] and the role of newly discovered genetic subtype-specific microRNAs in ALL.

Targeted Therapies

Several new targeted therapies may contribute to a further improvement in treatment results in childhood and adolescent ALL (**Table 4**). The ultimate target of therapy is the leukemogenic fusion product. The best example is the *BCR/ABL* fusion product leading to an abnormal *ABL* tyrosine kinase activity. Imatinib is an effective inhibitor of this kinase,[95] but resistance rapidly occurs when it is used as a single agent, mainly because of the selection or development of leukemic subclones with *BCR-ABL* point mutations. It therefore seems that imatinib must be combined with standard antileu-kemic agents to treat *BCR-ABL*–positive ALL effectively. A European randomized study currently is attempting to assess the efficacy and toxicity of the addition of imatinib to all chemotherapy blocks. Resistance to imatinib is caused mainly by the outgrowth of subclones with mutations in the kinase domain of *BCR-ABL* that interfere

Table 4
New targeted therapies for childhood and adolescent acute lymphoblastic leukemia

Drug	Target	Type of ALL
Imatinib	*ABL* tyrosine kinase	*BCR-ABL* fusion, *NUP214-ABL1* fusion
Dasatinib, nilotinib	*ABL* tyrosine kinase (also many mutations), *SRC* kinases	*BCR-ABL* fusion
PKC412, CEP701, other FLT3 inhibitors	Mutated *FLT3*, wild type over-expressed *FLT3*	*MLL* gene–rearranged ALL, hyperdiploid ALL
Demethylating agents	Hypermethylation	*MLL* gene–rearranged ALL, other subtypes?
Rituximab	CD20	CD20 + (B-lineage) ALL
Epratuzumab	CD22	CD22 + (B-lineage) ALL
Gemtuzumab ozogamicin	CD33	CD33 + ALL
Alemtuzumab	CD52	CD52 + ALL
Forodesine	PNP (purine nucleoside phosphorylase)	T-ALL
Nelarabine		T-ALL

with imatinib binding. For most mutations, this resistance can be overcome with dasatinib[96] or nilotinib.[97] A pediatric phase I-II study with dasatinib is underway. The very rare subset of T-ALL with *NUP214-ABL1* fusion also may be a suitable group for targeted therapies using these compounds.

The recent finding that half of T-ALL cases have activating mutations of the *NOTCH1* gene provides a rationale for targeted therapies of the NOTCH pathway. Cleavage of the trans-membrane receptor *NOTCH1* by gamma secretase leads to release of the intracellular domain of *NOTCH1* (ICN1), followed by translocation to the nucleus and transcription activation. Inhibitors of ICN1 production and activity seemed to be toxic for T-ALL cells in vitro and have led to a clinical trial of a gamma secretase inhibitor in patients who had refractory T-ALL; however, this trial was stopped because of gastrointestinal side effects. Targeting the enzyme purine nucleoside phosphorylase in T-ALL, especially by forodesine,[98] is another strategy that will be tested in childhood ALL in the forthcoming years. Nelarabine is a nucleoside analogue that is converted intracellularly to cytarabine with promising activity as single agent in T-ALL.[99,100]

Overexpression of wild-type *FLT3*, especially in *MLL*-rearranged ALL and hyperdiploid ALL, also provides an opportunity for targeted therapies with *FLT3* inhibitors. Another opportunity may be found in the hypermethylation state of *MLL*-rearranged ALL, where the tumor-suppressor gene *FHIT* is silenced by hypermethylation. Re-expression leads to the killing of infant *MLL*-rearranged ALL cells, and demethylation agents have the same effect.[101]

Finally, different monoclonal antibodies, directed against different antigens (CD20, CD22, and CD52), with or without conjugated toxins, are in early clinical studies in childhood ALL.

Host Pharmacogenetics

There is no doubt that host polymorphisms in drug-metabolizing genes alter drug levels and target engagement. The ultimate goal of host pharmacogenetic studies is to optimize drug dosing for each patient to achieve maximum treatment efficacy with a minimum toxicity. Germline SNPs determine the toxicity of different antileukemic drugs[102] The most extensively studied is the gene encoding for thiopurine methyltransferase (*TPMT*) involved in the metabolism of 6-MP. Genetic polymorphisms in *TPMT* correlate with enzyme activity and with both 6-MP toxicity and outcome in ALL. Many other genes are subject to genetic polymorphisms, and the development of tools such as SNP arrays facilitates the studies of many of these polymorphisms simultaneously.

SUMMARY

More than 80% of children who have ALL are cured with contemporary intensive chemotherapy protocols. In the forthcoming decades it will be of great importance to tailor therapy for individual patients according to early response to therapy (mainly by detecting MRD) so that the intensity of therapy can be reduced or augmented. Also, more specific therapy schedules will be developed for immunophenotypic and genetic subclasses of ALL, because it now is apparent that ALL is not a single disease entity but in fact includes different diseases with differing underlying biology and clinical courses. New genomic techniques will lead to the discovery of new molecular genetic abnormalities that will provide more insights into the biology of the different ALL subtypes. New targeted therapy approaches will be developed, and it will be important to investigate how new agents can be incorporated in existing regimens.

REFERENCES

1. Greaves M. Infection, immune responses and the aetiology of childhood leukaemia. Nat Rev Cancer 2006;6(3):193–203.
2. Fischer S, Mann G, Konrad M, et al. Screening for leukemia- and clone-specific markers at birth in children with T cell precursor ALL suggests a predominantly postnatal origin. Blood 2007;110:3036–8.
3. Conter V, Arico M, Valsecchi MG, et al. Long-term results of the Italian Association of Pediatric Hematology and Oncology (AIEOP) acute lymphoblastic leukemia studies, 1982–1995. Leukemia 2000;14(12):2196–204.
4. Schrappe M, Reiter A, Zimmerman M, et al. Long-term results of four consecutive trials in childhood ALL performed by the ALL-BFM study group from 1981 to 1995. Berlin-Frankfurt-Munster. Leukemia 2000;14(12):2205–22.
5. Gaynon PS, Trigg ME, Heerema NA, et al. Children's Cancer Group trials in childhood acute lymphoblastic leukemia: 1983–1995. Leukemia 2000;14(12):2223–33.
6. Harms DO, Janka-Schaub GE. Co-operative Study Group for Childhood Acute Lymphoblastic Leukemia (COALL): long-term follow-up of trials 82, 85, 89 and 92. Leukemia 2000;14(12):2234–9.
7. Kamps WA, Veerman AJ, van Wering ER, et al. Long-term follow-up of Dutch Childhood Leukemia Study Group (DCLSG) protocols for children with acute lymphoblastic leukemia, 1984–1991. Leukemia 2000;14(12):2240–6.
8. Silverman LB, Declerck L, Gelber RD, et al. Results of Dana-Farber Cancer Institute Consortium protocols for children with newly diagnosed acute lymphoblastic leukemia (1981–1995). Leukemia 2000;14(12):2247–56.
9. Vilmer E, Suciu S, Ferster A, et al. Long-term results of three randomized trials (58831, 58832, 58881) in childhood acute lymphoblastic leukemia: a CLCG-EORTC report. Children Leukemia Cooperative Group. Leukemia 2000;14(12):2257–66.

10. Gustafsson G, Schmiegelow K, Forestier E, et al. Improving outcome through two decades in childhood ALL in the Nordic countries: the impact of high-dose methotrexate in the reduction of CNS irradiation. Nordic Society of Pediatric Haematology and Oncology (NOPHO). Leukemia 2000;14(12):2267–75.

11. Pui CH, Boyett JM, Rivera GK, et al. Long-term results of total therapy studies 11, 12 and 13A for childhood acute lymphoblastic leukemia at St Jude Children's Research Hospital. Leukemia 2000;14(12):2286–94.

12. Aricò M, Valsecchi MG, Camitta B, et al. Outcome of treatment in children with Philadelphia chromosome-positive acute lymphoblastic leukemia. N Engl J Med 2000;342(14):998–1006.

13. Szczepański T, Orfão A, van der Velden VH, et al. Minimal residual disease in leukaemia patients. Lancet Oncol 2001;2(7):409–17.

14. Pieters R, den Boer ML, Durian M, et al. Relation between age, immunophenotype and in vitro drug resistance in 395 children with acute lymphoblastic leukemia—implications for treatment of infants. Leukemia 1998;12(9):1344–8.

15. Ramakers-van Woerden NL, Pieters R, Hoelzer D, et al. In vitro drug resistance profile of Philadelphia positive acute lymphoblastic leukemia is heterogeneous and related to age: a report of the Dutch and German Leukemia Study Groups. Med Pediatr Oncol 2002;38(6):379–86.

16. Biondi A, Cimino G, Pieters R, et al. Biological and therapeutic aspects of infant leukemia. Blood 2000;96(1):24–33.

17. Pieters R, Schrappe M, De Lorenzo P, et al. A treatment protocol for infants younger than 1 year with acute lymphoblastic leukaemia (Interfant-99): an observational study and a multicentre randomised trial. Lancet 2007; 370(9583):240–50.

18. Hilden JM, Dinndorf PA, Meerbaum SO, et al. Analysis of prognostic factors of acute lymphoblastic leukemia in infants: report on CCG 1953 from the Children's Oncology Group. Blood 2006;108(2):441–51.

19. Rots MG, Pieters R, Peters GJ, et al. Role of folylpolyglutamate synthetase and folylpolyglutamate hydrolase in methotrexate accumulation and polyglutamylation in childhood leukemia. Blood 1999;93(5):1677–83.

20. Heerema NA, Sather HN, Sensel MG, et al. Prognostic impact of trisomies of chromosomes 10, 17, and 5 among children with acute lymphoblastic leukemia and high hyperdiploidy (>50 chromosomes). J Clin Oncol 2000; 18(9):1876–87.

21. Kaspers GJ, Smets LA, Pieters R, et al. Favorable prognosis of hyperdiploid common acute lymphoblastic leukemia may be explained by sensitivity to antimetabolites and other drugs: results of an in vitro study. Blood 1995;85(3):751–6.

22. Ramakers-van Woerden NL, Pieters R, Loonen AH, et al. TEL/AML1 gene fusion is related to in vitro drug sensitivity for L-asparaginase in childhood acute lymphoblastic leukemia. Blood 2000;96(3):1094–9.

23. Stams WA, den Boer ML, Holleman A, et al. Asparagine synthetase expression is linked with L-asparaginase resistance in TEL-AML1-negative but not TEL-AML1-positive pediatric acute lymphoblastic leukemia. Blood 2005; 105(11):4223–5.

24. Stams WA, den Boer ML, Beverloo HB, et al. Sensitivity to L-asparaginase is not associated with expression levels of asparagine synthetase in t(12;21)+ pediatric ALL. Blood 2003;101(7):2743–7.

25. Frost BM, Froestier E, Gustafsson G, et al. Translocation t(12;21) is related to in vitro cellular drug sensitivity to doxorubicin and etoposide in childhood acute lymphoblastic leukemia. Blood 2004;104(8):2452–7.

26. Pui CH, Gaynon PS, Boyett JM, et al. Outcome of treatment in childhood acute lymphoblastic leukaemia with rearrangements of the 11q23 chromosomal region. Lancet 2002;359(9321):1909–15.

27. Jansen MW, Corral L, van der Velden VH, et al. Immunobiological diversity in infant acute lymphoblastic leukemia is related to the occurrence and type of MLL gene rearrangement. Leukemia 2007;21(4):633–41.

28. Armstrong SA, Staunton JE, Silverman LB, et al. MLL translocations specify a distinct gene expression profile that distinguishes a unique leukemia. Nat Genet 2002;30(1):41–7.

29. Dordelmann M, Reiter A, Borkhardt A, et al. Prednisone response is the strongest predictor of treatment outcome in infant acute lymphoblastic leukemia. Blood 1999;94(4):1209–17.

30. Ramakers-van Woerden NL, Beverloo HB, Veerman AJ, et al. In vitro drug-resistance profile in infant acute lymphoblastic leukemia in relation to age, MLL rearrangements and immunophenotype. Leukemia 2004;18(3):521–9.

31. Stam RW, den Boer ML, Meijerink JP, et al. Differential mRNA expression of Ara-C-metabolizing enzymes explains Ara-C sensitivity in MLL gene-rearranged infant acute lymphoblastic leukemia. Blood 2003;101(4):1270–6.

32. Ramakers-van Woerden NL, Pieters R, Rots MG, et al. Infants with acute lymphoblastic leukemia: no evidence for high methotrexate resistance. Leukemia 2002;16(5):949–51.

33. Stam RW, van den Heuvel-Eibrink MM, den Boer ML, et al. Multidrug resistance genes in infant acute lymphoblastic leukemia: Ara-C is not a substrate for the breast cancer resistance protein. Leukemia 2004;18(1):78–83.

34. Thompson PA, Murry DJ, Rosner GL, et al. Methotrexate pharmacokinetics in infants with acute lymphoblastic leukemia. Cancer Chemother Pharmacol 2007;59(6):847–53.

35. Schrappe M, Arico M, Harbott J, et al. Philadelphia chromosome-positive (Ph+) childhood acute lymphoblastic leukemia: good initial steroid response allows early prediction of a favorable treatment outcome. Blood 1998;92(8):2730–41.

36. Graux C, Cools J, Michaux L, et al. Cytogenetics and molecular genetics of T-cell acute lymphoblastic leukemia: from thymocyte to lymphoblast. Leukemia 2006;20(9):1496–510.

37. Breit S, Stanulla M, Flohr T, et al. Activating NOTCH1 mutations predict favorable early treatment response and long-term outcome in childhood precursor T-cell lymphoblastic leukemia. Blood 2006;108(4):1151–7.

38. Moorman AV, Richards SM, Robinson HM, et al. Prognosis of children with acute lymphoblastic leukemia (ALL) and intrachromosomal amplification of chromosome 21 (iAMP21). Blood 2007;109(6):2327–30.

39. Nachman JB, Heerema NA, Sather H, et al. Outcome of treatment in children with hypodiploid acute lymphoblastic leukemia. Blood 2007;110(4):1112–5.

40. Bassal M, La MK, Whitlock JA, et al. Lymphoblast biology and outcome among children with Down syndrome and ALL treated on CCG-1952. Pediatr Blood Cancer 2005;44(1):21–8.

41. Whitlock JA, Sather HN, Gaynon P, et al. Clinical characteristics and outcome of children with Down syndrome and acute lymphoblastic leukemia: a Children's Cancer Group study. Blood 2005;106(13):4043–9.

42. Tubergen DG, Gilchrist GS, O'Brien RT, et al. Improved outcome with delayed intensification for children with acute lymphoblastic leukemia and intermediate presenting features: a Childrens Cancer Group phase III trial. J Clin Oncol 1993;11:527–37.

43. Bostrom BC, Sensel MR, Sather HN, et al. Dexamethasone versus prednisone and daily oral versus weekly intravenous mercaptopurine for patients with standard-risk acute lymphoblastic leukemia: a report from the Children's Cancer Group. Blood 2003;101(10):3809–17.
44. Mitchell CD, Richards SM, Kinsey SE, et al. Benefit of dexamethasone compared with prednisolone for childhood acute lymphoblastic leukaemia: results of the UK Medical Research Council ALL97 randomized trial. Br J Haematol 2005;129(6):734–45.
45. Igarashi S, Manabe A, Ohara A, et al. No advantage of dexamethasone over prednisolone for the outcome of standard- and intermediate-risk childhood acute lymphoblastic leukemia in the Tokyo Children's Cancer Study Group L95-14 protocol. J Clin Oncol 2005;23(27):6489–98.
46. Kaspers GJ, Veerman AJ, Popp-Snijders C, et al. Comparison of the antileukemic activity in vitro of dexamethasone and prednisolone in childhood acute lymphoblastic leukemia. Med Pediatr Oncol 1996;27(2):114–21.
47. Ito C, Evans WE, McNinch L, et al. Comparative cytotoxicity of dexamethasone and prednisolone in childhood acute lymphoblastic leukemia. J Clin Oncol 1996;14(8):2370–6.
48. Duval M, Suciu S, Ferster A, et al. Comparison of Escherichia coli-asparaginase with Erwinia-asparaginase in the treatment of childhood lymphoid malignancies: results of a randomized European Organisation for Research and Treatment of Cancer-Children's Leukemia Group phase 3 trial. Blood 2002; 99(8):2734–9.
49. Moghrabi A, Levy DE, Asselin B, et al. Results of the Dana-Farber Cancer Institute ALL Consortium Protocol 95-01 for children with acute lymphoblastic leukemia. Blood 2007;109(3):896–904.
50. Appel IM, Pinheiro JP, den Boer ML, et al. Lack of asparagine depletion in the cerebrospinal fluid after one intravenous dose of PEG-asparaginase: a window study at initial diagnosis of childhood ALL. Leukemia 2003;17(11):2254–6.
51. Pession A, Valsecchi MG, Masera G, et al. Long-term results of a randomized trial on extended use of high dose L-asparaginase for standard risk childhood acute lymphoblastic leukemia. J Clin Oncol 2005;23(28):7161–7.
52. Rizzari C, Vasecchi MG, Arico M, et al. Effect of protracted high-dose L-asparaginase given as a second exposure in a Berlin-Frankfurt-Munster-based treatment: results of the randomized 9102 intermediate-risk childhood acute lymphoblastic leukemia study–a report from the Associazione Italiana Ematologia Oncologia Pediatrica. J Clin Oncol 2001;19(5):1297–303.
53. Amylon MD, Shuster J, Pullen J, et al. Intensive high-dose asparaginase consolidation improves survival for pediatric patients with T cell acute lymphoblastic leukemia and advanced stage lymphoblastic lymphoma: a Pediatric Oncology Group study. Leukemia 1999;13(3):335–42.
54. Avramis VI, Sencer C, Periclou AP, et al. A randomized comparison of native Escherichia coli asparaginase and polyethylene glycol conjugated asparaginase for treatment of children with newly diagnosed standard-risk acute lymphoblastic leukemia: a Children's Cancer Group study. Blood 2002;99(6):1986–94.
55. Silverman LB, Gelber RD, Dalton VK, et al. Improved outcome for children with acute lymphoblastic leukemia: results of Dana-Farber Consortium Protocol 91-01. Blood 2001;97(5):1211–8.
56. Clarke M, Gaynon P, Hann I, et al. CNS-directed therapy for childhood acute lymphoblastic leukemia: childhood ALL Collaborative Group overview of 43 randomized trials. J Clin Oncol 2003;21(9):1798–809.

57. Matloub Y, Lindemulder S, Gaynon PS, et al. Intrathecal triple therapy decreases central nervous system relapse but fails to improve event-free survival when compared with intrathecal methotrexate: results of the Children's Cancer Group (CCG) 1952 study for standard-risk acute lymphoblastic leukemia, reported by the Children's Oncology Group. Blood 2006;108(4):1165–73.

58. Harms DO, Gobel U, Spaar HJ, et al. Thioguanine offers no advantage over mercaptopurine in maintenance treatment of childhood ALL: results of the randomized trial COALL-92. Blood 2003;102(8):2736–40.

59. Vora A, Mitchell CD, Lennard L, et al. Toxicity and efficacy of 6-thioguanine versus 6-mercaptopurine in childhood lymphoblastic leukaemia: a randomised trial. Lancet 2006;368(9544):1339–48.

60. Relling MV, Hancock ML, Boyett JM, et al. Prognostic importance of 6-mercaptopurine dose intensity in acute lymphoblastic leukemia. Blood 1999;93(9): 2817–23.

61. Lilleyman JS, Lennard L. Mercaptopurine metabolism and risk of relapse in childhood lymphoblastic leukaemia. Lancet 1994;343(8907):1188–90.

62a. McLeod HL, Relling MV, Liu Q, et al. Polymorphic thiopurine methyltransferase in erythrocytes is indicative of activity in leukemic blasts from children with acute lymphoblastic leukemia. Blood 1995;85(7):1897–902.

62b. Aricó M, Baruchel A, Bertrand Y, et al. The seventh international childhood acute lymphoblastic leukemia workshop report: palermo, Italy, January 29–30, 2005. Leukemia 2005;19(7):1145–52.

63. Duration and intensity of maintenance chemotherapy in acute lymphoblastic leukaemia: overview of 42 trials involving 12,000 randomised children. Childhood ALL Collaborative Group. Lancet 1996;347(9018):1783–8.

64. Lange BJ, Bostrom BC, Cherlow JM, et al. Double-delayed intensification improves event-free survival for children with intermediate-risk acute lymphoblastic leukemia: a report from the Children's Cancer Group. Blood 2002; 99(3):825–33.

65. Nachman JB, Sather HN, Sensel MG, et al. Augmented post-induction therapy for children with high-risk acute lymphoblastic leukemia and a slow response to initial therapy. N Engl J Med 1998;338(23):1663–71.

66. Kamps WA, Bokkerink JP, Hahlen K, et al. Intensive treatment of children with acute lymphoblastic leukemia according to ALL-BFM-6 without cranial radiotherapy: results of Dutch Childhood Leukemia Study Group Protocol ALL-7 (1988–1991). Blood 1999;94(4):1226–36.

67. Toyoda Y, Manabe A, Tsuchida M, et al. Six months of maintenance chemotherapy after intensified treatment for acute lymphoblastic leukemia of childhood. J Clin Oncol 2000;18(7):1508–16.

68. Conter V, Valsecchi MG, Silvestri D, et al. Pulses of vincristine and dexamethasone in addition to intensive chemotherapy for children with intermediate-risk acute lymphoblastic leukaemia: a multicentre randomised trial. Lancet 2007; 369(9556):123–31.

69. Veerman AJ, Hahlen K, Kamps WA, et al. High cure rate with a moderately intensive treatment regimen in non-high-risk childhood acute lymphoblastic leukemia. Results of protocol ALL VI from the Dutch Childhood Leukemia Study Group. J Clin Oncol 1996;14(3):911–8.

70. Balduzzi A, Valsecchi MG, Uderzo C, et al. Chemotherapy versus allogeneic transplantation for very-high-risk childhood acute lymphoblastic leukaemia in first complete remission: comparison by genetic randomisation in an international prospective study. Lancet 2005;366(9486):635–42.

71. Ribera JM, Ortega JJ, Oriol A, et al. Comparison of intensive chemotherapy, allogeneic, or autologous stem-cell transplantation as postremission treatment for children with very high risk acute lymphoblastic leukemia: PETHEMA ALL-93 Trial. J Clin Oncol 2007;25(1):16–24.

72. Schrauder A, Reiter A, Gadner H, et al. Superiority of allogeneic hematopoietic stem-cell transplantation compared with chemotherapy alone in high-risk childhood T-cell acute lymphoblastic leukemia: results from ALL-BFM 90 and 95. J Clin Oncol 2006;24(36):5742–9.

73. Boissel N, Auclerc MF, Lheritier V, et al. Should adolescents with acute lymphoblastic leukemia be treated as old children or young adults? Comparison of the French FRALLE-93 and LALA-94 trials. J Clin Oncol 2003;21(5):774–80.

74. de Bont JM, Holt B, Dekker AW, et al. Significant difference in outcome for adolescents with acute lymphoblastic leukemia treated on pediatric vs adult protocols in the Netherlands. Leukemia 2004;18(12):2032–5.

75. Deangelo DJ. The treatment of adolescents and young adults with acute lymphoblastic leukemia. Hematology Am Soc Hematol Educ Program 2005;123–30.

76. Ramanujachar R, Richards S, Hann I, et al. Adolescents with acute lymphoblastic leukaemia: outcome on UK national paediatric (ALL97) and adult (UKALLXII/E2993) trials. Pediatr Blood Cancer 2007;48(3):254–61.

77. Christensen MS, Heyman M, Mottonen M, et al. Treatment-related death in childhood acute lymphoblastic leukaemia in the Nordic countries: 1992–2001. Br J Haematol 2005;131(1):50–8.

78. Caruso V, Iacoviello L, Di Castelnuovo A, et al. Thrombotic complications in childhood acute lymphoblastic leukemia: a meta-analysis of 17 prospective studies comprising 1752 pediatric patients. Blood 2006;108(7):2216–22.

79. Carroll WL, Bhojwani D, Min DJ, et al. Childhood acute lymphoblastic leukemia in the age of genomics. Pediatr Blood Cancer 2006;46(5):570–8.

80. Yeoh EJ, Ross ME, Shurtleff SA, et al. Classification, subtype discovery, and prediction of outcome in pediatric acute lymphoblastic leukemia by gene expression profiling. Cancer Cell 2002;1(2):133–43.

81. Ross ME, Zhou X, Song G, et al. Classification of pediatric acute lymphoblastic leukemia by gene expression profiling. Blood 2003;102(8):2951–9.

82. Holleman A, Cheok MH, den Boer ML, et al. Gene-expression patterns in drug-resistant acute lymphoblastic leukemia cells and response to treatment. N Engl J Med 2004;351(6):533–42.

83. Lugthart S, Cheok MH, den Boer ML, et al. Identification of genes associated with chemotherapy crossresistance and treatment response in childhood acute lymphoblastic leukemia. Cancer Cell 2005;7(4):375–86.

84. Wei G, Twomey D, Lamb J, et al. Gene expression-based chemical genomics identifies rapamycin as a modulator of MCL1 and glucocorticoid resistance. Cancer Cell 2006;10(4):331–42.

85. Bhojwani D, Kang H, Moskowitz NP, et al. Biologic pathways associated with relapse in childhood acute lymphoblastic leukemia: a Children's Oncology Group study. Blood 2006;108(2):711–7.

86. Armstrong SA, Kung AL, Mabon ME, et al. Inhibition of FLT3 in MLL. Validation of a therapeutic target identified by gene expression based classification. Cancer Cell 2003;3(2):173–83.

87. Stam RW, den Boer ML, Schneider P, et al. Targeting FLT3 in primary MLL-gene-rearranged infant acute lymphoblastic leukemia. Blood 2005;106(7):2484–90.

88. Stam RW, Schneider P, de Lorenzo P, et al. Prognostic significance of high-level FLT3 expression in MLL-rearranged infant acute lymphoblastic leukemia. Blood 2007;110(7):2774–5.
89. Mullighan CG, Goorha S, Radtke I, et al. Genome-wide analysis of genetic alterations in acute lymphoblastic leukaemia. Nature 2007;446(7137):758–64.
90. Lahortiga I, De Keersmaecker K, Van Vlierberghe P, et al. Duplication of the MYB oncogene in T cell acute lymphoblastic leukemia. Nat Genet 2007;39(5): 593–5.
91. van Vlierberghe P, Meijerink JP, Lee C, et al. A new recurrent 9q34 duplication in pediatric T-cell acute lymphoblastic leukemia. Leukemia 2006;20(7):1245–53.
92. Van Vlierberghe P, van Grotel M, Beverloo HB, et al. The cryptic chromosomal deletion del(11)(p12p13) as a new activation mechanism of LMO2 in pediatric T-cell acute lymphoblastic leukemia. Blood 2006;108(10):3520–9.
93. Cheok MH, Evans WE. Acute lymphoblastic leukaemia: a model for the pharmacogenomics of cancer therapy. Nat Rev Cancer 2006;6(2):117–29.
94. Lu J, Getz G, Miska EA, et al. MicroRNA expression profiles classify human cancers. Nature 2005;435(7043):834–8.
95. Champagne MA, Capdeville R, Krailo M, et al. Imatinib mesylate (STI571) for treatment of children with Philadelphia chromosome-positive leukemia: results from a Children's Oncology Group phase 1 study. Blood 2004;104(9):2655–60.
96. Talpaz M, Shah NP, Kantarjian H, et al. Dasatinib in imatinib-resistant Philadelphia chromosome-positive leukemias. N Engl J Med 2006;354(24):2531–41.
97. Kantarjian H, Giles F, Wunderle L, et al. Nilotinib in imatinib-resistan CML and Philadelphia chromosome-positive ALL. N Engl J Med 2006;354(24):2542–51.
98. Gandhi V, Kilpatrick JM, Plunkett W, et al. A proof-of-principle pharmacokinetic, pharmacodynamic, and clinical study with purine nucleoside phosphorylase inhibitor immucillin-H (BCX-1777, forodesine). Blood 2005;106(13):4253–60.
99. Kurtzberg J, Ernst TJ, Keating MJ, et al. Phase I study of 506U78 administered on a consecutive 5-day schedule in children and adults with refractory hematologic malignancies. J Clin Oncol 2005;23(15):3396–403.
100. Berg SL, Blaney SM, Devidas M, et al. Phase II study of nelarabine (compound 506U78) in children and young adults with refractory T-cell malignancies: a report from the Children's Oncology Group. J Clin Oncol 2005;23(15): 3376–82.
101. Stam RW, den Boer ML, Passier MM, et al. Silencing of the tumor suppressor gene FHIT is highly characteristic for MLL gene rearranged infant acute lymphoblastic leukemia. Leukemia 2006;20(2):264–71.
102. Kishi S, Cheng C, French D, et al. Ancestry and pharmacogenetics of antileukemic drug toxicity. Blood 2007;109(10):4151–7.

Acute Leukemias in Children with Down Syndrome

C. Michel Zwaan, MD, PhD[a,*], Dirk Reinhardt, PD[b],
Johann Hitzler, FRCP(C), FAAP[c,d], Paresh Vyas, FRCPath, DPHil[e]

KEYWORDS

• Down syndrome • Leukemia • Children

Childhood leukemias often originate from a premalignant clone, a generally asymptomatic condition that can only be detected by demonstrating leukemia-specific genetic changes in peripheral blood, including that obtained from Guthrie cards or in cord-blood.[1] Subsequently, secondary genetic events cause outgrowth of this dormant clone and result in frank leukemia. However, the likelihood of developing leukemia in children who carry premalignant clones, harboring genetic aberrations such as TEL-AML or AML1-ETO is low. Because of the very low transformation into frank leukemia, prevention strategies are generally considered not feasible.

Children with Down syndrome (DS) (for a review on DS, see Roizen and Patterson in[2]) have an increased risk of developing leukemias, which was already recognized in the 1950s,[3] although their risk of cancer in general is not increased because of a reduced propensity for solid tumors.[3,4] This increased risk of leukemia includes both acute lymphoblastic leukemia as well as myeloid leukemia. Approximately 10% of newborns with DS develop a preleukemic clone, originating from myeloid progenitors in the fetal liver that are characterized by a somatic mutation in the gene encoding for the

A version of this article was previously published in the *Pediatric Clinics of North America*, 55:1. None of the authors have direct financial interests to disclose. P. Vyas receives research support from the Leukemia Research Fund; C.M. Zwaan receives research support from Stichting Kinderen Kankervrij.

[a] Department of Pediatric Oncology/Hematology, Erasmus MC/Sophia Children's Hospital, Dr Molewaterplein 60, 3015GJ Rotterdam, The Netherlands
[b] Acute Myeloid Leukemia–Berlin-Frankfurt-Münster Study Group, Pediatric Hematology/Oncology, Hannover Medical School, Carl-Neuberg-Straße 1, D-30625 Hannover, Germany
[c] Division of Hematology/Oncology, The Hospital for Sick Children, 555 University Avenue, Toronto, ON M5G 1X8, Canada
[d] Developmental and Stem Cell Biology, The Hospital for Sick Children Research Institute, University of Toronto, Toronto, ON M5G 1X8, Canada
[e] Medical Research Council Molecular Haematology Unit, John Radcliffe Hospital and the Weatherall Institute of Molecular Medicine, University of Oxford, Oxford OX3 9DS, UK
* Corresponding author.
E-mail address: c.m.zwaan@erasmusmc.nl (C.M. Zwaan).

hematopoietic transcription factor GATA1, which is localized on the X-chromosome. Mutations in this transcription factor lead to a truncated mutant protein GATA1short or GATA1s.[5,6] This preleukemia is referred to as transient leukemia (TL), transient myeloproliferative disease (TMD), or transient abnormal myelopoiesis (TAM).

Transient leukemia is associated with a variable clinical presentation, ranging from a symptomatic to severe complications, which may even be fatal.[7,8] As TL originates in the liver, peripheral blood blast counts are usually higher than the bone marrow blast count. Subsequently, approximately 20% of children who have been diagnosed with TL develop myeloid leukemia of Down syndrome (ML DS; this term has been introduced to refer to the unique subtype of AML that develops in children with DS, as explained later in this article), usually with an onset before the age of 5 years.[7] Studying TL and ML DS may contribute significantly to our understanding of the stepwise process of leukemogeneis.[9] However, so far the genetic factors that drive this progression are unknown. Mutations in the GATA1 gene are present both in both TL and ML DS, and are therefore not sufficient to explain this progression.[10]

Of interest, children with DS are also predisposed to develop acute lymphoblastic leukemia (ALL), which is not associated with an overt preleukemic phase. Both ML and ALL in patients with DS are biologically distinct when compared with their non-DS counterparts, and are characterized by a different clinical behavior.[11–14] For children with DS who develop ALL, this does not lead to improved outcome, as is observed for children with DS who develop ML. This article reviews the current knowledge and research questions regarding TL and the DS-associated acute leukemias.

HEMATOLOGIC ABNORMALITIES IN CHILDREN WITH DOWN SYNDROME

Tunstall-Pedoe and colleagues[15] studied hematopoiesis in fetal bood, bone marrow, and liver cells from 16 fetuses with DS with a gestational age of 15 to 37 weeks. GATA1 mutations were not detected in the hematopoietic cells of these fetuses, although minor clones may have been missed, as explained later in this article. A marked increase in the megakaryocyte-erythrocyte progenitors in the fetal liver was found, as well as dysmegakaryopoiesis and dyserythropoiesis in the peripheral blood, but not in the bone marrow, when compared with non-DS fetuses. The investigators conclude that trisomy 21 by itself affects fetal hematopoiesis, and that the expansion of fetal liver progenitors creates a cellular substrate for GATA1 mutations to occur, which subsequently gives rise to TL (see later in this article and **Fig. 1**).

In DS newborns (n = 158), peripheral blood abnormalities in the first week of life included neutrophilia in 80% of children, thrombocytopenia in 66% (6% had platelets less than $50 \times 10^9/l$) and polycythemia in 33%.[16] Anemia, neutropenia, and thrombocytosis were present in less than 1% of DS newborns. In 6% of children, TL was diagnosed. Widness and colleagues[17] suggested that the observed polycythemia may be caused by increased erythopoietin levels when compared with non-DS newborns.

After the first week of life, the main peripheral blood abnormalities consist of red blood cell macrocytosis and thrombocytosis, although this study was limited to DS children who were younger than 1 year of age.[18]

De Hingh and colleagues[19] have studied T- and B-lymphocyte counts in children with DS and compared these to children without trisomy 21. Over time, the T-lymphocyte subpopulation gradually reached normal levels, but the B-lymphocyte population appeared severely decreased (88% of values were below the tenth percentile, and 61% below the fifth percentile of normal). These abnormalities may at least in part explain the increased susceptibility to infections, which children with DS may experience.

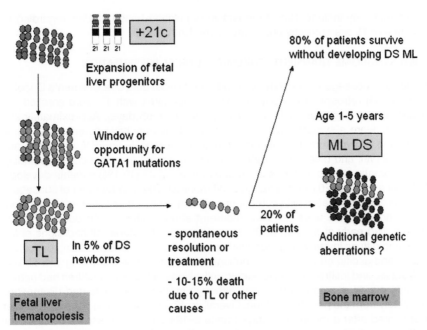

Fig. 1. Stepwise development of ML DS following TL. Transient leukemia arises from expanded fetal liver progenitors as a result of constitutional trisomy 21, providing a window of opportunity for the occurrence of acquired mutations in the hematopoietic transcription factor GATA1. In most cases TL spontaneously disappears, but some children may need treatment because of severe TL-related symptoms. Approximately 20% of children with TL subsequently develop ML DS, which requires additional hits.

HOW FREQUENT IS TRANSIENT LEUKEMIA IN DOWN SYNDROME CHILDREN?

The frequency of TL is estimated to be around 10% in DS children, although this was studied in a selected (hospitalized) population.[18] Most investigators assume that the true frequency is higher, but recent data suggest that his may not be the case. In The Netherlands, children with DS are registered in different nation-wide registries (the Dutch Pediatric Surveillance Unit and the National Dutch Neonatal and Obstetrical Registry), which provide population-based data. After matching these databases, it was assessed that 322 children (95% confidence interval 303–341) with DS were born in 2003, resulting in a prevalence of 16 out of 10,000 live-born babies.[20] To date, five children with DS who were born in 2002 and 2003 have been diagnosed with myeloid leukemia (by the Dutch Childhood Oncology Group, E.R. van Wering, personal communication, 2007). As ML in patients with DS typically occurs before the age of 5 years, with a median age of approximately 2 years, and the frequency for progression from TL to ML DS is well established at 20%, these data suggest that the true frequency of TL is in the 3% to 5% range.

This is further supported by a recent study from Pine and colleagues,[21] who screened Guthrie cards from 590 infants with DS for mutations in the GATA1 gene and found a mutation in 3.8% of children. However, GATA1 mutations may have been missed in those patients with minor preleukemic clones, subclonal mutations, low numbers of cells on Guthrie cards, or extramedullary TL without circulating blasts. In addition, one has to consider that some fetuses with DS may die in utero from causes that may include TL.[22] Prospective population-based studies regarding the incidence of TL are currently underway in The Netherlands.

DOWN SYNDROME TRANSIENT LEUKEMIA: CLINICAL PRESENTATION

Massey and colleagues[7] recently published the clinical data of a Children's Oncology Group (COG) retrospective study in which 48 neonates with TL were enrolled. The median age at diagnosis of TL was 7 days (range 1–65 days). Approximately 25% of patients were a-symptomatic, although this study may have been biased toward registration of symptomatic patients. Hepatosplenomagaly (in 56% of cases), effusions (in 21%), and bleeding or petechiae (in 25%) were the most common findings in symptomatic infants. In terms of outcome, 9 out of 47 (19.1%) patients developed ML DS at a mean of 20 months (range 9–38 months). The development of subsequent leukemia was associated with cytogenetic abnormalities other than the constitutional +21, although there were no clear recurrent abnormalities. Eight out of 47 (17%) patients died early at a mean of 90 days. These eight children all had signs of liver failure and diffuse intravascular coagulation, as well as effusions (including pericardial, pleural, and ascitic effusions). Four patients had liver biopsies showing liver fibrosis, cholestasis, and infiltration with leukemic cells. None of the eight children had normalized their blood counts before death, although in three the blasts had disappeared completely from the peripheral blood. Overall, in 42 out of 47 (89%) patients the blasts disappeared after a mean of 58 days (range 2–194 days). Of these 42 children, four developed subsequent leukemia and three died early because of complications. The other 35 children did not have detectable hematologic abnormalities at follow-up, and normalized their blood counts at a mean of 84 days (range 2–201 days). See **Fig. 2**A for an example of a blood smear of a TL patient.

The study from Massey and colleagues was recently confirmed by two other series, one from Japan and one from the AML-Berlin Frankfurt Münster Study Group (AML-BFM SG). The Japanese study evaluated 70 children with TL, and reported an early death rate of 23% and development of ML DS in 17% of surviving children.[23] The AML-BFM SG registered 148 children with TMD between 1993 and 2006, mainly consisting of children with symptomatic TL (D. Reinhardt, unpublished data, 2007). Median white blood cell count at diagnosis was 40.3×10^9 per liter. Complete remission was achieved spontaneously in 66% of children; 19% of children were treated with low-dose cytarabine to relieve symptoms and achieved remission. Two children progressed to ML DS after 9 and 13 months of follow-up, without clearing their peripheral blood TL cells in the meantime. In total, 24 children died, including 21 in the first 23 months of life. Death was attributed to TL in 13 of these children, including seven cases with liver fibrosis. In most children (85%) blasts were cleared from the peripheral blood after 4 weeks. Of the 124 surviving children, 29 developed ML DS (23.4%) after a median remission of 1.5 years (0.5–3.0 years).

One of the most relevant questions unanswered to date is whether the development of ML DS following TL can be inhibited by treating children for TL. The AML BFM SG and the Dutch COG are currently performing a study to prospectively investigate this.

CLINICAL FEATURES OF DOWN SYNDROME LEUKEMIAS
Myeloid Leukemia of Down Syndrome: Clinical Characteristics and Classification

According to the World Health Organization (WHO) classification, AML requires the presence of at least 20% blasts in the bone marrow or peripheral blood.[24] However, the pediatric literature suggests that this 20% threshold does not apply to ML in patients with DS.[25] Overt leukemia in these children is preceded in 20% to 60% of

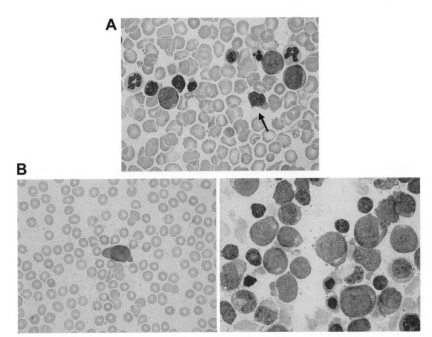

Fig. 2. Peripheral blood and bone marrow smears of patients with TL and with ML DS. (*A*) Peripheral blood smear (63×, May-Grünwald-Giemsa staining), from a baby with DS admitted at the neonatal intensive care for meconium aspiration. A high white blood cell count (56 × 10^9/l, after correction for normoblasts) was found. The smear shows transient leukemia, with four identifiable blasts, one with typical blebs (*arrow*), among several other normal blood cells. (*B*) Peripheral blood (*left panel*) and bone marrow (*right panel*) smear (63×, May-Grünwald-Giemsa staining), from a child that was diagnosed previously with TL (white blood cell count at birth 88 × 10^9/l with 37% blasts, which normalized within 3 months) and developed thrombocytopenia at the age of 1.5 years. Peripheral blood showed 3% blasts. Bone marrow examination showed 24% blasts, and was morphologically classified as French-American-British (FAB) M0.

cases by an indolent prephase of myelodysplasia (MDS), characterized by thrombocytopenia and dysplastic changes in the bone marrow, often with accompanying marrow fibrosis.[26,27] This MDS may last several months or even years before progressing to overt leukemia. In contrast to MDS in non-DS children, which requires stem-cell transplantation for cure, MDS in children with DS shows a highly favorable response to chemotherapy alone.[26–28] Therefore, Hasle and colleagues[25] suggested that all cases of MDS and overt myeloid leukemia in DS, children should be classified as one disease entity, and referred to as "myeloid leukemia of Down syndrome" or ML DS. As this is a unique disease, it should be classified separately from other cases of AML in the WHO-classification.

The presenting characteristics of DS patients with ML differ from those with non-DS AML.[14,26,27,29] In general, patients with ML DS are younger than 5 years of age at diagnosis, have a low diagnostic white blood cell count, and do not show meningeal involvement. Roughly two-thirds of cases are classified as acute megakaryoblastic leukemia (FAB M7), with the other patients being classified as FAB M0, M2, and M6 (see **Fig.** 2B). Cytogenetic abnormalities, such as t(8;21) or inv(16), which can frequently be found in the blasts of non-DS AML patients, typically do not occur in patients with DS who develop ML. In contrast, somatic mutations of GATA1 are specific for ML DS. Additional copies of chromosome 8 and 21 (in addition to the constitutional trisomy 21) are the most frequently occurring cytogenetic abnormalities, and are found in approximately 10% to 15% each. Cytogenetic findings associated with a high rate of relapse in non-DS AML, such as monosomy 7 and −5/5q- also occur in DS patients (together in approximately 10%–20% of cases), but do not seem to have a negative impact on prognosis, although numbers are small.[14,30]

Myeloid Leukemia in Down Syndrome: Treatment Outcome

DS children with ML have a superior outcome when compared with children without DS who develop AML. This was first recognized by investigators from the Pediatric Oncology Group (POG),[31] and the Nordic Society for Pediatric Hematology and Oncology (NOPHO).[32] However, to obtain excellent outcome rates it is crucial that high intensity treatment, which is required for cure of non-DS AML, is avoided, as this results in unacceptable high induction and treatment-related mortality rates in children with DS.[14,27,33] This observation has led to specific treatment guidelines for children with DS who develop ML, mostly with reduced treatment intensity regimens.[13,14,29] Recent results from several collaborative groups confirm the favorable outcome for this patient population. The 10-year overall survival (OS) for 61 patients treated according to the NOPHO between 1984 and 2001 was 74%.[29] Similarly, the 5-year OS for 161 patients treated according to the Children's Cancer Group study CCG 2891 between 1989 and 1999 was 79%.[14] Finally, the 3-year OS for 67 children treated between 1998 and 2003, according to the AML-BFM 98 study, was 91%.[13] Together, these data confirm a fairly favorable outcome for DS patients who develop myeloid leukemia.

Based on the excellent results in the AML-BFM 98 study, a prospective European treatment protocol was recently opened. DS patients with ML will receive the standard BFM chemotherapy regimen, with significant dose-reductions for cytarabine (28 g/m^2 versus 41 g/m^2 –47 g/m^2 for non-DS patients) and anthracyclines (230 mg/m^2 versus 320 mg/m^2–450 mg/m^2 for non-DS patients). Moreover, DS patients will not receive maintenance therapy, nor cranial radiation, nor stem-cell transplantation.[13,34] The COG has chosen a different approach in their 2971A trial, in which several drugs (etoposide and dexamethasone), as well as the 3-month maintenance period, were eliminated from the standard chemotherapy schedule used in the 2891 AML trial. In contrast to the European approach, there are no dose-reductions of the remaining drugs in the COG study, and the cumulative anthracycline and cytarabine dosages will be 320 mg/m^2 and 44 g/m^2, respectively.[30] Preliminary analysis shows outcome data (3-year probability of OS 84%) which are comparable to the CCG 2891 standard timing arm.[28]

The potential for reduced treatment intensity is based on the unique hypersensitivity of myeloid leukemia cells of DS patients to chemotherapy, when compared with AML cells from non-DS individuals, as demonstrated by various investigators.[35–38] This increased sensitivity to chemotherapy extends to agents with different mechanisms of action. Zwaan and colleagues[35] have reported that myeloid blasts were significantly more sensitive to cytarabine (median, 12-fold), anthracyclines (2- to 7-fold), mitoxantrone (9-fold), amsacrine (16-fold), etoposide (20-fold), 6-thioguanine (3-fold), busulfan (5-fold) and vincristine (23-fold), than non-DS AML cells. Taub and colleagues have provided evidence for specific mechanisms to explain the observed differences in drug sensitivity, and linked sensitivity to a gene-dosage effect of chromosome 21 localized genes.[39,40] For instance, cytarabine sensitivity may be caused by increased expression levels of the cystathionine-beta-synthase gene, which is located on chromosome 21.[41,42] Other studies from this group have shown the impact of GATA1s on cytidine deaminase levels and cytarabine sensitivity.[43] However, the fact that enhanced in-vitro sensitivity was described for drugs that exert therapeutic effect by different mechanisms of action may suggest a more general mechanism of enhanced chemotherapy susceptibility, such as a propensity to undergo apoptosis.[35] Interestingly, ALL cells from DS patients do not differ in drug sensitivity when compared with those of patients without constitutional trisomy 21. This further supports the notion that ML in DS is a unique disease, and that sensitivity is cell-lineage specific rather than associated with a gene-dosage effect of genes located on chromosome 21.[35,37]

It is currently unknown to what extent treatment intensity can be reduced in DS children with ML. In a small case series, a 77% overall survival in a selected group of patients (n = 18) was reported with a regimen consisting of cytarabine 10 mg/m^2 per dose subcutaneously, twice daily for 7 days every 2 weeks; vincristine 1 mg/m^2 intravenously every 2 weeks; and retinylpalmitate 250,000 units/m^2 per day orally.[44] The NOPHO reported that approximately half of the patients included in their AML-93 protocol had dose-reductions of 75% and 67% of anthracyclines and cytarabine, respectively, which did not influence the relapse rate in those patients.[45] These data suggest that further treatment reduction may be possible, at least in some patients. However, most studies have also reported resistant or relapsed cases of ML DS. Therefore, it would be helpful if investigators could identify subgroups of patients with ML DS, at low risk of resistant or relapsed disease, for whom further dose-reduction of treatment intensity is feasible.

So far, such prognostic subgroups have not been described, and most published series lack the statistical power to identify prognostic factors because of small patient numbers.[30] Gamis and colleagues reported that children older than 4 years of age with ML DS had a poorer outcome than younger children. The older children, however, may have suffered from non-DS AML rather than typical DS associated ML, which occurs almost invariably in children younger than 5 years of age.[14,33] Indeed, Hasle and colleagues[46] have shown that only 2 out of 12 DS children over 4 years of age, with myeloid leukemia, had a GATA1 mutation. Hence, the authors suggest that ML occurring in children with DS may be classified based on GATA1 mutations as its unique molecular genetic basis. Cases lacking this mutation may benefit from treatment according to a protocol developed for non-DS AML, rather than treatment according to the less dose-intensive protocols developed for GATA1-mutation positive ML DS. It is still unclear whether real-time quantitative polymerase chain reaction (PCR) analysis for mutated GATA1 will be able to successfully measure minimal residual disease (MRD) levels, and therefore could be used for further risk stratification of ML in DS patients.[47] The disadvantage of this assay is that it is laborious, given that GATA1 mutations are private. Alternative methods for MRD-detection that could be employed include flowcytometry or reverse transcription-PCR for the Wilms tumor gene WT1.[48]

Acute Lymphoblastic Leukemia in Patients with Down Syndrome

In contrast to children with ML DS, children with ALL do not have a superior outcome when compared with their non-DS counterparts.[11,12,29,49–52] Whitlock and colleagues,[11] summarizing the CCG data on ALL in patients with DS treated between 1983 and 1995, reported that DS patients stratified to the standard risk ALL arm had a poorer outcome than those who did not have DS, while this difference was not present for those treated according to the high-risk ALL arm. This suggests that DS children with ALL may be under-treated when stratified in a standard risk arm, based on classical National Cancer Institute risk criteria (age 1–9 years and white blood cell count less than or equal to 50 $\times 10^9$/l). This was confirmed in the CCG 1952 study, which enrolled patients between 1996 and 2000.[12] Another possible explanation for this observation could be that physicians may have dose-reduced DS children with ALL in fear of enhanced toxicity (see later in this article). This may also have contributed to the observed higher relapse rate in these reports, although details on dose intensity were not provided. In the BFM 2000 study, which used MRD-based stratification using T-cell receptor and immunoglobulin gene rearrangements, there were no significant differences between DS and non-DS ALL patients in MRD-based risk-group assignment, nor in day-15 marrow response or in antileukemic efficacy between DS and non-DS ALL.[50] However, there was an increased rate of toxic deaths in the DS patients. At 5-years of follow-up, probability for event free survival was equivalent with 82% (standard error 5%) for DS children and 82% (standard error 1%) for non-DS children.

Despite a similar distribution over MRD-subgroups in the BFM study, there are clear biologic differences between DS and non-DS ALL cases.[12] When considering favorable prognostic factors, the frequency of hyperdiploid (more than 50 chromosomes) ALL is lower in DS patients.[11,12,29,49,50] The prognostically favorable trisomies, such as trisomy of chromosome 4, 10, and 17, are considerably less frequent in DS patients with ALL.[12] Several,[12,50,53] but not all[54] investigators report a lower frequency of TEL-AML1 rearranged ALL in children with DS. Considering the unfavorable prognostic factors, there are neither cases of infant ALL with DS, nor CD10-negative pro-B ALL cases, while the frequency of T-cell ALL is lower in children with DS. In addition, unfavorable cytogenetic abnormalities, such as t(1;19), the Philadelphia chromosome, or MLL-gene rearrangements occur less frequently in DS ALL,[11,12,29,51] although this was not confirmed by all groups.[50] It needs to be stressed however, that the definitions for favorable and unfavorable characteristics in all these studies were based on ALL in non-DS patients. It is unknown whether these abnormalities have the same impact in the context of constitutional trisomy 21.

Similar to ML treatment, an optimal balance between antileukemic efficacy and treatment-related toxicity needs to be established for children with DS and ALL, who lack the typical enhanced chemotherapy sensitivity that characterizes the myeloid blasts in DS patients. There are two studies describing in vitro cellular drug resistance profiles of ALL lymphoblasts in DS, and both studies did not report enhanced sensitivity of DS lymphoblasts when compared with non-DS lymphoblasts.[35,37] However, the data in these studies were not corrected for the differences in genetic make-up of DS and non-DS ALL, and therefore need to be interpreted with caution. Dördelmann and colleagues[49] reported a tendency for ALL to have a better initial steroid response in DS patients. However this was not confirmed in the BFM 2000 study, which showed a nonsignificant difference of 5.8% nonresponders in non-DS ALL, and 3.2% in DS ALL cases.[50]

INCREASED RISK FOR TOXICITY IN CHILDREN WITH DOWN SYNDROME

In children with DS, there is a delicate balance between the antileukemic efficacy of intensive chemotherapy and the increased toxic morbidity and mortality rates with which chemotherapy in these vulnerable children is associated.[12–14,29,30] Given the enhanced sensitivity of myeloid leukemic cells in these patients, dose-reductions in ML regimens for DS patients are easier accepted than for ALL regimens. For instance, in the CCG 2891 AML study, excessive toxicity resulted in poor prognosis and subsequent exclusion of children with ML and DS from the intensively timed induction regimen and stem cell transplantation.[14] Moreover, the excellent results of study AML BFM-98 were in part achieved by a significant reduction of induction mortality (the early death rate in the AML-BFM 93 study was 11%, in the subsequent AML-BFM 98-study, 0%).[13] Similarly, in the ALL 2000 study, children with DS experienced life-threatening adverse events in 23% of subjects, versus 6% in non-DS children.[50] The main side effects include mucositis, and an increased susceptibility to infections.[14,30,50,55,56] Mucositis is mainly associated with high-dose methotrexate (MTX), and probably caused by altered MTX pharmacokinetics in children with DS.[55] It needs to be mentioned, however, that many of these studies only comprised small numbers of patients, and were performed in an era preceding modern supportive care with well-established leucovorin rescue regimens. In addition, the reduced folate carrier (RFC), which is responsible for MTX transport into the cell, is localized on chromosome 21, and may be involved in an enhanced sensitivity for MTX, including gastrointestinal toxicity, although RFC transcript levels were not increased in the DS myeloblasts that were studied by Taub and colleagues.[39,41] Unfortunately, a consensus regarding MTX-dosing in children with DS and ALL is currently lacking.

An important aspect in treating children with DS is whether they have an increased risk of long-term cardiotoxicity following anthracycline exposure, given the fact that a significant proportion of DS children may have a compromised cardiac function because of congenital abnormalities to begin with. O'Brien and colleagues report on 57 DS patients treated on POG 9421, of whom 33% had a structural cardiac abnormality at inclusion.[57,58] One patient with an uncorrected tetralogy of Fallot died early because of a cardiac event as a consequence of fatal hypoxia during septicemia. Of the 54 patients in first complete remission, one patient with an atrioventricular canal was taken off study for congestive heart failure (CHF), and another patient died from CHF. At later follow-up, 21% of patients had documented CHF, requiring diuretics or inotropes. The cumulative anthracycline dose in this study was 135 mg/m^2 of daunorubicin and 80 mg/m^2 of mitoxantrone (cumulative dose of 535 mg/m^2 daunorubicin equivalents when assuming a ratio of 1:5). Creutzig and colleagues[59] describe the cardiotoxicity in DS patients (n = 121) treated according to protocol AML BFM 93 and -98, and report early cardiac toxicity in 4% and late cardiac toxicity in 5% of the subjects. In this study, there was no increased cardiotoxicity in DS children, but these children were treated with reduced dosages of anthracyclines (approximately 200 mg/m^2 –300 mg/m^2 daunorubicin dose equivalents).

GATA1 MUTATIONS

GATA1 is a double zinc finger DNA-binding transcription factor that has a critical role in promoting specification and terminal maturation of myeloid progenitor cells to red cells and megakaryocytes, that has been conserved through evolution.[60] Acquired mutations in the hemopoietic transcription factor GATA1 in ML DS were initially described by Wechsler and colleagues,[61] and subsequently by a number of groups. Three studies have studied the function of N-terminal region of GATA1 in murine megakaryopoiesis.[6,62,63] Expression of the mutated GATA1 protein GATA1s in embryonic and fetal megakaryocyte progenitors results in excessive megakaryocyte proliferation, and to a lesser extent abnormal differentiation of megakaryocytes into platelets.[6,62,63]

GATA1 mutations occur both in TL and ML in DS, as well as in blood and fetal liver samples from DS neonates.[64–71] GATA1 mutations are disease specific, as they are not detectable in remission samples. As GATA1 is encoded on the X-chromosome, the mutant clone expresses only the mutant allele in both males and females (because of X-inactivation). Over 100 different somatic genomic GATA1 mutations have been reported, which uniformly result in the expression of the amino-terminal truncated mutated GATA1 protein GATA1s (**Fig. 3**). Reports of newborns with multiple

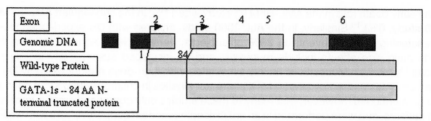

Fig. 3. Mutations in GATA1 in ML DS and TL. The GATA1 gene is composed of six exons with noncoding (*blue*) and coding (*brown*) regions. Two translational start sites (*arrows*) are present, one in exon 2, the other in exon 3. Protein translated from the second ATG, GATA1s, lacks the first 84 amino acids. Mutations in TL and ML DS are principally in exons 2 and 3 and introduce stop codons in the first 84 amino acids, or abrogate splicing of exon 2 to 3.

oligoclonal GATA1 mutations suggest that GATA1 mutations are a frequent event in hematopoietic cells of DS children.[69] Given the high frequency of GATA1 mutations in fetal blood cells trisomic for chromosome 21, and the fact that DS children are not prone to cancer in general, it has been suggested that GATA1 mutations impart a selective advantage, rather than trisomy 21 being a mutator phenotype.[69] The mutations occur principally in the 5' end of the gene, in exon 2, and less commonly in exon 3. Most are small insertions, duplications, deletions, or point mutations, though rare cases of large deletions have been reported. Given this, most mutations can be detected by PCR amplification of GATA1 exons 2 and 3, followed by direct sequencing or analysis by direct high pressure liquid chromatography (DHPLC). The ability to detect mutations depends on the proportion of mutant cells in the sample. In general, for direct sequencing, approximately 20% of the sample has to contain mutant cells. The sensitivity of DHPLC is higher, at approximately 2% to 5%. Once a mutation has been identified, mutation-specific probes and primers for mutation detection by real-time PCR can be designed that allow for more sensitive detection of mutant cells, which may be indicted for MRD detection.[47]

Expression profile analysis of GATA1s and the full-length GATA1-expressing murine fetal megakaryocytes showed that GATA1s fails to repress a number of transcription factor genes (GATA2, Ikaros, MYB and MYC), that have a proproliferative effect on hemopoietic cell growth.[6,63]

COOPERATING GENETIC EVENTS INVOLVED IN PROGRESSION FROM TRANSIENT LEUKEMIA TO MYELOID LEUKEMIA OF DOWN SYNDROME

AML is hypothesized to result from at least two types of cooperating genetic events, including growth promoting mutations (referred to as type 1 genetic aberrations) in, for example, receptor tyrosine kinases (such as FLT3 or KIT) or the RAS-oncogene, as well as translocations—such as t(8;21) or t(15;17)—that mainly impair differentiation (type 2 abnormalities).[72] In agreement with this hypothesis, recent studies have shown that GATA1s is insufficient to induce leukemia without other cooperating events.[6,73]

Little is known about the proliferation-enhancing type 1 mutations that are frequently encountered in non-DS AMLs, and their role in TL and ML DS. However, several articles have recently reported a potential role for mutations in the gene encoding for the non-receptor tyrosine kinase family of Janus kinases, (ie, JAK2 and JAK3).[74–79] These mutations were first identified in cell-lines using a proteomic approach.[77,79] So far, JAK2 gene mutations have not been found in the 38 primary samples from children with DS and TL or ML studied to date.[75,78] JAK3 mutations, however, were found in 13 out of 68 (19%) samples studied, suggesting a role in TL and ML in DS.[74–78] Given the fact that mutations were detected both in TL and ML DS, it is suggested that they are not sufficient for disease progression. Moreover, their contribution to DS malignancies still needs to be proven. No mutations in the gene encoding for well-known tyrosine kinases involved in non-DS AML, such as FLT3 or KIT, the RAS oncogene, or the gene encoding for the thrombopoietin receptor c-MPL were identified in any TL or ML samples from DS patients.[75,76,78]

Expression profiles from whole bone marrow or peripheral blood samples obtained from DS patients with ML showed that they have a quite distinct expression signature from other myeloid malignancies, including increased expression of GATA2, MYC (as in the mouse studies above), KIT and GATA1 itself.[80] Moreover, the chromosome 21 encoded transcription factor BACH1, which has been implicated as a repressor of megakaryocyte differentiation, was overexpressed, as well as SON, a gene with homology to the MYC family.[80] In contrast, expression of the chromosome 21 encoded transcription factor RUNX1, the most commonly mutated gene in non-DS AML, was reduced. This is an intriguing finding, as in most human AML cases reduced RUNX1 function is leukemogenic. ETS2 and ERG were not differentially expressed, despite their localization on chromosome 21. These genes are involved in megakaryocytic differentiation, and ERG-overexpression can frequently be found in AML cells from non-DS individuals, in particular in normal karyotype AML.[81,82] Whether ERG contributes to the development of TL awaits further study.[83]

These findings suggest a complex network of deregulated expression of key genes controlling the cell fate of megakaryocyte-erythroid lineage cells. A major caveat in attributing an oncogenic effect to these deregulated genes is that these gene expression profiles are not compared with relevant nonmalignant cell populations. Thus, it is impossible to assess if the observed gene expression profiles reflect the arrested differentiation of the leukemic cell population or in fact contribute to leukemogenesis.

SUMMARY

Constitutional trisomy 21 results in an enhanced risk of developing leukemias, both ALL as well as ML DS. TL and ML DS offer a unique model to obtain insight into the stepwise progression of leukemia, and of gene dosage effects mediated by aneuploidy. TL arises from expanded fetal liver progenitors as a result of constitutional trisomy 21, providing a window of opportunity for the occurrence of acquired mutations in the hematopoietic transcription factor GATA1. Many questions, however, remain unanswered. These include the true frequency of TL among infants with DS, the events involved in the subsequent development of ML in 20% of children diagnosed with TL, and the mechanisms underlying the spontaneous remission of TL. From a clinical point of view, studies assessing whether timely initiated cytarabine treatment may reduce the number of children dying early from TL-related complications (such as effusions, hydrops, or liver fibrosis), and whether the subsequent development of ML can be prevented by treating TL, are underway. Specific treatment protocols for children with ML DS have been designed, and show that treatment can safely be reduced, probably related to the unique hypersensitivity to chemotherapy of ML blasts in children with DS. Prospective studies need to identify to which extent and for which subgroups treatment can be further reduced, without an increase in recurrent disease. Recent attention has focused on ALL in patients with DS, which may be biologically distinct from non-DS ALL. ALL in DS is not characterized by increased sensitivity to chemotherapy. Given the enhanced sensitivity of DS children to the side effects of intensive chemotherapy, the development of new treatment modalities that confer less toxic side effects needs to be prioritized, and the recent discovery of mutations in JAK3 may be an example of a leukemia-specific target. Meanwhile, investigators will have to carefully assess the balance between the antileukemic efficacy and treatment-related mortality of current chemotherapy regimens. Several studies are currently in progress that will answer some of the questions raised above.

REFERENCES

1. Greaves M. In utero origins of childhood leukaemia. Early Hum Dev 2005;81(1): 123–9.
2. Roizen NJ, Patterson D. Down's syndrome. Lancet 2003;361(9365):1281–9.
3. Krivit W, Good RA. The simultaneous occurrence of leukemia and mongolism; report of four cases. AMA J Dis Child 1956;91(3):218–22.
4. Hasle H, Clemmensen IH, Mikkelsen M. Risks of leukaemia and solid tumours in individuals with Down's syndrome. Lancet 2000;355:165–9.
5. Hitzler JK, Zipursky A. Origins of leukaemia in children with Down syndrome. Nat Rev Cancer 2005;5(1):11–20.
6. Li Z, Godinho FJ, Klusmann JH, et al. Developmental stage-selective effect of somatically mutated leukemogenic transcription factor GATA1. Nat Genet 2005; 37(6):613–9.
7. Massey GV, Zipursky A, Chang MN, et al. A prospective study of the natural history of transient leukemia (TL) in neonates with Down syndrome (DS): a Children's Oncology Group (COG) study POG-9481. Blood 2006;107:4606–13.
8. Al Kasim F, Doyle JJ, Massey GV, et al. Incidence and treatment of potentially lethal diseases in transient leukemia of Down syndrome: Pediatric Oncology Group Study. J Pediatr Hematol Oncol 2002;24(1):9–13.
9. Vyas P, Roberts I. Down myeloid disorders: a paradigm for childhood preleukaemia and leukaemia and insights into normal megakaryopoiesis. Early Hum Dev 2006;82(12):767–73.
10. Vyas P, Crispino JD. Molecular insights into Down syndrome-associated leukemia. Curr Opin Pediatr 2007;19(1):9–14.
11. Whitlock JA, Sather HN, Gaynon P, et al. Clinical characteristics and outcome of children with down syndrome and acute lymphoblastic leukemia: a Children's Cancer Group study. Blood 2005;106:4043–9.
12. Bassal M, La MK, Whitlock JA, et al. Lymphoblast biology and outcome among children with Down syndrome and ALL treated on CCG-1952. Pediatr Blood Cancer 2005;44:21–8.
13. Creutzig U, Reinhardt D, Diekamp S, et al. AML patients with Down syndrome have a high cure rate with AML-BFM therapy with reduced dose intensity. Leukemia 2005;19(8):1355–60.
14. Gamis AS, Woods WG, Alonzo TA, et al. Increased age at diagnosis has a significantly negative effect on outcome in children with Down syndrome and acute myeloid leukemia: a report from the Children's Cancer Group Study 2891. J Clin Oncol 2003;21(18):3415–22.
15. Tunstall-Pedoe O, De la Fuente J, Bennet PR. Trisomy 21 expands the megakaryocyte-erytroid progenitor compartment in human fetal liver—implications for Down syndrome AMKL [abstract]. Blood 2006;108(11):170a.
16. Henry E, Walker D, Wiedmeier SE, et al. Hematological abnormalities during the first week of life among neonates with Down syndrome: data from a multihospital healthcare system. Am J Med Genet A 2007;143(1):42–50.

17. Widness JA, Pueschel SM, Pezzullo JC, et al. Elevated erythropoietin levels in cord blood of newborns with Down's syndrome. Biol Neonate 1994;66(1):50–5.
18. Kivivuori SM, Rajantie J, Siimes MA. Peripheral blood cell counts in infants with Down's syndrome. Clin Genet 1996;49(1):15–9.
19. De Hingh YC, Van der Vossen PW, Gemen EF, et al. Intrinsic abnormalities of lymphocyte counts in children with Down syndrome. J Pediatr 2005;147(6): 744–7.
20. Weijerman ME, Van Furth AM, Vonk-Noordegraaf A, et al. Prevalence, neonatal characteristics and first year mortality of Down syndrome: a national study. J Pediatr, in press.
21. Pine SR, Guo Q, Yin C, et al. Incidence and clinical implications of GATA1 mutations in newborns with Down syndrome. Blood 2007;110(6):2128–31.
22. Heald B, Hilden JM, Zbuk K, et al. Severe TMD/AMKL with GATA1 mutation in a stillborn fetus with Down syndrome. Nat Clin Pract Oncol 2007;4(7):433–8.
23. Muramatsu H, Watanabe N, Matsumoto K, et al. A retrospective analysis of 70 cases of transient leukemia in neonates with Down syndrome [abstract]. Blood 2006;108(11):301b.
24. Vardiman JW, Harris NL, Brunning RD. The World Health Organization (WHO) classification of the myeloid neoplasms. Blood 2002;100(7):2292–302.
25. Hasle H, Niemeyer CM, Chessells JM, et al. A pediatric approach to the WHO classification of myelodysplastic and myeloproliferative diseases. Leukemia 2003;17(2):277–82.
26. Creutzig U, Ritter J, Vormoor J, et al. Myelodysplasia and acute myelogenous leukemia in Down's syndrome. A report of 40 children of the AML-BFM Study Group. Leukemia 1996;10(11):1677–86.
27. Lange BJ, Kobrinsky N, Barnard DR, et al. Distinctive demography, biology, and outcome of acute myeloid leukemia and myelodysplastic syndrome in children with Down syndrome: Children's Cancer Group Studies 2861 and 2891. Blood 1998;91(2):608–15.
28. Gamis AS, Alonzo T, Hiden JM, et al. Outcome of Down syndrome children with acute myeloid leukemia (AML) or myelodysplasia (MDS) treated with a uniform prospective trial—initial report of the COG trial A2971 [abstract]. Blood 2006; 108(11):9a.
29. Zeller B, Gustafsson G, Forestier E, et al. Acute leukaemia in children with Down syndrome: a population-based Nordic study. Br J Haematol 2005;128(6): 797–804.
30. Gamis AS. Acute myeloid leukemia and Down syndrome evolution of modern therapy—state of the art review. Pediatr Blood Cancer 2005;44(1):13–20.
31. Ravindranath Y, Abella E, Krischer JP, et al. Acute myeloid leukemia (AML) in Down's syndrome is highly responsive to chemotherapy: experience on Pediatric Oncology Group AML Study 8498. Blood 1992;80(9):2210–4.
32. Lie SO, Jonmundsson G, Mellander L, et al. A population-based study of 272 children with acute myeloid leukaemia treated on two consecutive protocols with different intensity: best outcome in girls, infants, and children with Down's syndrome. Nordic Society of Paediatric Haematology and Oncology (NOPHO). Br J Haematol 1996;94(1):82–8.
33. Ravindranath Y. Down syndrome and acute myeloid leukemia: the paradox of increased risk for leukemia and heightened sensitivity to chemotherapy. J Clin Oncol 2003;21(18):3385–7.
34. Creutzig U, Zimmermann M, Lehrnbecher T, et al. Less toxicity by optimizing chemotherapy, but not by addition of granulocyte colony-stimulating factor in

children and adolescents with acute myeloid leukemia: results of AML-BFM 98. J Clin Oncol 2006;24(27):4499–506.

35. Zwaan CM, Kaspers GJL, Pieters R, et al. Different drug sensitivity profiles of acute myeloid and lymphoblastic leukemia and normal peripheral blood mononuclear cells, in children with and without Down syndrome. Blood 2002;99:245–51.

36. Taub JW, Stout ML, Buck SA, et al. Myeloblasts from Down syndrome children with acute myeloid leukemia have increased in vitro sensitivity to cytosine arabinoside and daunorubicin. Leukemia 1997;11(9):1594–5.

37. Frost BM, Gustafsson G, Larsson R, et al. Cellular cytotoxic drug sensitivity in children with acute leukemia and Down's syndrome: an explanation to differences in clinical outcome? [letter]. Leukemia 2000;14(5):943–4.

38. Yamada S, Hongo T, Okada S, et al. Distinctive multidrug sensitivity and outcome of acute erythroblastic and megakaryoblastic leukemia in children with Down syndrome. Int J Hematol 2001;74(4):428–36.

39. Taub JW, Ge Y. Down syndrome, drug metabolism and chromosome 21. Pediatr Blood Cancer 2005;44(1):33–9.

40. Taub JW, Matherly LH, Stout ML, et al. Enhanced metabolism of 1-beta-D-arabinofuranosylcytosine in Down syndrome cells: a contributing factor to the superior event free survival of Down syndrome children with acute myeloid leukemia. Blood 1996;87(8):3395–403.

41. Taub JW, Huang X, Matherly LH, et al. Expression of chromosome 21-localized genes in acute myeloid leukemia: differences between Down syndrome and non-Down syndrome blast cells and relationship to in vitro sensitivity to cytosine arabinoside and daunorubicin. Blood 1999;94(4):1393–400.

42. Taub JW, Huang X, Ge Y, et al. Cystathionine-beta-synthase cDNA transfection alters the sensitivity and metabolism of 1-beta-D-arabinofuranosylcytosine in CCRF-CEM leukemia cells in vitro and in vivo: a model of leukemia in Down syndrome. Cancer Res 2000;60(22):6421–6.

43. Ge Y, Jensen TL, Stout ML, et al. The role of cytidine deaminase and GATA1 mutations in the increased cytosine arabinoside sensitivity of Down syndrome myeloblasts and leukemia cell lines. Cancer Res 2004;64(2):728–35.

44. Al Ahmari A, Shah N, Sung L, et al. Long-term results of an ultra low-dose cytarabine-based regimen for the treatment of acute megakaryoblastic leukaemia in children with Down syndrome. Br J Haematol 2006;133(6):646–8.

45. Abildgaard L, Ellebaek E, Gustafsson G, et al. Optimal treatment intensity in children with Down syndrome and myeloid leukaemia: data from 56 children treated on NOPHO-AML protocols and a review of the literature. Ann Hematol 2006;85(5): 275–80.

46. Hasle H, Niemeyer C, O'Marcaigh A, et al. Myeloid leukemia in children 4 years or older with Down syndrome. A BFM, DCOG, MRC, NOPHO collaborative study. [abstract]. Presented at the 5th Bi-annual Symposium on Childhood Leukemia. Noordwijkerhout, the Netherlands, April 30–May 2, 2006.

47. Pine SR, Guo Q, Yin C, et al. GATA1 as a new target to detect minimal residual disease in both transient leukemia and megakaryoblastic leukemia of Down syndrome. Leuk Res 2005;29(11):1353–6.

48. Hasle H, Lund B, Nyvold CG, et al. WT1 gene expression in children with Down syndrome and transient myeloproliferative disorder. Leuk Res 2006;30(5):543–6.

49. Dördelmann M, Schrappe M, Reiter A, et al. Down's syndrome in childhood acute lymphoblastic leukemia: clinical characteristics and treatment outcome in four consecutive BFM trials. Berlin-Frankfurt-Münster Group. Leukemia 1998;12(5): 645–51.

50. Möricke A, Zimmermann M, Schwarz C, et al. Excellent event-free survival despite higher incidence of treatment related toxicity and mortality in Down syndrome patients with ALL as compared to patients without Down syndrome: data from the ALL-BFM 2000 trial [abstract]. Presented at the 5th Bi-annual Symposium on Childhood Leukemia. Noordwijkerhout, the Netherlands, April 30–May 2, 2006.
51. Pui CH, Raimondi SC, Borowitz MJ, et al. Immunophenotypes and karyotypes of leukemic cells in children with Down syndrome and acute lymphoblastic leukemia. J Clin Oncol 1993;11(7):1361–7.
52. Chessells JM, Harrison CJ, Kempski H, et al. Clinical features, cytogenetics and outcome in acute lymphoblastic and myeloid leukaemia of infancy: report from the MRC Childhood Leukaemia Working Party. Leukemia 2002;16(5):776–84.
53. Lanza C, Volpe G, Basso G, et al. The common TEL/AML1 rearrangement does not represent a frequent event in acute lymphoblastic leukaemia occuring in children with Down syndrome. Leukemia 1997;11(6):820–1.
54. Steiner M, Attarbaschi A, Konig M, et al. Equal frequency of TEL/AML1 rearrangements in children with acute lymphoblastic leukemia with and without Down syndrome. Pediatr Hematol Oncol 2005;22(3):229–34.
55. Garré ML, Relling MV, Kalwinsky D, et al. Pharmacokinetics and toxicity of methotrexate in children with Down syndrome and acute lymphocytic leukemia. J Pediatr 1987;111(4):606–12.
56. Whitlock JA. Down syndrome and acute lymphoblastic leukaemia. Br J Haematol 2006;135(5):595–602.
57. Becton D, Dahl GV, Ravindranath Y, et al. Randomized use of Cyclosporin A (CSA) to modulate P-glycoprotein in children with AML in remission: Pediatric Oncology Group study 9421. Blood 2006;107:1315–24.
58. O'Brien M, Taub J, Stine K, et al. Excessive cardiotxocity despite excellent leukemia-free survival for pediatric patients with Down syndrome and acute myeloid leukemia: results from POG (Pediatric Oncology Group) protocol 9421 [abstract]. Blood 2006;108(11):168a–9a.
59. Creutzig U, Diekamp S, Zimmermann M, et al. Longitudinal evaluation of early and late anthracycline cardiotoxicity in children with AML. Pediatr Blood Cancer 2007;48(7):651–62.
60. Cantor AB. GATA transcription factors in hematologic disease. Int J Hematol 2005;81(5):378–84.
61. Wechsler J, Greene M, McDevitt MA, et al. Acquired mutations in GATA1 in the megakaryoblastic leukemia of Down syndrome. Nat Genet 2002;32(1):148–52.
62. Kuhl C, Atzberger A, Iborra F, et al. GATA1-mediated megakaryocyte differentiation and growth control can be uncoupled and mapped to different domains in GATA1. Mol Cell Biol 2005;25(19):8592–606.
63. Muntean AG, Crispino JD. Differential requirements for the activation domain and FOG-interaction surface of GATA-1 in megakaryocyte gene expression and development. Blood 2005;106(4):1223–31.
64. Hitzler JK, Cheung J, Li Y, et al. GATA1 mutations in transient leukemia and acute megakaryoblastic leukemia of Down syndrome. Blood 2003;101(11):4301–4.
65. Mundschau G, Gurbuxani S, Gamis AS, et al. Mutagenesis of GATA1 is an initiating event in Down syndrome leukemogenesis. Blood 2003;101(11):4298–300.
66. Rainis L, Bercovich D, Strehl S, et al. Mutations in exon 2 of GATA1 are early events in megakaryocytic malignancies associated with trisomy 21. Blood 2003;102:981–6.

67. Groet J, McElwaine S, Spinelli M, et al. Acquired mutations in GATA1 in neonates with Down's syndrome with transient myeloid disorder. Lancet 2003;361(9369): 1617–20.
68. Xu G, Nagano M, Kanezaki R, et al. Frequent mutations in the GATA-1 gene in the transient myeloproliferative disorder of Down syndrome. Blood 2003;102(8): 2960–8.
69. Ahmed M, Sternberg A, Hall G, et al. Natural history of GATA1 mutations in Down syndrome. Blood 2004;103(7):2480–9.
70. Shimada A, Xu G, Toki T, et al. Fetal origin of the GATA1 mutation in identical twins with transient myeloproliferative disorder and acute megakaryoblastic leukemia accompanying Down syndrome [letter]. Blood 2004;103(1):366.
71. Taub JW, Mundschau G, Ge Y, et al. Prenatal origin of GATA1 mutations may be an initiating step in the development of megakaryocytic leukemia in Down syndrome. Blood 2004;104(5):1588–9.
72. Deguchi K, Gilliland DG. Cooperativity between mutations in tyrosine kinases and in hematopoietic transcription factors in AML. Leukemia 2002;16(4):740–4.
73. Hollanda LM, Lima CS, Cunha AF, et al. An inherited mutation leading to production of only the short isoform of GATA-1 is associated with impaired erythropoiesis. Nat Genet 2006;38(7):807–12.
74. De Vita S, Mulligan C, McElwaine S, et al. Loss-of-function JAK3 mutations in TMD and AMKL of Down syndrome. Br J Haematol 2007;137(4):337–41.
75. Klusmann JH, Reinhardt D, Hasle H, et al. Janus kinase mutations in the development of acute megakaryoblastic leukemia in children with and without Down's syndrome. Leukemia 2007;21(7):1584–7.
76. Kiyoi H, Yamaji S, Kojima S, et al. JAK3 mutations occur in acute megakaryoblastic leukemia both in Down syndrome children and non-Down syndrome adults. Leukemia 2007;21(3):574–6.
77. Walters DK, Mercher T, Gu TL, et al. Activating alleles of JAK3 in acute megakaryoblastic leukemia. Cancer Cell 2006;10(1):65–75.
78. Norton A, Fisher C, Liu H, et al. Analysis of JAK3, JAK2, and C-MPL mutations in transient myeloproliferative disorder and myeloid leukemia of Down syndrome blasts in children with Down syndrome. Blood 2007;110(3):1077–9.
79. Mercher T, Wernig G, Moore SA, et al. JAK2T875N is a novel activating mutation that results in myeloproliferative disease with features of megakaryoblastic leukemia in a murine bone marrow transplantation model. Blood 2006;108(8): 2770–9.
80. Bourquin JP, Subramanian A, Langebrake C, et al. Identification of distinct molecular phenotypes in acute megakaryoblastic leukemia by gene expression profiling. Proc Natl Acad Sci USA 2006;103:3339–44.
81. Marcucci G, Baldus CD, Ruppert AS, et al. Overexpression of the ETS-related gene, ERG, predicts a worse outcome in acute myeloid leukemia with normal karyotype: a Cancer and Leukemia Group B study. J Clin Oncol 2005;23(36): 9234–42.
82. Rainis L, Toki T, Pimanda JE, et al. The proto-oncogene ERG in megakaryoblastic leukemias. Cancer Res 2005;65(17):7596–602.
83. Izraeli S, Rainis L, Hertzberg L, et al. Trisomy of chromosome 21 in leukemogenesis. Blood Cells Mol Dis 2007;39(2):156–9.

Acute Myeloid Leukemia

Jeffrey E. Rubnitz, MD, PhD[a,*], Brenda Gibson, MD[b],
Franklin O. Smith, MD[c]

KEYWORDS

- Myeloid • Leukemia • Childhood

Acute myeloid leukemia (AML) is a heterogeneous group of leukemias that arise in precursors of myeloid, erythroid, megakaryocytic, and monocytic cell lineages. These leukemias result from clonal transformation of hematopoietic precursors through the acquisition of chromosomal rearrangements and multiple gene mutations. New molecular technologies have allowed a better understanding of these molecular events, improved classification of AML according to risk, and the development of molecularly targeted therapies. As a result of highly collaborative clinical research by pediatric cooperative cancer groups worldwide, disease-free survival (DFS) has improved significantly during the past 3 decades.[1–15] Further improvements in the outcome of children who have AML probably will reflect continued progress in understanding the biology of AML and the concomitant development of new molecularly targeted agents for use in combination with conventional chemotherapy drugs.

EPIDEMIOLOGY AND RISK FACTORS

Approximately 6500 children and adolescents in the United States develop acute leukemia each year.[16] AML comprises only 15% to 20% of these cases but accounts for a disproportionate 30% of deaths from acute leukemia. The incidence of pediatric AML is estimated to be between five and seven cases per million people per year, with a peak incidence of 11 cases per million at 2 years of age.[17–19] Incidence reaches a low point at age approximately 9 years, then increases to nine cases per million during adolescence and remains relatively stable until age 55 years. There is no

A version of this article was previously published in the *Pediatric Clinics of North America*, 55:1.
JER was supported, in part, by the American Lebanese Syrian Associated Charities (ALSAC).
[a] Department of Oncology, St. Jude Children's Research Hospital, MS 260, 262 Danny Thomas Place, Memphis, TN 38105, USA
[b] Department of Paediatric Haematology, Royal Hospital for Sick Children, Yorkhill, G3 8SJ, Glasgow, Scotland, UK
[c] Division of Hematology/Oncology, University of Cincinnati College of Medicine, Cincinnati Children's Hospital Medical Center
* Corresponding author.
E-mail address: jeffrey.rubnitz@stjude.org (J.E. Rubnitz).

difference in incidence between male and female or black and white populations.[16] There is, however, evidence suggesting that incidence is highest in Hispanic children, intermediate in black children (5.8 cases per million), and slightly lower in white children (4.8 cases per million).[20–23] The French-American-British (FAB) classification subtypes of AML are equally represented across ethnic and racial groups with the exception of acute promyelocytic leukemia (APL), which has a higher incidence among children of Latin and Hispanic ancestry.

During the years between 1977 and 1995, the overall incidence of AML remained stable, but there was a disturbing increase in the incidence of secondary AML as the result of prior exposure to chemotherapy and radiation.[24–30] This risk remains particularly high among individuals exposed to alkylating agents (cyclophosphamide, nitrogen mustard, ifosfamide, melphalan, and chlorambucil) and intercalating topoisomerase II inhibitors, including the epipodophyllotoxins (etoposide).

Most children who have de novo AML have no identifiable predisposing environmental exposure or inherited condition, although a number of environmental exposures, inherited conditions, and acquired disorders are associated with the development of AML. Myelodysplastic syndrome and AML reportedly are associated with exposure to chemotherapy and ionizing radiation and also to chemicals that include petroleum products and organic solvents (benzene), herbicides, and pesticides (organophosphates).[31–36]

A large number of inherited conditions predispose children to the development of AML. Among these are Down syndrome, Fanconi anemia, severe congenital neutropenia (Kostmann syndrome), Shwachman-Diamond syndrome, Diamond-Blackfan syndrome, neurofibromatosis type 1, Noonan syndrome, dyskeratosis congenita, familial platelet disorder with a predisposition to AML (FDP/AML), congenital amegakaryocytic thrombocytopenia, ataxia-telangiectasia, Klinefelter's syndrome, Li-Fraumeni syndrome, and Bloom syndrome.[37–40]

Finally, AML has been associated with several acquired conditions including aplastic anemia,[41,42] myelodysplastic syndrome, acquired amegakaryocytic thrombocytopenia,[43,44] and paroxysmal nocturnal hemoglobinuria.

PATHOGENESIS

AML is the result of distinct but cooperating genetic mutations that confer a proliferative and survival advantage and that impair differentiation and apoptosis.[45–47] This multistep mechanism for the pathogenesis of AML is supported by murine models,[48,49] the analysis of leukemia in twins,[50–53] and the analysis of patients who have FDP/AML syndrome.[54] Mutations in a number of genes that confer a proliferative and/or survival advantage to cells but do not affect differentiation (Class I mutations) have been identified in AML, including mutations of *FLT3*, *ALM*, oncogenic *Ras* and *PTPN11*, and the *BCR/ABL* and *TEL/PDGFβR* gene fusions. Similarly, gene mutations and translocation-associated fusions that impair differentiation and apoptosis (Class II mutations) in AML include the *AML/ETO* and *PML/RARα* fusions, *MLL* rearrangements, and mutations in *CEBPA*, *CBF*, *HOX* family members, *CBP/P300*, and co-activators of *TIF1*. AML results when hematopoietic precursor cells acquire both Class I and Class II genetic abnormalities. Although only one cytogenetic or molecular abnormality has been reported in many cases of AML, new molecular tools now are identifying multiple genetic mutations in such cases.

Accumulating data suggest that the leukemic stem cell arises at different stages of differentiation and involves heterogeneous, complex patterns of abnormality in myeloid precursor cells.[55–60] The leukemic stem cell, also called the "self-renewing leukemia-initiating cell," is located within both the CD34$^+$ and CD34$^-$ cell compartments and is rare (0.2–200 per 10^6 mononuclear cells).[61–64] A recent study of pediatric AML suggested that patients who have *FLT3* abnormalities in less mature CD34$^+$ CD38$^-$ precursor cells are less likely to survive than patients who have *FLT3* mutations in more mature CD34$^+$ CD38$^+$ cells (11% versus 100% at 4 years; P = .002).[65] Although sample sizes in this study were small, this result demonstrates the heterogeneity of genetic abnormalities in various stem cell compartments and suggests a worse outcome when less mature precursor cells harbor these abnormalities.

CLINICAL PRESENTATION AND DIAGNOSIS

The presentation of childhood AML reflects signs and symptoms that result from leukemic infiltration of the bone marrow and extramedullary sites. Replacement of normal bone marrow hematopoietic cells results in neutropenia, anemia, and thrombocytopenia. Children commonly present with signs and symptoms of pancytopenia, including fever, fatigue, pallor, bleeding, bone pain, and infections. Disseminated intravascular coagulation may be observed at presentation of all AML subtypes but is much more frequent in childhood APL. Infiltration of extramedullary sites can result in lymphadenopathy, hepatosplenomegaly, chloromatous tumors (myeloblastomas and granulocytic sarcomas), disease in the skin (leukemia cutis), orbit, and epidural space, and, rarely, testicular involvement. The central nervous system is involved at diagnosis in approximately 15% of cases.[66] Patients who have high white blood cells counts may present with signs or symptoms of leukostasis, most often affecting the lung and brain.

A diagnosis is suggested by a complete blood cell count showing pancytopenia and blast cells and is confirmed by examination of the bone marrow. The diagnosis and subtype classification of AML is based on morphologic, cytochemical, cytogenetic, and fluorescent in situ hybridization analyses, flow cytometric immunophenotyping, and molecular testing (eg, *FLT3* mutation analysis).

TREATMENT OF CHILDHOOD ACUTE MYELOID LEUKEMIA

The prognosis of children who have AML has improved greatly during the past 3 decades (**Fig. 1**). Rates of complete remission (CR) as high as 80% to 90% and overall survival (OS) rates of 60% now are reported. (**Table 1**)[1] This success reflects the use of

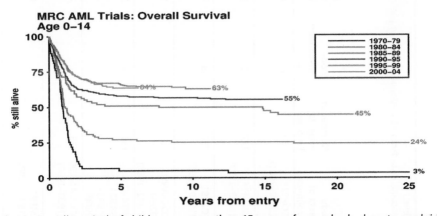

Fig. 1. Overall survival of children younger than 15 years of age who had acute myeloid leukemia treated in MRC trials during the past 3 decades.

Table 1
Outcome data from 13 national groups for patients younger than 15 years of age who had acute myeloid leukemia

Study (Years of Enrollment)	Number of Patients Enrolled	Non-Responders (%)	Early Death Rate (%)	Complete Response (%)	% 5-Year Event-free Survival (SE)	% 5-Year Overall Survival (SE)	Death Rate in Complete Response (%)	Cumulative Doses of ara-C, Etoposide, and Anthracyclines[a]	% of Total Number of Patients Who Underwent Allogeneic Stem cell Transplantation
AIEOP92 (1992–2001)	160	5	6	89	54 (4)	60 (4)	7	No strict protocol guidelines	29
AML-BFM93 (1993–1998)	427	10	7	83	51 (3)	58 (2)	4	41.1 g/m^2 950 mg/m^2 300–400 mg/m^2	7
CCG2891 (1989–1995)	750	18	4	78	34 (3)	47 (4)	15	14.6 g/m^2 1100 mg/m^2 180 mg/m^2	25
DCOG-ANLL 92/94 (1992–1998)	78	8	10	82	42 (6)	42 (6)	16	33.2 g/m^2 950 mg/m^2 400 mg/m^2	27
EORTC-CLG 58,921 (1993–2000)	166	13	2	84	48 (4)	62 (4)	6	23.32–29.32 g/m^2 1350 mg/m^2 380 mg/m^2	20
GATLA-AML90 (1990–1997)	179	11	20	70	31 (4)	41 (4)	7	41.1 g/m^2 1450 mg/m^2 300 mg/m^2	3
LAME91 (1991–1998)	247	5	4	91	48 (4)	62 (4)	6	9.8–13.4 g/m^2 400 mg/m^2 460 mg/m^2	30

Study								
NOPHO-AML93 (1993–2001)	223	5	2	92	50 (3)	66 (3)	2	49.6–61.3 g/m² 1600 mg/m² 300–375 mg/m²	25
PINDA-92 (1992–1998)	151	5	26	68	36	36	4	7.64 g/m² 450 mg/m² 350 mg/m²	—
POG8821 (1988–1993)	511	19	4	77	31 (2)	42 (2)	8	55.7 g/m² 2250 mg/m² 360 mg/m²	13
PPLLSG98 (1998–2002)	104	13	8	80	47 (5)	50 (5)	10	7.0–15.1 g/m² 450–950 mg/m² 420–600 mg/m²	Not reported
St Jude-AML91 (1991–1997)	62	16	3	79	44 (15)	57 (11)	?	3.8 g/m² 1200 mg/m² 270 mg/m²	Not given
UK MRC AML10 (1988–1995)	303	3	4	93	49	58	10	10.6 g/m² 500–1500 mg/m² 550 mg/m²	20
UK MRC AML12 (1995–2002)	455	4	4	92	56	66	6	4.6–34.6 g/m² 1500 mg/m² 300–610 mg/m²	8

Abbreviations: AIEOP, Associazione Italiana Ematologia Oncologia Pediatrica; BFM, Berlin-Frankfurt-Münster; CCG, Children's Cancer Group; DCOG, Dutch Childhood Oncology Group; EORTC-CLG, European Organization for the Research and Treatment of Cancer–Children Leukemia Group; GATLA, The Argentine Group for the Treatment of Acute Leukemia; LAME, Leucemie Aigue Myeloblastique Enfant); NOPHO, Nordic Society of Pediatric Haematology and Oncology; PINDA, the National Program for Antineoplastic Drugs for Children; POG, Pediatric Oncology Group; PPLLSG, Polish Pediatric Leukemia/Lymphoma Study Group; UK MRC, United Kingdom Medical Research Council.

[a] Cumulative dose of anthracyclines was calculated by applying the following arbitrary conversion factors to obtain daunorubicin equivalents: idarubicin, 5×; mitoxantrone, 5×; doxorubicin, 1×. Some groups (Leucemie Aique Myeloide Enfant and the Medical Research Council in the United Kingdom) also administered amsacrine, which is not included in calculated total anthracycline exposure.

increasingly intensive induction chemotherapy followed by postremission treatment with additional anthracyclines and high-dose cytarabine or myeloablative regimens followed by stem cell transplantation (SCT). The drugs used in the treatment of AML have changed little, but refinement of their delivery and striking advances in supportive care have allowed administration of optimally intensive therapy with less morbidity and mortality. Better postrelapse salvage therapy also has contributed to the improvement in OS.

Treatment of AML in children generally is based on an anthracycline, cytarabine, and etoposide regimen given as a minimum of four cycles of chemotherapy. A recent report compared the results of anthracycline, cytarabine, and etoposide regimens used by 13 national study groups.[1] The regimens differed in many ways, including the cumulative doses of drugs, the choice of anthracycline, the number and intensity of blocks of treatment, and the intrathecal chemotherapy used for central nervous system (CNS) prophylaxis. Treatment generally was risk stratified, although the definition of risk groups varied, as did the indications for SCT. Despite the varying strategies, results are relatively similar (see **Table 1**).[2] Many groups now achieve CR rates of 80% to 90%, relapse rates of 30% to 40%, event-free survival (EFS) rates of 50%, and OS rates of 60%.[3–15]

Because of the small number of pediatric patients who have AML, many important questions have not been addressed in the context of randomized trials. The unresolved issues include the optimal intensity of chemotherapy, the optimal anthracycline, the optimal dose of cytarabine, the cumulative dose of anthracycline that minimizes cardiotoxicity without compromising outcome, the role of allogeneic SCT in first CR, and the use of risk-directed therapy.

Induction and Consolidation Therapy

The most favorable outcomes are achieved by the use of a relatively high cumulative dose of either anthracycline or cytarabine (see **Table 1**).[1,2] The schedule and timing of intensification also are important. The Children's Cancer Group (CCG) reported that intensively timed induction therapy (the second cycle delivered 10 days after the first cycle) was more advantageous than standard therapy (the second cycle delivered 14 or more days after the first cycle, dependent on bone marrow status and cell-count recovery).[4,67] Both the CR and EFS rates were significantly higher with intensively timed dosing, regardless of postremission therapy, suggesting that the depth of remission may profoundly affect survival. The benefit derived from early intensification, whether achieved by time sequencing or by adjusting cytarabine and etoposide doses to achieve a targeted plasma level, may be lost, however, if prolonged neutropenia and thrombocytopenia cause unacceptable delays in subsequent treatment.[9,13] The intensification of early therapy beyond a certain threshold therefore is unlikely to improve outcome and may even be detrimental to OS.[13]

In a Medical Research Council (MRC) study, an additional course of postremission chemotherapy (four versus five courses in total) provided no advantage to patients already receiving intensive treatment,[5] suggesting a plateau in the benefit of conventional postremission chemotherapy. If such a plateau is confirmed, it is likely that any additional antileukemic effect will have to come from alternative approaches, such as targeted or cellular therapies.

Certain anthracyclines are favored for their perceived greater antileukemic effect and/or their lower cardiotoxicity, but no anthracycline agent has been demonstrated to be superior. The MRC found daunorubicin and mitoxantrone to be equally efficacious but mitoxantrone to be more myelosuppressive.[5] Idarubicin is used commonly because in vitro and preclinical studies suggest that it offers a greater clinical benefit because of its faster cellular uptake, increased retention, and lower susceptibility to multidrug resistant glycoprotein.[68,69] In addition, its main metabolite, idarubicinol, has a prolonged plasma half-life (54 hours) and has antileukemic activity in the cerebrospinal fluid.[70] In the Berlin-Frankfurt-Münster (BFM) AML 93 trial, induction therapy with idarubicin, cytarabine, and etoposide (AIE) resulted in significantly greater blast-cell clearance at day 15 than induction with daunorubicin, cytarabine, and etoposide (ADE) (P = .01) but did not improve 5-year OS (51% with AIE versus 50% with ADE; P = .72) or EFS (60% for AIE versus 57% for ADE; P = .55).[71] Similarly, the Australian and New Zealand Children's Cancer Study Group reported that idarubicin and daunorubicin were equally efficacious, but idarubicin was more toxic.[72] The addition of cyclosporin A to induction chemotherapy to inhibit P-glycoprotein–mediated anthracycline efflux did not prolong the duration of remission or improve OS in children.[73]

Another important question is whether the cumulative dose of anthracyclines can be reduced safely without compromising survival. Although cumulative doses above 375 mg/m^2 increase the risk of cardiotoxicity, EFS is lower in protocols that use lower doses of anthracycline.[1,2] Optimal results may be achievable with a cumulative dose of approximately 375 to 550 mg/m^2 if high-dose cytarabine is used in postremission therapy.[1,2] The full impact of cardiotoxicity, particularly late cardiotoxicity, also is poorly defined. In the MRC AML10 protocol, which delivered a high cumulative anthracycline dose (550 mg/m^2), 9 of 341 registered patients died of acute cardiotoxicity (all after a cumulative dose of 300 mg/m^2); 7 of the 9 deaths occurred during an episode of sepsis. Subclinical deficits in cardiac function would have gone undetected in the absence of cardiac monitoring.[74] Minimizing cardiotoxicity is important, however, and cardioprotectant agents and liposomal anthracyclines with reduced cardiotoxicity are being tested.

The use of high-dose cytarabine in postremission therapy seems to be important in improving survival, but the optimal dose has not been determined. Core binding factor (CBF) leukemias may respond particularly well to multiple courses of high-dose cytarabine.[75]

Central Nervous System–directed Therapy

The impact of CNS involvement on EFS is not well defined.[8,9,11,13,76,77] Most pediatric clinical trial groups use intrathecal chemotherapy for CNS prophylaxis, employing either one or three agents and various doses. Not all pediatric groups routinely use intrathecal CNS prophylaxis,[9] however, and few adult groups do. The correlation between the type of CNS treatment given and the incidence of CNS relapse is not clear. The CNS relapse rate seems to be around 2% for isolated CNS relapse and between 2% and 9% for combined CNS and bone marrow relapse.[2,4–10] The low rate of CNS relapse may reflect both the use of intrathecal chemotherapy and the CNS protection afforded by high-dose cytarabine and by idarubicin, both of which can penetrate the CNS.[70] Cranial irradiation, because of its sequelae, is not widely used as prophylaxis. It is used currently only by the BFM Study Group, which observed an increase in CNS and systemic relapse in patients who did not receive cranial irradiation in the AML BFM 87 trial.[78] The current AML BFM 98 trial is exploring reduction of the dose of cranial irradiation to limit late sequelae. The necessity of cranial irradiation for patients who have CNS involvement at presentation or CNS relapse is unproven. Many groups reserve cranial irradiation for patients whose CNS is not cleared of leukemic cells by intrathecal and intensive systemic chemotherapy.[4,11,13]

Maintenance Therapy

Maintenance therapy is no longer used in the treatment of AML, having failed to demonstrate benefit except in BFM studies. Patients who have APL, however, do seem to benefit from antimetabolite maintenance treatment given with all-trans retinoic acid (ATRA). In patients who have non-APL AML, maintenance treatment showed no benefit in two randomized studies (Leucemie Aigue Myeloblastique Enfant 91 and CCG 213); these studies even suggested that maintenance therapy may be deleterious when intensive chemotherapy is used and may contribute to clinical drug resistance and treatment failure after relapse.[9,79]

Stem Cell Transplantation

SCT is the most successful curative treatment for AML; it produces a strong graft-versus-leukemia effect and can cure even relapsed AML. Its potential benefit, however, must be weighed against the risk of transplantation-related mortality and the late sequelae of transplantation. SCT has become a less attractive option as the outcomes of increasingly intensive chemotherapy and postrelapse salvage therapy have improved. Furthermore, although SCT is reported to provide a survival advantage for patients in first CR, studies so far have used matched sibling donors, who are available to only about one in four patients. Although experienced groups have reported comparable outcomes with alternative donors, it is too early to determine whether their wider use will result in greater transplantation-related mortality.

The role of allogeneic SCT, particularly whether it should be done during first CR or reserved for second remission, remains the most controversial issue in pediatric AML. Competing factors, particularly risk group, may tip the balance in favor of SCT or intensive chemotherapy. Most groups agree that children who have APL, AML and Down syndrome or AML and the t(8;21) or inv(16) are not candidates for SCT in first CR, but opinions differ about patients in the standard-risk and high-risk categories. The trend in Europe[79] is to reduce the use of SCT in first CR, but in the United States[80] SCT in first CR is supported. Both views have been reported recently.[80–82]

In the absence of randomized, controlled trials comparing allogeneic SCT with postremission intensive chemotherapy, "biologic randomization" or "donor versus no donor" studies are accepted as the least biased comparison methods, but even these are open to criticism. Much of the trial data used to support the benefits of SCT and intensive chemotherapy are old and do not reflect current improvements in SCT and intensive chemotherapy. A meta-analysis[83] of studies enrolling patients younger than 21 years of age between 1985 and 2000 that recommended SCT if a histocompatible family donor were available found that SCT from a matched sibling donor reduced the risk of relapse significantly and improved DFS and OS.

The MRC AML10 (included in the meta-analysis) and AML12 studies combined (relapse risk did not differ between the trials; $P = .3$) showed a significant reduction in relapse risk ($2P = 0.02$) but no significant improvement in DFS ($2P = 0.06$) or OS ($2P = 0.1$).[5] MRC AML10 is typical of a number of trials in which SCT significantly reduced the risk of relapse, but the resulting improvement in survival was not statistically significant (68% versus 59%; $P = .3$). The small number of pediatric patients in AML10 hinders meaningful interpretation, but at 7 years' follow-up SCT recipients (children and adults) who had a suitable donor showed a significant reduction in relapse risk (36%, versus 52% in patients who did not have a suitable donor; $P = .0001$) and a significant improvement in DFS (50%, versus 42% in patients who did not have a suitable donor; $P = .001$) but no significant improvement in OS (55% versus 50%; $P = .1$).[84] The reduction in relapse risk was seen in all risk and age groups, but the significant benefit in DFS was seen only in the cytogenetic intermediate-risk group (50% versus 39%; $P = .004$). The 86 children who had a donor, 61 of whom (71%) underwent SCT, had no survival advantage, and children who did not undergo SCT were salvaged more easily.[5]

The lack of benefit found for pediatric SCT in the MRC trials mirrors the experience of the BFM.[3,85] CCG trial 2891, however, showed a significant survival advantage for patients who underwent allogeneic SCT versus autologous SCT (60% versus 53%; $P = .002$) or chemotherapy (60% versus 48%; $P = .05$) as postremission treatment, although autologous SCT provided no advantage over intensive chemotherapy.[86] The benefit was most marked in patients who had received intensively timed induction chemotherapy. The CCG analysis was not a true intent-to-treat comparison, however. Although it included patients whether or not they received SCT, it did not include all patients who lacked a donor; instead, it included only patients who lacked a donor and who were randomly assigned to autologous SCT instead of chemotherapy,[86] and favorable cytogenetics were overrepresented among patients who had a donor (38% versus 23%). The MRC AML10 (5-year OS, 58%) and CCG 2891 (5-year OS, 47%; 49% for the intensive arm) studies enrolled patients during approximately the same time period, although the patient populations may not have been comparable. It is possible that the improved outcomes achieved by intensive chemotherapy may diminish the role of SCT in first CR of AML and that SCT provides a benefit only when compared with relatively less intensive treatment.

Randomized studies analyzed according to intent to treat have failed to show that autologous SCT provides a survival advantage over intensive chemotherapy,[87-89] and a meta-analysis concluded that data were insufficient to determine whether autologous SCT is superior to nonmyeloablative chemotherapy.[83]

The controversy continues. In some groups, all patients who have a matched sibling donor proceed to SCT, whereas in others SCT is reserved for patients at high risk, although high risk is not defined consistently. In the MRC, SCT has not been demonstrated to reduce the risk of relapse even in children at high risk.[90] Unless it is demonstrated to reduce the risk of relapse, transplantation can offer no benefit. SCT may have a role in the treatment of pediatric AML in first CR if the graft-versus-leukemia effect can be expanded by pre- and posttransplantation graft manipulation, which may include the use of killer-cell immunoglobulin receptor–incompatible donors and donor lymphocyte infusions.

There is also a need to improve risk-group stratification and to identify better the children who may benefit from SCT. This goal may be achieved by identifying better prognostic indicators and by using minimal residual disease (MRD) monitoring, both of which are discussed in later sections.

Special Subgroups

Acute myeloid leukemia in children who have Down syndrome
Children who have Down syndrome who develop AML generally do so between 1 and 4 years of age. This subset of cases of AML is very responsive to therapy but carries a significant risk of early mortality. Children treated during the past decade have had a reported EFS estimate of 83%,[91] with relapse rates as low as 3%.[92] The recommendation is to limit the cumulative anthracycline dose to 240 to 250 mg/m^2[93] or to reduce overall dose intensity rather than the absolute dose.[94]

Acute promyelocytic leukemia
Children who have APL are treated with special APL protocols that combine ATRA with intensive chemotherapy. Although ATRA can cause considerable (but

manageable) toxicity in some children, this approach induces a stable and continuous remission without the early hemorrhagic deaths that previously characterized this type of leukemia. APL is the only subtype of AML in which maintenance chemotherapy is believed to be of benefit.[95] SCT in first CR is not indicated for a disease that responds so well to chemotherapy. Regimens increasingly based on alternatives to traditional chemotherapy, including ATRA and arsenic trioxide, are being tested.[96]

Relapsed acute myeloid leukemia

After relapse, chemotherapy alone is unlikely to be curative, and the survival rate is only 21% to 33% in recent reports.[77,97–101] In these reports, the length of first remission was the best predictor of survival.[97–100] Various remission induction regimens, including fludarabine plus cytarabine and mitoxantrone plus cytarabine, seem to give similar results. The addition of liposomal daunorubicin to fludarabine plus cytarabine is being tested currently to try to improve CR rates while minimizing cardiotoxicity. It is important to reduce the toxicity of reinduction to a level that allows SCT to proceed, because children who receive SCT can have a 5-year survival probability of 60% (56% after early relapse; 65% after late relapse).[102]

The targeted immunotherapy agents gemtuzumab ozogamicin and clofarabine have shown activity against relapsed AML. Gemtuzumab ozogamicin has been shown to be safe and well tolerated in children and, as a single agent, has induced responses in 30% of patients who have recurrent CD33$^+$ AML.[103] Clofarabine has demonstrated activity against refractory and relapsed AML.[104] Both of these drugs may be more useful when given in combination with other chemotherapeutic agents.

A second allograft seems to offer a benefit to patients who experience relapse after SCT during first CR. Despite a high rate of transplantation-related mortality and second relapse, more than one third of patients are reported to be long-term survivors. Patients who undergo SCT during remission may have an even better outcome.[105] Therefore every effort should be made to induce remission before the second SCT.

Prognostic Factors

Although clinical measures of tumor burden, such as leukocyte count and hepatosplenomegaly, largely have been replaced by genetic factors in the risk-classification schemes of contemporary treatment protocols, several clinical features are still prognostically important. In both adult and pediatric patients who have AML, age at diagnosis is associated inversely with the probability of survival.[106,107] In an analysis of 424 patients less than 21 years of age, an age greater than 10 years at diagnosis was significantly associated with a worse outcome, even after controlling for cytogenetics, leukocyte count, and FAB subtype.[107] The effect of age was important only among patients treated in contemporary trials, reinforcing the view that the effect of any prognostic factor ultimately depends on the therapy given. Two recent studies suggest that another clinically apparent feature—ethnicity—may be an important predictor of outcome.[108,109] Among more than 1600 children who had AML treated on the CCG 2891 and 2961 trials, black children treated with chemotherapy had a significantly worse outcome than white children treated with chemotherapy, a disparity that the authors suggest may reflect pharmacogenetic differences.[109] Body mass index, another easily measured clinical feature, also may affect the outcome of children who have AML.[110] In the CCG 2961 trial, underweight and overweight patients were less likely to survive than normoweight patients because of a greater risk of treatment-related death.[110]

In addition to clinical features, certain pathologic features, such as M0 and M7 subtypes, seem to carry prognostic importance in AML.[111,112] The present authors and others have demonstrated that non–Down syndrome patients who have megakaryoblastic leukemia have significantly worse outcomes than patients who have other subtypes of AML.[111,113,114] The EFS estimates for patients who have megakaryoblastic leukemia treated in the CCG 2891 trial or in the St Jude trial were only 22% and 14%, respectively.[111,113] In the St Jude study[111] and in a report from the European Group for Blood and Marrow Transplantation,[115] patients who underwent SCT during first remission had a better outcome than those who received chemotherapy, suggesting that SCT should be recommended for these patients. A study by French investigators, however, suggested that children who had megakaryoblastic leukemia with the t(1;22), but without Down syndrome, had a better outcome than similar children who did not have the t(1;22), indicating that this subgroup may not need transplantation.[114] In addition, the BFM study group reported an improved outcome for patients who had megakaryoblastic leukemia treated in recent, more intensive trials.[116] SCT did not provide a benefit to patients treated in these trials. Thus, the role of SCT for patients who have megakaryoblastic leukemia remains controversial.

Conventional cytogenetic studies have demonstrated that the karyotype of leukemic blast cells is one of the best predictors of outcome.[117,118] An analysis of more than 1600 patients enrolled in the MRC AML 10 trial revealed that t(8;21) and inv(16) were associated with a favorable outcome (5-year OS estimates, 69% and 61%, respectively), whereas a complex karyotype, -5, del(5q), -7, and abnormalities of 3q predicted a poor outcome.[117] On the basis of these observations, the MRC investigators proposed a cytogenetics-based risk classification system that is used by many cooperative groups today.[117] Among the 340 patients in the MRC study who were less than 15 years old, those with a favorable karyotype had a 3-year survival estimate of 78%, compared with 55% for the intermediate-risk group and 42% for the high-risk group. Other cooperative groups have confirmed the MRC findings, with slightly different results for some subgroups that probably reflect differences in therapy. For example, in the Pediatric Oncology Group 8821 trial, patients who had t(8;21) had a 4-year OS estimate of 52% and those who had inv(16) had an estimate of 75%.[118] Similarly, among adults who had AML treated in Cancer and Leukemia Group B trials, patients who had these karyotypes had a better outcome than others and had a particularly good outcome when treated with multiple courses of high-dose cytarabine.[75,119,120]

Because both t(8;21) and inv(16) disrupt the CBF, they are often referred to as "CBF leukemias" and are grouped together in risk-classification systems. Several studies, however, have demonstrated that CBF leukemia is a heterogeneous group of diseases in adults and therefore probably is heterogeneous in children as well.[121,122] An analysis of 312 adults who had CBF AML demonstrated that, although CR and relapse rates were similar for patients who had t(8;21) and inv(16), OS was significantly worse for those who had t(8;21), primarily because of a lower salvage rate after relapse.[121] In addition, race was prognostically important among patients who had t(8;21), whereas sex and secondary cytogenetic changes were predictive of outcome among patients who had inv(16). A similar analysis of 370 adults who had CBF AML confirmed the heterogeneity of this type of AML and confirmed the poor outcome after relapse among patients who had t(8;21).[122] Not surprisingly, in both studies, outcome depended on treatment intensity.

Other prognostically important cytogenetic abnormalities include rearrangements of the MLL gene, located at chromosome band 11q23. The abnormality is usually a reciprocal translocation between MLL and one of more than 30 other genes in distinct chromosomal loci.[123] MLL rearrangements are seen in as many as 20% of cases of AML, although the reported frequency varies among studies.[124,125] In general, children and adults whose leukemic cells contain 11q23 abnormalities are considered at intermediate risk, and their outcome does not differ significantly from that of patients without these translocations (3-year OS estimate, 50% in the MRC AML 10 trial).[117] Some studies, however, suggest that t(9;11) confers a favorable outcome.[124] Among patients treated for AML at St Jude, those who had t(9;11) had a better outcome (5-year EFS estimate, 65%) than did patients in all other cytogenetic or molecular subgroups. This finding may be attributable to the use of epipodophyllotoxins and cladribine, both of which are effective against monoblastic leukemia.

In the MRC AML 10 study mentioned previously, monosomy 7 was associated with a particularly poor outcome (5-year OS, 10%) but was detected in only 4% of cases.[117]

Because of the rarity of this abnormality, an international collaborative study was undertaken to characterize further the impact of -7 and del(7q) in children and adolescents who have AML.[126] In this study, which included 172 patients who had -7 (with or without other abnormalities) and 86 patients who had del(7q) (also with or without other changes), patients who had -7 had lower CR rates (61% versus 89%) and worse outcome (5-year survival, 30% versus 51%) than those who had del(7q). Patients who had del(7q) and a favorable genetic abnormality had a good outcome (5-year survival, 75%), suggesting that the del(7q) does not alter the impact of the favorable feature. By contrast, patients who had -7 and inv(3), -5/del(5q), or +21 had a dismal outcome (5-year survival, 5%) that was not improved by SCT.[126]

During the past 10 years, molecular studies have demonstrated heterogeneity within cytogenetically defined subgroups of AML and have identified new, prognostically important subgroups. Mutations of c-kit, ras, and FLT3 have been detected in cases of childhood and adult AML; c-kit mutations may be particularly important in cases of CBF leukemia.[127–131] Several studies demonstrated that among adult patients who had t(8;21), those who had mutations at c-kit codon 816 had a significantly higher relapse rate and worse outcome than those who had wild-type c-kit.[127–129] In some studies, mutations of c-kit also seem to confer a worse outcome among patients who have inv(16).[132] Although c-kit mutations have been detected in 3% to 11% of pediatric AML cases, their prognostic impact is uncertain.[130,133] One study found c-kit mutations in 37% of cases of CBF leukemia, but these cases did not differ from others in outcome.[130] In contrast, the Japanese Childhood AML Cooperative Study Group found that c-kit mutations, in 8 of 46 patients who had t(8;21), were associated with significantly worse OS, DFS, and relapse rates.[131]

The impact of FLT3 mutations in childhood and adult AML has been established by dozens of studies, only a few of which are summarized here. In one of the first studies reported, the estimated 5-year OS rate was only 14% for adult patients who had internal tandem duplications (ITD) of FLT3, and the presence of these mutations was the strongest prognostic factor in multivariate analysis.[134] Similarly, in an analysis of 106 adults who had AML treated in MRC trials, 13 of the 14 patients who had FLT3 ITD died within 18 months of diagnosis.[135] A subsequent study of 854 patients treated in the MRC AML trials demonstrated a FLT3 ITD, present in 27% of cases, was associated with an increased risk of relapse and a lower probability of DFS, EFS, and OS.[136] Other reports have confirmed the presence of FLT ITD in 20% to 30% of adult AML cases, but some studies suggest that its negative prognostic impact may depend on the absence of the wild-type allele or the ratio of the mutant to the wild-type allele.[137–139]

Studies of childhood AML identify FLT3 ITD in only 10% to 15% of cases, but still it is associated with a poor outcome.[140–143] Among 91 pediatric patients who had AML treated in CCG trials, the 8-year EFS estimate was only 7% for patients who had FLT3

ITD, whereas among 234 patients treated on Dutch AML protocols, the 5-year EFS for these patients estimate was only 29%.[140,141] In both studies, multivariate analysis demonstrated that *FLT3*-ITD was the strongest predictor of relapse. A more recent study of 630 patients treated in contemporary CCG trials confirmed the poor outcome associated with *FLT3* ITD and demonstrated that survival decreased with an increasing allelic ratio of *FLT* ITD to *FLT3* wild-type.[143] The estimated progression-free survival was considerably lower with a ratio greater than 0.4 than with a lower ratio (16% versus 72%). CCG investigators also compared the outcome of patients who had *FLT3* ITD in CD34⁺/CD33⁻ precursors with that of patients who had the mutated gene in only the more mature CD34⁺/CD33⁺ progenitors.[65] Patients who had the mutation in the less mature precursors had dramatically worse outcomes, confirming the heterogeneity within *FLT3* ITD–positive cases of AML and suggesting that only a subset of these patients have a poor prognosis. Data from studies by the Pediatric Oncology Group suggest that gene expression profiles also may be used to identify patients who have a good prognosis despite *FLT3* mutations.[144]

Other molecular alterations reported to be prognostic factors in AML include expression of ATP-binding cassette transporters,[145–147] *CEBPA* mutations,[148,149] *DCC* expression,[150] secretion of vascular endothelial growth factor,[151] expression of apoptosis-related genes,[152–154] expression of *BAALC*,[155] expression of *ERG*,[156,157] *NPM1* mutations,[158–160] partial tandem duplications (PTD) of the *MLL* gene,[161,162] and global gene expression patterns.[163–167] The clinical relevance of these alterations has been reviewed comprehensively[168] and is discussed only briefly here. Mutations of the nucleophosmin member 1 (*NPM1*) gene have been detected in about 50% of cases of adult AML with a normal karyotype[159] but occur much less commonly in childhood AML.[160] In both populations, *NPM1* mutations are associated with *FLT3* ITD; however, in patients who have wild-type *FLT3*, *NPM1* mutations are associated with a favorable outcome.[168] *MLL* PTD occur in about 5% to 10% of adult AML cases and, like *NPM1* mutations, commonly are associated with *FLT3* ITD.[168] *MLL* PTD seem to be an adverse prognostic factor, but it is not clear whether the negative impact is related to the association with *FLT3* ITD. High expression of the *BAALC* gene and the *ERG* gene are additional factors that have independent negative prognostic significance among adult patients who have a normal karyotype, whereas mutations of the *CEBPA* gene are associated with a favorable outcome.[168] A risk-classification scheme for adults who have a normal AML karyotype that incorporates the status of *FLT3*, *NPM1*, *BAALC*, *MLL*, and *CEBPA* has been proposed and may be used in future clinical trials.[168] *MLL* PTD, *BAALC*, and *CEBPA* have not been studied extensively in childhood AML. Nevertheless, it is likely that forthcoming pediatric clinical trials will use gene-expression profiling to identify important prognostic subgroups that may benefit from more intensive or novel therapies.[144,169]

MINIMAL RESIDUAL DISEASE

The heterogeneity within cytogenetically and even molecularly defined subgroups indicates that other methods are needed to optimize risk classification. Many studies of ALL and AML have demonstrated the prognostic importance of early response to therapy (ie, reduction or elimination of leukemic cells in the bone marrow), which may be a more powerful predictor of outcome than genetic features.[170] Response to therapy can be measured by morphologic[171,172] or cytogenetic[173] examination of bone marrow, but these methods cannot detect levels of residual leukemia below 1% (1 leukemic cell in 100 mononuclear bone marrow cells). In contrast, MRD assays provide objective and sensitive measurement of low levels of leukemic cells[170,174] in childhood[175–178] and adult[179–183] AML. Methods of assessing MRD include DNA-based polymerase chain reaction (PCR) analysis of clonal antigen-receptor gene rearrangements (applicable to less than 10% of AML cases), RNA-based PCR analysis of leukemia-specific gene fusions (applicable to less than 50% of AML cases), and flow cytometric detection of aberrant immunophenotype (applicable to more than 90% of AML cases). Among 252 children evaluated for MRD in the CCG-2961 trial, occult leukemia (defined as more than 0.5% bone marrow blast cells with an aberrant phenotype) was detected in 16% of the children considered to be in remission.[176] Multivariate analysis demonstrated that patients who had detectable MRD were 4.8 times more likely to experience relapse (P<.0001) and 3.1 times more likely to die (P<.0001) than patients who were MRD negative. A study at St Jude Children's Research Hospital yielded similar findings: the 2-year survival estimate for patients who had detectable MRD at the end of induction therapy was 33%, compared with 72% for MRD-negative patients (P = .022).[177] Recent studies in adults have confirmed that the level of residual leukemia cells detected immunophenotypically after induction or consolidation therapy is associated strongly with the risk of relapse.[181–183]

Quantitative reverse transcription PCR assays of leukemia-specific fusion transcripts is an alternative method of MRD detection that can be used in AML cases that harbor these gene fusions.[113,184–190] Several studies have indicated that quantification of AML1-ETO and CBFβ-MYH11 fusion transcripts at the time of diagnosis and during therapy is a useful predictor of outcome. Similarly, there is emerging evidence that quantitative PCR assessment of WT1 transcripts also may prove useful for monitoring MRD and predicting outcome in patients who have AML.[191–193]

PHARMACOGENOMICS OF THERAPY FOR ACUTE MYELOID LEUKEMIA

Patient factors, such as pharmacodynamics and pharmacogenomics, significantly affect the outcome of treatment in many types of cancer, including AML.[194,195] The effect of such factors is demonstrated clearly by the chemosensitivity and excellent outcome of AML in children who have Down syndrome, who have cure rates of 80% to 100%.[196] Increased levels of cystathionine-β-synthetase (CBS), a high frequency of CBS genetic polymorphisms, low levels of cytidine deaminase, and altered expression of other GATA1 target genes in these patients' leukemic blast cells contribute to the high cure rates.[197–200] Polymorphisms or altered expression of other proteins involved in cytarabine metabolism, such as deoxycytidine kinase, DNA polymerase, and es nucleoside transporter, also may play a role in leukemic blast cell sensitivity to this agent.[201–203] In addition, polymorphisms may influence toxicity. For example, homozygous deletions of the glutathione S-transferase theta (GSTT1) gene have been reported to be associated with a higher frequency of early toxic death and a lower likelihood of survival.[204,205] Recently, polymorphisms of the XPD gene (XPD751), which is involved in DNA repair, were shown to be associated with a lower likelihood of survival and a higher risk of therapy-related leukemia in elderly patients who had AML.[206] XPD751 does not seem to influence outcome in children who have AML, however.[207]

COMPLICATIONS AND SUPPORTIVE CARE

At the time of diagnosis, patients who have AML may have life-threatening complications, including bleeding, leukostasis, tumor lysis syndrome, and infection. The first three are managed through the use of platelet transfusions, leukapheresis or exchange transfusion, aggressive hydration, oral phosphate binders and recombinant urate oxidase, and the prompt initiation of chemotherapy. Infectious complications at the time of diagnosis and during therapy remain a major cause of morbidity and mortality.[74,208–211] Viridans streptococci, which commonly colonize the oral, gastrointestinal, and vaginal mucosa, are particularly troublesome in patients undergoing therapy for AML.[208,210,212,213] Because of the high risk of sepsis, most clinicians agree that all patients who have AML and who have febrile neutropenia should be hospitalized and treated with broad-spectrum intravenous antibiotics, such as a third- or fourth-generation cephalosporin, as well as vancomycin. Patients who have evidence of sepsis or infection with *Pseudomonas aeruginosa* should receive an aminoglycoside, and patients who have severe abdominal pain, evidence of typhlitis, or known infection with *Bacillus cereus* should be treated with a carbapenem (imipenem or meropenem) rather than a cephalosporin. In addition, patients who have AML are at high risk of fungal infection[213] and therefore should receive empiric antifungal therapy with traditional amphotericin B, lipid formulations of amphotericin B, an azole (voriconazole or posaconazole), or an echinocandin (caspofungin or micafungin). Cytokines such as granulocyte-macrophage colony stimulating factor and granulocyte colony-stimulating factor also should be considered in cases of proven sepsis or fungal infection, but there is little evidence that their prophylactic use significantly reduces morbidity.[214–216]

Because of the high incidence of bacterial and fungal infections, the present authors recently tested several prophylactic antimicrobial regimens in 78 children receiving chemotherapy for AML at St Jude Children's Research Hospital. Oral cephalosporins were ineffective, but intravenous cefepime completely prevented viridans streptococcal sepsis and reduced the odds of bacterial sepsis by 91%. Similarly, intravenous vancomycin given with oral ciprofloxacin reduced the odds of viridans streptococcal sepsis by 98% and the odds of any bacterial sepsis by 94%. All patients received antifungal prophylaxis with oral voriconazole, which contributed to a low rate of disseminated fungal infection (1.0/000 patient-days). Most important, there were no deaths from bacterial or fungal infection among patients who received prophylactic antibiotics and voriconazole. Because of the relatively small number of patients studied, these prophylactic antibiotic regimens must be evaluated in a multi-institutional setting before recommendations can be made.

FUTURE DIRECTIONS

As a result of highly collaborative clinical trials, the outcome for children who have AML has improved continuously over the past several decades, but approximately half of all children diagnosed as having AML still die of the disease or of complications of treatment. Further advances will require a greater understanding of the biology of AML, improved risk stratification and risk-directed therapies, improved treatment of high-risk disease, and the development of molecularly targeted agents or better cellular therapies. Targeted therapies may cause less toxicity, but they may be clinically applicable only to well-defined molecular subgroups, as with the use of ATRA and arsenic trioxide for APL.[95,217] Agents under investigation include gemtuzumab ozogamicin.[218] proteasome inhibitors,[219,220] histone deacetylase inhibitors,[221,222] and tyrosine kinases inhibitors.[223–225] Clofarabine, a purine nucleoside analogue that was designed to integrate the qualities of fludarabine and cladribine, also has activity against AML.[226–228] Recently, cellular therapy with haploidentical natural killer cells has been shown to exert antitumor activity with minimal toxicity in patients who have relapsed AML.[229] Timely evaluation of these and other therapies will require novel clinical trial designs with new statistical models that allow the testing of new treatment approaches in increasingly small subgroups of patients. In addition, future clinical trials will require international collaboration among the pediatric cooperative oncology groups.

ACKNOWLEDGMENTS

The authors thank Sharon Naron for expert editorial review.

REFERENCES

1. Kaspers G, Creutzig U. Pediatric AML: long term results of clinical trials from 13 study groups worldwide. Leukemia 2005;19:2025–146.
2. Kaspers GJ, Creutzig U. Pediatric acute myeloid leukemia: international progress and future directions. Leukemia 2005;19(12):2025–9.
3. Creutzig U, Zimmermann M, Ritter J, et al. Treatment strategies and long-term results in paediatric patients treated in four consecutive AML-BFM trials. Leukemia 2005;19(12):2030–42.
4. Smith FO, Alonzo TA, Gerbing RB, et al. Long-term results of children with acute myeloid leukemia: a report of three consecutive phase III trials by the Children's Cancer Group: CCG 251, CCG 213 and CCG 2891. Leukemia 2005;19(12):2054–62.
5. Gibson BE, Wheatley K, Hann IM, et al. Treatment strategy and long-term results in paediatric patients treated in consecutive UK AML trials. Leukemia 2005;19(12):2130–8.
6. Pession A, Rondelli R, Basso G, et al. Treatment and long-term results in children with acute myeloid leukaemia treated according to the AIEOP AML protocols. Leukemia 2005;19(12):2043–53.
7. Kardos G, Zwaan CM, Kaspers GJ, et al. Treatment strategy and results in children treated on three Dutch Childhood Oncology Group acute myeloid leukemia trials. Leukemia 2005;19(12):2063–71.
8. Entz-Werle N, Suciu S, van der Werff ten Bosch J, et al. Results of 58872 and 58921 trials in acute myeloblastic leukemia and relative value of chemotherapy vs allogeneic bone marrow transplantation in first complete remission: the EORTC Children Leukemia Group report. Leukemia 2005;19(12):2072–81.
9. Perel Y, Auvrignon A, Leblanc T, et al. Treatment of childhood acute myeloblastic leukemia: dose intensification improves outcome and maintenance therapy is of no benefit—multicenter studies of the French LAME (Leucemie Aigue Myeloblastique Enfant) Cooperative Group. Leukemia 2005;19(12):2082–9.
10. Lie SO, Abrahamsson J, Clausen N, et al. Long-term results in children with AML: NOPHO-AML Study Group–report of three consecutive trials. Leukemia 2005;19(12):2090–100.
11. Ravindranath Y, Chang M, Steuber CP, et al. Pediatric Oncology Group (POG) studies of acute myeloid leukemia (AML): a review of four consecutive childhood AML trials conducted between 1981 and 2000. Leukemia 2005;19(12):2101–16.
12. Dluzniewska A, Balwierz W, Armata J, et al. Twenty years of Polish experience with three consecutive protocols for treatment of childhood acute myelogenous leukemia. Leukemia 2005;19(12):2117–24.
13. Ribeiro RC, Razzouk BI, Pounds S, et al. Successive clinical trials for childhood acute myeloid leukemia at St Jude Children's Research Hospital, from 1980 to 2000. Leukemia 2005;19(12):2125–9.
14. Armendariz H, Barbieri MA, Freigeiro D, et al. Treatment strategy and long-term results in pediatric patients treated in two consecutive AML-GATLA trials. Leukemia 2005;19(12):2139–42.

15. Quintana J, Advis P, Becker A, et al. Acute myelogenous leukemia in Chile PINDA protocols 87 and 92 results. Leukemia 2005;19(12):2143–6.
16. Smith MA, Ries LAG, Gurney JG, et al. Leukemia. In: Ries LAG, Smith MA, Gurney JG, et al, editors. Cancer incidence and survival among children and adolescents: United States SEER Progam 1975–1995. NIH Pub. No. 99–4649. Bethesda (MD): National Cancer Institute, SEER Program; 1999. p. 17–34.
17. Glavel J, Goubin A, Auclerc MF, et al. Incidence of childhood leukaemia and non-Hodgkin's lymphoma in France: National Registry of Childhood Leukaemia and Lymphoma, 1990–1999. Eur J Cancer Prev 2004;13:97–103.
18. Hjalgrim LL, Rostgaard K, Schmiegelow K, et al. Age- and sex-specific incidence of childhood leukemia by immunophenotype in the Nordic countries. J Natl Cancer Inst 2003;95(20):1539–44.
19. Xie Y, Davies SM, Xiang Y, et al. Trends in leukemia incidence and survival in the United States (1973–1998). Cancer 2003;97(9):2229–35.
20. Gurney JG, Severson RK, Davis S, et al. Incidence of cancer in children in the United States. Sex-, race-, and 1-year age-specific rates by histologic type. Cancer 1995;75(8):2186–95.
21. Bhatia S, Neglia JP. Epidemiology of childhood acute myelogenous leukemia. see comments. J Pediatr Hematol Oncol 1995;17(2):94–100.
22. Ross JA, Davies SM, Potter JD, et al. Epidemiology of childhood leukemia, with a focus on infants. Epidemiol Rev 1994;16(2):243–72.
23. Sandler DP, Ross JA. Epidemiology of acute leukemia in children and adults. Semin Oncol 1997;24(1):3–16.
24. Linassier C, Barin C, Calais G, et al. Early secondary acute myelogenous leukemia in breast cancer patients after treatment with mitoxantrone, cyclophosphamide, fluorouracil and radiation therapy. Ann Oncol 2000;11(10): 1289–94.
25. Micallef IN, Lillington DM, Apostolidis J, et al. Therapy-related myelodysplasia and secondary acute myelogenous leukemia after high-dose therapy with autologous hematopoietic progenitor-cell support for lymphoid malignancies. J Clin Oncol 2000;18(5):947–55.
26. Smith MA, McCaffrey RP, Karp JE. The secondary leukemias: challenges and research directions. J Natl Cancer Inst 1996;88(7):407–18.
27. Sandoval C, Pui CH, Bowman LC, et al. Secondary acute myeloid leukemia in children previously treated with alkylating agents, intercalating topoisomerase II inhibitors, and irradiation. J Clin Oncol 1993;11(6):1039–45.
28. Relling MV, Yanishevski Y, Nemec J, et al. Etoposide and antimetabolite pharmacology in patients who develop secondary acute myeloid leukemia. Leukemia 1998;12(3):346–52.
29. Pui CH, Ribeiro RC, Hancock ML, et al. Acute myeloid leukemia in children treated with epipodophyllotoxins for acute lymphoblastic leukemia. N Engl J Med 1991;325(24):1682–7.
30. Le Deley MC, Leblanc T, Shamsaldin A, et al. Risk of secondary leukemia after a solid tumor in childhood according to the dose of epipodophyllotoxins and anthracyclines: a case-control study by the Societe Francaise d'Oncologie Pediatrique. J Clin Oncol 2003;21(6):1074–81.
31. Korte JE, Hertz-Picciotto I, Schulz MR, et al. The contribution of benzene to smoking-induced leukemia. Environ Health Perspect 2000;108(4):333–9.
32. McBride ML. Childhood cancer and environmental contaminants. Can J Public Health 1998;89(Suppl 1):S53–68.

33. Yin SN, Hayes RB, Linet MS, et al. An expanded cohort study of cancer among benzene-exposed workers in China. Benzene Study Group. Environ Health Perspect 1996;104(Suppl 6):1339–41.
34. Yin SN, Hayes RB, Linet MS, et al. A cohort study of cancer among benzene-exposed workers in China: overall results. Am J Ind Med 1996;29(3):227–35.
35. Linet MS, Bailey PE. Benzene, leukemia, and the Supreme Court. J Public Health Policy 1981;2(2):116–35.
36. Mills PK, Zahm SH. Organophosphate pesticide residues in urine of farmworkers and their children in Fresno County, California. Am J Ind Med 2001; 40(5):571–7.
37. Rosenberg PS, Greene MH, Alter BP. Cancer incidence in persons with Fanconi anemia. Blood 2003;101(3):822–6.
38. German J. Bloom's syndrome. XX. The first 100 cancers. Cancer Genet Cytogenet 1997;93(1):100–6.
39. Bader JL, Miller RW. Neurofibromatosis and childhood leukemia. J Pediatr 1978; 92(6):925–9.
40. Bader-Meunier B, Tchernia G, Mielot F, et al. Occurrence of myeloproliferative disorder in patients with Noonan syndrome. J Pediatr 1997;130(6):885–9.
41. Socie G, Henry-Amar M, Bacigalupo A, et al. Malignant tumors occurring after treatment of aplastic anemia. European Bone Marrow Transplantation-Severe Aplastic Anaemia Working Party. N Engl J Med 1993;329(16):1152–7.
42. Imashuku S, Hibi S, Nakajima F, et al. A review of 125 cases to determine the risk of myelodysplasia and leukemia in pediatric neutropenic patients after treatment with recombinant human granulocyte colony-stimulating factor. Blood 1994; 84(7):2380–1.
43. Xue Y, Zhang R, Guo Y, et al. Acquired amegakaryocytic thrombocytopenic purpura with a Philadelphia chromosome. Cancer Genet Cytogenet 1993; 69(1):51–6.
44. Geissler D, Thaler J, Konwalinka G, et al. Progressive preleukemia presenting amegakaryocytic thrombocytopenic purpura: association of the 5q- syndrome with a decreased megakaryocytic colony formation and a defective production of Meg-CSF. Leuk Res 1987;11(8):731–7.
45. Gilliland DG. Molecular genetics of human leukemia. Leukemia 1998;12(Suppl 1):S7–12.
46. Dash A, Gilliland DG. Molecular genetics of acute myeloid leukaemia. Best Pract Res Clin Haematol 2001;14(1):49–64.
47. Gilliland DG, Tallman MS. Focus on acute leukemias. Cancer Cell 2002;1(5): 417–20.
48. Castilla LH, Garrett L, Adya N, et al. The fusion gene Cbfb-MYH11 blocks myeloid differentiation and predisposes mice to acute myelomonocytic leukaemia. Nat Genet 1999;23:144–6.
49. Higuchi M, O'Brien D, Kumaravelu P, et al. Expression of a conditional AML1-ETO oncogene bypasses embryonic lethality and establishes a murine model of human t(8;21) acute myeloid leukemia. Cancer Cell 2002;1(1):63–74.
50. Ford AM, Ridge SA, Cabrera ME, et al. In utero rearrangements in the trithorax-related oncogene in infant leukaemias. Nature 1993;363:358–60.
51. Gill Super HJ, Rothberg PG, Kobayashi H, et al. Clonal, nonconstitutional rearrangements of the MLL gene in infant twins with acute lymphoblastic leukemia: in utero chromosome rearrangement of 11q23. Blood 1994;83(3):641–4.
52. Megonigal MD, Rappaport EF, Jones DH, et al. t(11;22)(q23;q11.2) In acute myeloid leukemia of infant twins fuses MLL with hCDCrel, a cell division cycle

gene in the genomic region of deletion in DiGeorge and velocardiofacial syndromes. Proc Natl Acad Sci U S A 1998;95(11):6413–8.

53. Wiemels JL, Ford AM, Van Wering ER, et al. Protracted and variable latency of acute lymphoblastic leukemia after TEL-AML1 gene fusion in utero. Blood 1999; 94(3):1057–62.

54. Song WJ, Sullivan MG, Legare RD, et al. Haploinsufficiency of CBFA2 causes familial thrombocytopenia with propensity to develop acute myelogenous leukaemia. Nat Genet 1999;23(2):166–75.

55. Bonnet D, Dick JE. Human acute myeloid leukemia is organized as a hierarchy that originates from a primitive hematopoietic cell. Nat Med 1997;3(7):730–7.

56. Caligiuri MA, Strout MP, Gilliland DG. Molecular biology of acute myleloid leukemia. Semin Oncol 1997;24:32–44.

57. Sabbath KD, Ball ED, Larcom P, et al. Heterogeneity of clonogenic cells in acute myeloblastic leukemia. J Clin Invest 1985;75:746–53.

58. Lapidot T, Sirard C, Vormoor J, et al. A cell initiating human acute myeloid leukaemia after transplantation into SCID mice. Nature 1994;367(6464): 645–8.

59. Mehrotra B, George TI, Kavanau K, et al. Cytogenetically aberrant cells in the stem cell compartment (CD34+lin-) in acute myeloid leukemia. Blood 1995; 86(3):1139–47.

60. Sirard C, Lapidot T, Vormoor J, et al. Normal and leukemic SCID-repopulating cells (SRC) coexist in the bone marrow and peripheral blood from CML patients in chronic phase, whereas leukemic SRC are detected in blast crisis. Blood 1996;87(4):1539–48.

61. Hope KJ, Jin L, Dick JE. Human acute myeloid leukemia stem cells. Arch Med Res 2003;34(6):507–14.

62. Hope KJ, Jin L, Dick JE. Acute myeloid leukemia originates from a hierarchy of leukemic stem cell classes that differ in self-renewal capacity. Nat Immunol 2004;5(7):738–43.

63. Warner JK, Wang JC, Hope KJ, et al. Concepts of human leukemic development. Oncogene 2004;23(43):7164–77.

64. Terpstra W, Prins A, Ploemacher RE, et al. Long-term leukemia-initiating capacity of a CD34-subpopulation of acute myeloid leukemia. Blood 1996; 87(6):2187–94.

65. Pollard JA, Alonzo TA, Gerbing RB, et al. FLT3 internal tandem duplication in CD34+/. Blood 2006;108(8):2764–9.

66. Pui CH, Dahl GV, Kalwinsky DK, et al. Central nervous system leukemia in children with acute nonlymphoblastic leukemia. Blood 1985;66(5):1062–7.

67. Woods WG, Kobrinsky N, Buckley JD, et al. Time-sequential induction therapy improves postremission outcome in acute myeloid leukemia: a report from the Children's Cancer Group. Blood 1996;87(12):4979–89.

68. Carella AM, Berman E, Maraone MP, et al. Idarubicin in the treatment of acute leukemias. An overview of preclinical and clinical studies. Haematologica 1990;75(2):159–69.

69. Berman E, McBride M. Comparative cellular pharmacology of daunorubicin and idarubicin in human multidrug-resistant leukemia cells. Blood 1992;79(12): 3267–73.

70. Reid JM, Pendergrass TW, Krailo MD, et al. Plasma pharmacokinetics and cerebrospinal fluid concentrations of idarubicin and idarubicinol in pediatric leukemia patients: a Children's Cancer Study Group report. Cancer Res 1990; 50(20):6525–8.

71. Creutzig U, Ritter J, Zimmermann M, et al. Idarubicin improves blast cell clearance during induction therapy in children with AML: results of study AML-BFM 93. AML-BFM Study Group. Leukemia 2001;15(3):348–54.

72. O'Brien TA, Russell SJ, Vowels MR, et al. Results of consecutive trials for children newly diagnosed with acute myeloid leukemia from the Australian and New Zealand Children's Cancer Study Group. Blood 2002;100(8):2708–16.

73. Becton D, Dahl GV, Ravindranath Y, et al. Randomized use of cyclosporin A (CsA) to modulate P-glycoprotein in children with AML in remission: Pediatric Oncology Group Study 9421. Blood 2006;107(4):1315–24.

74. Riley LC, Hann IM, Wheatley K, et al. Treatment-related deaths during induction and first remission of acute myeloid leukaemia in children treated on the Tenth Medical Research Council acute myeloid leukaemia trial (MRC AML10). The MCR Childhood Leukaemia Working Party. Br J Haematol 1999;106(2):436–44.

75. Byrd JC, Dodge RK, Carroll A, et al. Patients with t(8;21)(q22;q22) and acute myeloid leukemia have superior failure-free and overall survival when repetitive cycles of high-dose cytarabine are administered. J Clin Oncol 1999;17(12):3767–75.

76. Abbott BL, Rubnitz JE, Tong X, et al. Clinical significance of central nervous system involvement at diagnosis of pediatric acute myeloid leukemia: a single institution's experience. Leukemia 2003;17(11):2090–6.

77. Johnston DL, Alonzo TA, Gerbing RB, et al. Risk factors and therapy for isolated central nervous system relapse of pediatric acute myeloid leukemia. J Clin Oncol 2005;23(36):9172–8.

78. Creutzig U, Ritter J, Zimmermann M, et al. Does cranial irradiation reduce the risk for bone marrow relapse in acute myelogenous leukemia? Unexpected results of the Childhood Acute Myelogenous Leukemia Study BFM-87. J Clin Oncol 1993;11(2):279–86.

79. Wells RJ, Woods WG, Buckley JD, et al. Treatment of newly diagnosed children and adolescents with acute myeloid leukemia: a Children's Cancer Group study. J Clin Oncol 1994;12(11):2367–77.

80. Creutzig U, Reinhardt D. Current controversies: which patients with acute myeloid leukaemia should receive a bone marrow transplantation? A European view. Br J Haematol 2002;118(2):365–77.

81. Chen AR, Alonzo TA, Woods WG, et al. Current controversies: which patients with acute myeloid leukaemia should receive a bone marrow transplantation? An American view. Br J Haematol 2002;118(2):378–84.

82. Wheatley K. Current controversies: which patients with acute myeloid leukaemia should receive a bone marrow transplantation? A statistician's view. Br J Haematol 2002;118(2):351–6.

83. Bleakley M, Lau L, Shaw PJ, et al. Bone marrow transplantation for paediatric AML in first remission: a systematic review and meta-analysis. Bone Marrow Transplant 2002;29(10):843–52.

84. Burnett AK, Wheatley K, Goldstone AH, et al. The value of allogeneic bone marrow transplant in patients with acute myeloid leukaemia at differing risk of relapse: results of the UK MRC AML 10 trial. Br J Haematol 2002;118(2):385–400.

85. Creutzig U, Reinhardt D, Zimmermann M, et al. Intensive chemotherapy versus bone marrow transplantation in pediatric acute myeloid leukemia: a matter of controversies. Blood 2001;97(11):3671–2.

86. Woods WG, Neudorf S, Gold S, et al. A comparison of allogeneic bone marrow transplantation, autologous bone marrow transplantation, and aggressive

chemotherapy in children with acute myeloid leukemia in remission. Blood 2001; 97(1):56–62.

87. Stevens RF, Hann IM, Wheatley K, et al. Marked improvements in outcome with chemotherapy alone in paediatric acute myeloid leukemia: results of the United Kingdom Medical Research Council's 10th AML trial. MRC Childhood Leukaemia Working Party. Br J Haematol 1998;101(1):130–40.

88. Ravindranath Y, Yeager AM, Chang MN, et al. Autologous bone marrow transplantation versus intensive consolidation chemotherapy for acute myeloid leukemia in childhood. Pediatric Oncology Group. N Engl J Med 1996; 334(22):1428–34.

89. Amadori S, Testi AM, Arico M, et al. Prospective comparative study of bone marrow transplantation and postremission chemotherapy for childhood acute myelogenous leukemia. The Associazione Italiana Ematologia ed Oncologia Pediatrica Cooperative Group. J Clin Oncol 1993;11(6):1046–54.

90. Gibson B, Hann I, Webb I, et al. Should stem cell transplantation (SCT) be recommended for a child with AML in 1st CR. Blood 2007;106:171.

91. Zeller B, Gustafsson G, Forestier E, et al. Acute leukaemia in children with Down syndrome: a population-based Nordic study. Br J Haematol 2005;128(6): 797–804.

92. Ao A, Hills R, Stiller C, et al. Treatment for myeloid leukaemia of Down syndrome: population-based experience in the UK and results from the Medical Research Council AML10 and AML 12 trials. Br J Haematol 2005;132:576–83.

93. Creutzig U, Ritter J, Vormoor J, et al. Myelodysplasia and acute myelogenous leukemia in Down's syndrome. A report of 40 children of the AML-BFM Study Group. Leukemia 1996;10(11):1677–86.

94. Gamis AS, Woods WG, Alonzo TA, et al. Increased age at diagnosis has a significantly negative effect on outcome in children with Down syndrome and acute myeloid leukemia: a report from the Children's Cancer Group Study 2891. J Clin Oncol 2003;21(18):3415–22.

95. Testi AM, Biondi A, Lo CF, et al. GIMEMA-AIEOP AIDA protocol for the treatment of newly diagnosed acute promyelocytic leukemia (APL) in children. Blood 2005;106:447–53.

96. Ravindranath Y, Gregory J, Feusner J. Treatment of acute promyelocytic leukemia in children: arsenic or ATRA. Leukemia 2004;18(10):1576–7.

97. Webb DK, Wheatley K, Harrison G, et al. Outcome for children with relapsed acute myeloid leukaemia following initial therapy in the Medical Research Council (MRC) AML 10 trial. MRC Childhood Leukaemia Working Party. Leukemia 1999;13(1):25–31.

98. Stahnke K, Boos J, Bender-Gotze C, et al. Duration of first remission predicts remission rates and long-term survival in children with relapsed acute myelogenous leukemia. Leukemia 1998;12(10):1534–8.

99. Aladjidi N, Auvrignon A, Leblanc T, et al. Outcome in children with relapsed acute myeloid leukemia after initial treatment with the French Leucemie Aique Myeloide Enfant (LAME) 89/91 protocol of the French Society of Pediatric Hematology and Immunology. J Clin Oncol 2003;21(23):4377–85.

100. Wells RJ, Adams MT, Alonzo TA, et al. Mitoxantrone and cytarabine induction, high-dose cytarabine, and etoposide intensification for pediatric patients with relapsed or refractory acute myeloid leukemia: Children's Cancer Group Study 2951. J Clin Oncol 2003;21(15):2940–7.

101. Rubnitz JE, Razzouk BI, Lensing S, et al. Prognostic factors and outcome of recurrence in childhood acute myeloid leukemia. Cancer 2007;109(1):157–63.

102. Abrahamsson J, Clausen N, Gustafsson G, et al. Improved outcome after relapse in children with acute myeloid leukaemia. Br J Haematol 2007;136(2): 222–36.

103. Zwaan CM, Reinhardt D, Corbacioglu S, et al. Gemtuzumab ozogamicin: first clinical experiences in children with relapsed/refractory acute myeloid leukemia treated on compassionate-use basis. Blood 2003;101(10):3868–71.

104. Jeha S, Gandhi V, Chan KW, et al. Clofarabine, a novel nucleoside analog, is active in pediatric patients with advanced leukemia. Blood 2004;103(3):784–9.

105. Meshinchi S, Leisenring WM, Carpenter PA, et al. Survival after second hematopoietic stem cell transplantation for recurrent pediatric acute myeloid leukemia. Biol Blood Marrow Transplant 2003;9(11):706–13.

106. Appelbaum FR, Gundacker H, Head DR, et al. Age and acute myeloid leukemia. Blood 2006;107(9):3481–5.

107. Razzouk BI, Estey E, Pounds S, et al. Impact of age on outcome of pediatric acute myeloid leukemia: a report from 2 institutions. Cancer 2006;106(11): 2495–502.

108. Rubnitz JE, Lensing S, Razzouk BI, et al. Effect of race on outcome of white and black children with acute myeloid leukemia: the St. Jude experience. Pediatr Blood Cancer 2007;48(1):10–5.

109. Aplenc R, Alonzo TA, Gerbing RB, et al. Ethnicity and survival in childhood acute myeloid leukemia: a report from the Children's Oncology Group. Blood 2006; 108(1):74–80.

110. Lange BJ, Gerbing RB, Feusner J, et al. Mortality in overweight and underweight children with acute myeloid leukemia. J Am Med Assoc 2005;293(2):203–11.

111. Athale UH, Razzouk BI, Raimondi SC, et al. Biology and outcome of childhood acute megakaryoblastic leukemia: a single institution's experience. Blood 2001; 97(12):3727–32.

112. Barbaric D, Alonzo TA, Gerbing R, et al. Minimally differentiated acute myeloid leukemia (FAB AML-10) is associated with an adverse outcome in children: a report from the Children's Oncology Group, studies CCG-2891 and CCG-2961. Blood 2007;109(6):2314–21.

113. Barnard D, Alonzo TA, Gerbing R, et al. Comparison of childhood myelodysplastic syndrome, AML FAB M6 or M7, CCG 2891: report from the Children's Oncology Group. Pediatr Blood Cancer 2007;49:17–22.

114. Dastugue N, Lafage-Pochitaloff M, Pages MP, et al. Cytogenetic profile of childhood and adult megakaryoblastic leukemia (M7): a study of the Groupe Francais de Cytogenetique Hematologique (GFCH). Blood 2002;100(2): 618–26.

115. Garderet L, Labopin M, Gorin NC, et al. Hematopoietic stem cell transplantation for de novo acute megakaryocytic leukemia in first complete remission: a retrospective study of the European Group for Blood and Marrow Transplantation (EBMT). Blood 2005;105(1):405–9.

116. Reinhardt D, Diekamp S, Langebrake C, et al. Acute megakaryoblastic leukemia in children and adolescents, excluding Down's syndrome: improved outcome with intensified induction treatment. Leukemia 2005;19(8):1495–6.

117. Grimwade D, Walker H, Oliver F, et al. The importance of diagnostic cytogenetics on outcome in AML: analysis of 1,612 patients entered into the MRC AML 10 trial. The Medical Research Council Adult and Children's Leukaemia Working Parties. Blood 1998;92(7):2322–33.

118. Raimondi SC, Chang MN, Ravindranath Y, et al. Chromosomal abnormalities in 478 children with acute myeloid leukemia: clinical characteristics and treatment

outcome in a cooperative Pediatric Oncology Group study-POG 8821. Blood 1999;94(11):3707–16.

119. Bloomfield CD, Lawrence D, Byrd JC, et al. Frequency of prolonged remission duration after high-dose cytarabine intensification in acute myeloid leukemia varies by cytogenetic subtype. Cancer Res 1998;58(18):4173–9.

120. Byrd JC, Mrozek K, Dodge RK, et al. Pretreatment cytogenetic abnormalities are predictive of induction success, cumulative incidence of relapse, and overall survival in adult patients with de novo acute myeloid leukemia: results from Cancer and Leukemia Group B (CALGB 8461). Blood 2002;100(13): 4325–36.

121. Marcucci G, Mrozek K, Ruppert AS, et al. Prognostic factors and outcome of core binding factor acute myeloid leukemia patients with t(8;21) differ from those of patients with inv(16): a Cancer and Leukemia Group B Study. J Clin Oncol 2006;24:5705–17.

122. Appelbaum F, Kopecky KJ, Tallman M, et al. The clinical spectrum of adult acute myeloid leukaemia associated with core binding factor translocations. Br J Haematol 2006;135:165–73.

123. Dimartino JF, Cleary ML. MII rearrangements in haematological malignancies: lessons from clinical and biological studies. Br J Haematol 1999;106(3):614–26.

124. Rubnitz JE, Raimondi SC, Tong X, et al. Favorable impact of the t(9;11) in childhood acute myeloid leukemia. J Clin Oncol 2002;20(9):2302–9.

125. Schoch C, Schnittger S, Klaus M, et al. AML with 11q23/MLL abnormalities as defined by the WHO classification: incidence, partner chromosomes, FAB subtype, age distribution, and prognostic impact in an unselected series of 1897 cytogenetically analyzed AML cases. Blood 2003;102(7):2395–402.

126. Hasle H, Alonzo TA, Auvrignon A, et al. Monosomy 7 and deletion 7q in children and adolescents with acute myeloid leukemia: an international retrospective study. Blood 2007;109(11):4641–7.

127. Cairoli R, Beghini A, Grillo G, et al. Prognostic impact of c-KIT mutations in core binding factor leukemias: an Italian retrospective study. Blood 2007;107:3463–8.

128. Schnittger S, Kohl T, Haferlach T, et al. KIT-D816 mutations in AML1-ETO-positive AML are associated with impaired event-free and overall survival. Blood 2006;107:1791–9.

129. Paschka P, Marcucci G, Ruppert AS, et al. Adverse prognostic significance of KIT mutations in adult acute myeloid leukemia with inv(16) and t(8;21): a Cancer and Leukemia Group B Study. J Clin Oncol 2006;24(24):3904–11.

130. Goemans BF, Zwaan CM, Miller M, et al. Mutations in KIT and RAS are frequent events in pediatric core-binding factor acute myeloid leukemia. Leukemia 2005; 19(9):1536–42.

131. Shimada A, Taki T, Tabuchi K, et al. KIT mutations, and not FLT3 internal tandem duplication, are strongly associated with a poor prognosis in pediatric acute myeloid leukemia with t(8;21); a study of the Japanese Childhood AML Cooperative Study Group. Blood 2006;107:1806–9.

132. Boissel N, Leroy H, Brethon B, et al. Incidence and prognostic impact of c-Kit, FLT3, and Ras gene mutations in core binding factor acute myeloid leukemia (CBF-AML). Leukemia 2006;20(6):965–70.

133. Meshinchi S, Stirewalt DL, Alonzo TA, et al. Activating mutations of RTK/ras signal transduction pathway in pediatric acute myeloid leukemia. Blood 2003; 102(4):1474–9.

134. Kiyoi H, Naoe T, Nakano Y, et al. Prognostic implication of FLT3 and N-RAS gene mutations in acute myeloid leukemia. Blood 1999;93(9):3074–80.

135. Abu-Duhier FM, Goodeve AC, Wilson GA, et al. FLT3 internal tandem duplication mutations in adult acute myeloid leukaemia define a high-risk group. Br J Haematol 2000;111(1):190–5.
136. Kottaridis PD, Gale RE, Frew ME, et al. The presence of a FLT3 internal tandem duplication in patients with acute myeloid leukemia (AML) adds important prognostic information to cytogenetic risk group and response to the first cycle of chemotherapy: analysis of 854 patients from the United Kingdom Medical Research Council AML 10 and 12 trials. Blood 2001;98(6):1752–9.
137. Whitman SP, Archer KJ, Feng L, et al. Absence of the wild-type allele predicts poor prognosis in adult de novo acute myeloid leukemia with normal cytogenetics and the internal tandem duplication of FLT3: a cancer and leukemia group B study. Cancer Res 2001;61(19):7233–9.
138. Schnittger S, Schoch C, Dugas M, et al. Analysis of FLT3 length mutations in 1003 patients with acute myeloid leukemia: correlation to cytogenetics, FAB subtype, and prognosis in the AMLCG study and usefulness as a marker for the detection of minimal residual disease. Blood 2002;100(1):59–66.
139. Thiede C, Steudel C, Mohr B, et al. Analysis of FLT3-activating mutations in 979 patients with acute myelogenous leukemia: association with FAB subtypes and identification of subgroups with poor prognosis. Blood 2002; 99(12):4326–35.
140. Zwaan CM, Meshinchi S, Radich JP, et al. FLT3 internal tandem duplication in 234 children with acute myeloid leukemia: prognostic significance and relation to cellular drug resistance. Blood 2003;102(7):2387–94.
141. Meshinchi S, Woods WG, Stirewalt DL, et al. Prevalence and prognostic significance of Flt3 internal tandem duplication in pediatric acute myeloid leukemia. Blood 2001;97(1):89–94.
142. Iwai T, Yokota S, Nakao M, et al. Internal tandem duplication of the FLT3 gene and clinical evaluation in childhood acute myeloid leukemia. The Children's Cancer and Leukemia Study Group, Japan. Leukemia 1999;13(1):38–43.
143. Meshinchi S, Alonzo TA, Stirewalt DL, et al. Clinical implications of FLT3 mutations in pediatric AML. Blood 2006;108(12):3654–61.
144. Lacayo NJ, Meshinchi S, Kinnunen P, et al. Gene expression profiles at diagnosis in de novo childhood AML patients identify FLT3 mutations with good clinical outcomes. Blood 2004;104(9):2646–54.
145. Leith CP, Kopecky KJ, Chen IM, et al. Frequency and clinical significance of the expression of the multidrug resistance proteins MDR1/P-glycoprotein, MRP1, and LRP in acute myeloid leukemia: a Southwest Oncology Group Study. Blood 1999;94(3):1086–99.
146. Legrand O, Simonin G, Beauchamp-Nicoud A, et al. Simultaneous activity of MRP1 and Pgp is correlated with in vitro resistance to daunorubicin and with in vivo resistance in adult acute myeloid leukemia. Blood 1999;94(3):1046–56.
147. den Boer ML, Pieters R, Kazemier KM, et al. Relationship between major vault protein/lung resistance protein, multidrug resistance-associated protein, P-glycoprotein expression, and drug resistance in childhood leukemia. Blood 1998;91(6):2092–8.
148. Preudhomme C, Sagot C, Boissel N, et al. Favorable prognostic significance of CEBPA mutations in patients with de novo acute myeloid leukemia: a study from the Acute Leukemia French Association (ALFA). Blood 2002;100(8):2717–23.
149. Frohling S, Schlenk RF, Stolze I, et al. CEBPA mutations in younger adults with acute myeloid leukemia and normal cytogenetics: prognostic relevance and analysis of cooperating mutations. J Clin Oncol 2004;22(4):624–33.

150. Inokuchi K, Yamaguchi H, Hanawa H, et al. Loss of DCC gene expression is of prognostic importance in acute myelogenous leukemia. Clin Cancer Res 2002; 8(6):1882–8.

151. De Bont ES, Fidler V, Meeuwsen T, et al. Vascular endothelial growth factor secretion is an independent prognostic factor for relapse-free survival in pediatric acute myeloid leukemia patients. Clin Cancer Res 2002;8(9):2856–61.

152. Kohler T, Schill C, Deininger MW, et al. High Bad and Bax mRNA expression correlate with negative outcome in acute myeloid leukemia (AML). Leukemia 2002;16(1):22–9.

153. Karakas T, Miething CC, Maurer U, et al. The coexpression of the apoptosis-related genes Bcl-2 and Wt1 in predicting survival in adult acute myeloid leukemia. Leukemia 2002;16(5):846–54.

154. Del Poeta G, Venditti A, Del Principe MI, et al. Amount of spontaneous apoptosis detected by Bax/Bcl-2 ratio predicts outcome in acute myeloid leukemia (AML). Blood 2003;101(6):2125–31.

155. Baldus CD, Thiede C, Soucek S, et al. BAALC expression and FLT3 internal tandem duplication mutations in acute myeloid leukemia patients with normal cytogenetics: prognostic implications. J Clin Oncol 2006;24(5):790–7.

156. Marcucci G, Maharry K, Whitman SP, et al. High expression levels of the ETS-related gene, ERG, predict adverse outcome and improve molecular risk-based classification of cytogenetically normal acute myeloid leukemia: a Cancer and Leukemia Group B Study. J Clin Oncol 2007;25(22):3337–43.

157. Marcucci G, Baldus CD, Ruppert AS, et al. Overexpression of the ETS-related gene, ERG, predicts a worse outcome in acute myeloid leukemia with normal karyotype: a Cancer and Leukemia Group B study. J Clin Oncol 2005;23(36): 9234–42.

158. Boissel N, Renneville A, Biggio V, et al. Prevalence, clinical profile, and prognosis of NPM mutations in AML with normal karyotype. Blood 2005;106(10): 3618–20.

159. Thiede C, Koch S, Creutzig E, et al. Prevalence and prognostic impact of NPM1 mutations in 1485 adult patients with acute myeloid leukemia (AML). Blood 2006;107(10):4011–20.

160. Brown P, McIntyre E, Rau R, et al. The incidence and clinical significance of nucleophosmin mutations in childhood AML. Blood 2007;110(3):979–85.

161. Schnittger S, Kinkelin U, Schoch C, et al. Screening for MLL tandem duplication in 387 unselected patients with AML identify a prognostically unfavorable subset of AML. Leukemia 2000;14(5):796–804.

162. Dohner K, Tobis K, Ulrich R, et al. Prognostic significance of partial tandem duplications of the MLL gene in adult patients 16 to 60 years old with acute myeloid leukemia and normal cytogenetics: a study of the Acute Myeloid Leukemia Study Group Ulm. J Clin Oncol 2002;20(15):3254–61.

163. Yagi T, Morimoto A, Eguchi M, et al. Identification of a gene expression signature associated with pediatric AML prognosis. Blood 2003;102(5): 1849–56.

164. Valk PJ, Verhaak RG, Beijen MA, et al. Prognostically useful gene-expression profiles in acute myeloid leukemia. N Engl J Med 2004;350(16):1617–28.

165. Bullinger L, Dohner K, Bair E, et al. Use of gene-expression profiling to identify prognostic subclasses in adult acute myeloid leukemia. N Engl J Med 2004; 350(16):1605–16.

166. Radmacher MD, Marcucci G, Ruppert AS, et al. Independent confirmation of a prognostic gene-expression signature in adult acute myeloid leukemia with

a normal karyotype: a Cancer and Leukemia Group B study. Blood 2006;108(5): 1677–83.

167. Wilson CS, Davidson GS, Martin SB, et al. Gene expression profiling of adult acute myeloid leukemia identifies novel biologic clusters for risk classification and outcome prediction. Blood 2006;108(2):685–96.

168. Mrozek K, Marcucci G, Paschka P, et al. Clinical relevance of mutations and gene-expression changes in adult acute myeloid leukemia with normal cytogenetics: are we ready for a prognostically prioritized molecular classification? Blood 2007;109(2):431–48.

169. Ross ME, Mahfouz R, Onciu M, et al. Gene expression profiling of pediatric acute myelogenous leukemia. Blood 2004;104(12):3679–87.

170. Campana D. Determination of minimal residual disease in leukaemia patients. Br J Haematol 2003;121(6):823–38.

171. Creutzig U, Zimmermann M, Ritter J, et al. Definition of a standard-risk group in children with AML. Br J Haematol 1999;104(3):630–9.

172. Kern W, Haferlach T, Schoch C, et al. Early blast clearance by remission induction therapy is a major independent prognostic factor for both achievement of complete remission and long-term outcome in acute myeloid leukemia: data from the German AML Cooperative Group (AMLCG) 1992 Trial. Blood 2003;101(1):64–70.

173. Marcucci G, Mrozek K, Ruppert AS, et al. Abnormal cytogenetics at date of morphologic complete remission predicts short overall and disease-free survival, and higher relapse rate in adult acute myeloid leukemia: results from Cancer and Leukemia Group B study 8461. J Clin Oncol 2004;22(12):2410–8.

174. Szczepanski T, Orfao A, van DV, et al. Minimal residual disease in leukaemia patients. Lancet Oncol 2001;2(7):409–17.

175. Sievers EL, Lange BJ, Buckley JD, et al. Prediction of relapse of pediatric acute myeloid leukemia by use of multidimensional flow cytometry. J Natl Cancer Inst 1996;88(20):1483–8.

176. Sievers EL, Lange BJ, Alonzo TA, et al. Immunophenotypic evidence of leukemia after induction therapy predicts relapse: results from a prospective Children's Cancer Group study of 252 patients with acute myeloid leukemia. Blood 2003;101(9):3398–406.

177. Coustan-Smith E, Ribeiro RC, Rubnitz JE, et al. Clinical significance of residual disease during treatment in childhood acute myeloid leukaemia. Br J Haematol 2003;123(2):243–52.

178. Langebrake C, Creutzig U, Dworzak M, et al. Residual disease monitoring in childhood acute myeloid leukemia by multiparameter flow cytometry: the MRD-AML-BFM Study Group. J Clin Oncol 2006;24(22):3686–92.

179. San Miguel JF, Martinez A, Macedo A, et al. Immunophenotyping investigation of minimal residual disease is a useful approach for predicting relapse in acute myeloid leukemia patients. Blood 1997;90(6):2465–70.

180. San Miguel JF, Vidriales MB, Lopez-Berges C, et al. Early immunophenotypical evaluation of minimal residual disease in acute myeloid leukemia identifies different patient risk groups and may contribute to postinduction treatment stratification. Blood 2001;98(6):1746–51.

181. Buccisano F, Maurillo L, Gattei V, et al. The kinetics of reduction of minimal residual disease impacts on duration of response and survival of patients with acute myeloid leukemia. Leukemia 2006;20(10):1783–9.

182. Feller N, van der Pol MA, van Stijn A, et al. MRD parameters using immunophenotypic detection methods are highly reliable in predicting survival in acute myeloid leukaemia. Leukemia 2004;18(8):1380–90.

183. Kern W, Voskova D, Schoch C, et al. Determination of relapse risk based on assessment of minimal residual disease during complete remission by multiparameter flow cytometry in unselected patients with acute myeloid leukemia. Blood 2004;104(10):3078–85.

184. Tobal K, Newton J, Macheta M, et al. Molecular quantitation of minimal residual disease in acute myeloid leukemia with t(8;21) can identify patients in durable remission and predict clinical relapse. Blood 2000;95(3):815–9.

185. Schnittger S, Weisser M, Schoch C, et al. New score predicting for prognosis in PML-RARA+, AML1-ETO+, or CBFBMYH11+ acute myeloid leukemia based on quantification of fusion transcripts. Blood 2003;102(8): 2746–55.

186. Buonamici S, Ottaviani E, Testoni N, et al. Real-time quantitation of minimal residual disease in inv(16)-positive acute myeloid leukemia may indicate risk for clinical relapse and may identify patients in a curable state. Blood 2002; 99(2):443–9.

187. Guerrasio A, Pilatrino C, De Micheli D, et al. Assessment of minimal residual disease (MRD) in CBFbeta/MYH11-positive acute myeloid leukemias by qualitative and quantitative RT-PCR amplification of fusion transcripts. Leukemia 2002; 16(6):1176–81.

188. Viehmann S, Teigler-Schlegel A, Bruch J, et al. Monitoring of minimal residual disease (MRD) by real-time quantitative reverse transcription PCR (RQ-RT-PCR) in childhood acute myeloid leukemia with AML1/ETO rearrangement. Leukemia 2003;17(6):1130–6.

189. Krauter J, Gorlich K, Ottmann O, et al. Prognostic value of minimal residual disease quantification by real-time reverse transcriptase polymerase chain reaction in patients with core binding factor leukemias. J Clin Oncol 2003; 21(23):4413–22.

190. Perea G, Lasa A, Aventin A, et al. Prognostic value of minimal residual disease (MRD) in acute myeloid leukemia (AML) with favorable cytogenetics t(8;21) and inv(16). Leukemia 2006;20:87–94.

191. Trka J, Kalinova M, Hrusak O, et al. Real-time quantitative PCR detection of WT1 gene expression in children with AML: prognostic significance, correlation with disease status and residual disease detection by flow cytometry. Leukemia 2002;16(7):1381–9.

192. Cilloni D, Gottardi E, De Micheli D, et al. Quantitative assessment of WT1 expression by real time quantitative PCR may be a useful tool for monitoring minimal residual disease in acute leukemia patients. Leukemia 2002;16(10): 2115–21.

193. Lapillonne H, Renneville A, Auvrignon A, et al. High WT1 expression after induction therapy predicts high risk of relapse and death in pediatric acute myeloid leukemia. J Clin Oncol 2006;24(10):1507–15.

194. Evans WE, Relling MV. Moving towards individualized medicine with pharmacogenomics. Nature 2004;429(6990):464–8.

195. Monzo M, Brunet S, Urbano-Ispizua A, et al. Genomic polymorphisms provide prognostic information in intermediate-risk acute myeloblastic leukemia. Blood 2006;107(12):4871–9.

196. Gamis AS. Acute myeloid leukemia and Down syndrome evolution of modern therapy—state of the art review. Pediatr Blood Cancer 2005;44(1):13–20.

197. Ge Y, Jensen T, James SJ, et al. High frequency of the 844ins68 cystathionine-beta-synthase gene variant in Down syndrome children with acute myeloid leukemia. Leukemia 2002;16(11):2339–41.

198. Ge Y, Stout ML, Tatman DA, et al. GATA1, cytidine deaminase, and the high cure rate of Down syndrome children with acute megakaryocytic leukemia. J Natl Cancer Inst 2005;97(3):226–31.

199. Ge Y, Dombkowski AA, Lafiura KM, et al. Differential gene expression, GATA1 target genes, and the chemotherapy sensitivity of Down syndrome megakaryocytic leukemia. Blood 2006;107(4):1570–81.

200. Taub JW, Ge Y. Down syndrome, drug metabolism and chromosome 21. Pediatr Blood Cancer 2005;44(1):33–9.

201. Galmarini CM, Thomas X, Calvo F, et al. In vivo mechanisms of resistance to cytarabine in acute myeloid leukaemia. Br J Haematol 2002;117(4):860–8.

202. Gati WP, Paterson AR, Belch AR, et al. Es nucleoside transporter content of acute leukemia cells: role in cell sensitivity to cytarabine (AraC). Leuk Lymphoma 1998;32(1–2):45–54.

203. Galmarini CM, Thomas X, Graham K, et al. Deoxycytidine kinase and cN-II nucleotidase expression in blast cells predict survival in acute myeloid leukaemia patients treated with cytarabine. Br J Haematol 2003;122(1): 53–60.

204. Davies SM, Robison LL, Buckley JD, et al. Glutathione S-transferase polymorphisms and outcome of chemotherapy in childhood acute myeloid leukemia. J Clin Oncol 2001;19(5):1279–87.

205. Naoe T, Tagawa Y, Kiyoi H, et al. Prognostic significance of the null genotype of glutathione S- transferase-T1 in patients with acute myeloid leukemia: increased early death after chemotherapy. Leukemia 2002;16(2):203–8.

206. Allan JM, Smith AG, Wheatley K, et al. Genetic variation in XPD predicts treatment outcome and risk of acute myeloid leukemia following chemotherapy. Blood 2004;104(13):3872–7.

207. Mehta PA, Alonzo TA, Gerbing RB, et al. XPD Lys751Gln polymorphism in the etiology and outcome of childhood acute myeloid leukemia: a Children's Oncology Group report. Blood 2006;107(1):39–45.

208. Okamoto Y, Ribeiro RC, Srivastava DK, et al. Viridans streptococcal sepsis: clinical features and complications in childhood acute myeloid leukemia. J Pediatr Hematol Oncol 2003;25(9):696–703.

209. Creutzig U, Zimmermann M, Reinhardt D, et al. Early deaths and treatment-related mortality in children undergoing therapy for acute myeloid leukemia: analysis of the multicenter clinical trials AML-BFM 93 and AML-BFM 98. J Clin Oncol 2004;22(21):4384–93.

210. Lehrnbecher T, Varwig D, Kaiser J, et al. Infectious complications in pediatric acute myeloid leukemia: analysis of the prospective multi-institutional clinical trial AML-BFM 93. Leukemia 2004;18(1):72–7.

211. Rubnitz JE, Lensing S, Zhou Y, et al. Death during induction therapy and first remission of acute leukemia in childhood: the St. Jude experience. Cancer 2004;101(7):1677–84.

212. Gamis AS, Howells WB, DeSwarte-Wallace J, et al. Alpha hemolytic Streptococcal infection during intensive treatment for acute myeloid leukemia: a report from the Children's Cancer Group Study CCG-2891. J Clin Oncol 2000;18(9): 1845–55.

213. Sung L, Lange BJ, Gerbing RB, et al. Microbiologically documented infections and infection-related mortality in children with acute myeloid leukemia. Blood 2007;110:3532–9.

214. Godwin JE, Kopecky KJ, Head DR, et al. A double-blind placebo-controlled trial of granulocyte colony-stimulating factor in elderly patients with previously

untreated acute myeloid leukemia: a Southwest Oncology Group study (9031). Blood 1998;91(10):3607–15.

215. Heil G, Hoelzer D, Sanz MA, et al. A randomized, double-blind, placebo-controlled, phase III study of filgrastim in remission induction and consolidation therapy for adults with de novo acute myeloid leukemia. The International Acute Myeloid Leukemia Study Group. Blood 1997;90(12):4710–8.

216. Amadori S, Suciu S, Jehn U, et al. Use of glycosylated recombinant human G-CSF (lenograstim) during and/or after induction chemotherapy in patients 61 years of age and older with acute myeloid leukemia: final results of AML-13, a randomized phase 3 study of the European Organisation for Research and Treatment of Cancer and Gruppo Italiano Malattie Ematologiche dell'Adulto (EORTC/GIMEMA) Leukemia Groups. Blood 2005;106:27–34.

217. George B, Mathews V, Poonkuzhali B, et al. Treatment of children with newly diagnosed acute promyelocytic leukemia with arsenic trioxide: a single center experience. Leukemia 2004;18(10):1587–90.

218. Burnett A, Kell WJ, Goldstone A, et al. The addition of gemtuzumab ozogamicin to induction chemotherapy for AML improves disease free survival without extra toxicity: preliminary analysis of 1115 patients in the MRC AML15 trial. Blood 2006;108:13.

219. Guzman ML, Swiderski CF, Howard DS, et al. Preferential induction of apoptosis for primary human leukemic stem cells. Proc Natl Acad Sci U S A 2002;99(25):16220–5.

220. Adams J. The proteasome: a suitable antineoplastic target. Nat Rev Cancer 2004;4(5):349–60.

221. Insinga A, Monestiroli S, Ronzoni S, et al. Inhibitors of histone deacetylases induce tumor-selective apoptosis through activation of the death receptor pathway. Nat Med 2005;11(1):71–6.

222. Nebbioso A, Clarke N, Voltz E, et al. Tumor-selective action of HDAC inhibitors involves TRAIL induction in acute myeloid leukemia cells. Nat Med 2005;11(1):77–84.

223. Levis M, Allebach J, Tse KF, et al. A FLT3-targeted tyrosine kinase inhibitor is cytotoxic to leukemia cells in vitro and in vivo. Blood 2002;99(11):3885–91.

224. Brown P, Meshinchi S, Levis M, et al. Pediatric AML primary samples with FLT3/ITD mutations are preferentially killed by FLT3 inhibition. Blood 2004;104(6):1841–9.

225. Smith BD, Levis M, Beran M, et al. Single-agent CEP-701, a novel FLT3 inhibitor, shows biologic and clinical activity in patients with relapsed or refractory acute myeloid leukemia. Blood 2004;103(10):3669–76.

226. Parker WB, Shaddix SC, Chang CH, et al. Effects of 2-chloro-9-(2-deoxy-2-fluoro-beta-D-arabinofuranosyl)adenine on K562 cellular metabolism and the inhibition of human ribonucleotide reductase and DNA polymerases by its 5′-triphosphate. Cancer Res 1991;51(9):2386–94.

227. Xie KC, Plunkett W. Deoxynucleotide pool depletion and sustained inhibition of ribonucleotide reductase and DNA synthesis after treatment of human lymphoblastoid cells with 2-chloro-9-(2-deoxy-2-fluoro-beta-D-arabinofuranosyl) adenine. Cancer Res 1996;56(13):3030–7.

228. Gandhi V, Kantarjian H, Faderl S, et al. Pharmacokinetics and pharmacodynamics of plasma clofarabine and cellular clofarabine triphosphate in patients with acute leukemias. Clin Cancer Res 2003;9(17):6335–42.

229. Miller JS, Soignier Y, Panoskaltsis-Mortari A, et al. Successful adoptive transfer and in vivo expansion of human haploidentical NK cells in patients with cancer. Blood 2005;105(8):3051–7.

Neuroblastoma: Biology, Prognosis, and Treatment

Julie R. Park, MD[a],*, Angelika Eggert, MD[b], Huib Caron, MD, PhD[c]

KEYWORDS

• Neuroblastoma • Epidemiology • Treatment

Neuroblastoma, a neoplasm of the sympathetic nervous system, is the second most common extracranial malignant tumor of childhood and the most common solid tumor of infancy. Neuroblastoma is a heterogeneous malignancy with prognosis ranging from near uniform survival to high risk for fatal demise. Neuroblastoma serves as a paradigm for the prognostic utility of biologic and clinical data and the potential to tailor therapy for patient cohorts at low, intermediate, and high risk for recurrence. Overall survival is excellent for patients who have low- and intermediate-risk neuroblastoma with a general trend toward minimization of therapy. In contrast, a marked intensification of therapy has led to only incremental improvement in survival for high-risk disease because less than 40% of high-risk patients survive. Chemotherapy and radiotherapy resistance remain the hallmark of failure. This article summarizes our understanding of neuroblastoma biology and prognostic features and discusses their impact on current and proposed risk stratification schemas, risk-based therapeutic approaches, and the development of novel therapies for patients at high risk for failure.

EPIDEMIOLOGY AND CAUSE

The incidence of neuroblastoma per year is 10.5 per million children less than 15 years of age.[1] Neuroblastoma accounts for 8% to 10% of all childhood cancers and for approximately 15% of cancer deaths in children. There seems to be no significant geographical variation in the incidence between North America and Europe, and there are no differences between races. Neuroblastoma occurs slightly more frequently in

A version of this article was previously published in the *Pediatric Clinics of North America*, 55:1.
[a] Division of Hematology and Oncology, University of Washington School of Medicine and Seattle Children's Hospital, 4800 Sand Pt. Way NE, MS: B6553, Seattle, WA 98105-0371, USA
[b] Department of Hematology/Oncology, University Children's Hospital Essen, Hufelandstr. 55, 45122 Essen, Germany
[c] Department of Pediatric Oncology and Hematology, Emma Children's Hospital AMC, EKZ/AMC, PO Box 22700, 1100 DE, Amsterdam, the Netherlands
* Corresponding author.
E-mail address: julie.park@seattlechildrens.org (J.R. Park).

boys than girls (ratio 1.2:1). The incidence peaks at age 0 to 4 years, with a median age of 23 months. Forty percent of patients who present with clinical symptoms at diagnosis are under 1 year of age, and less than 5% with clinical symptoms are over the age of 10 years. Cases of familial neuroblastoma have been reported.[2] Environmental factors are implicated in the development of neuroblastoma (eg, paternal exposure to electromagnetic fields or prenatal exposure to alcohol, pesticides, or phenobarbital). A potential relationship with assisted pregnancies has also been made. None of these environmental factors has been confirmed in independent studies.[3,4]

Screening for neuroblastoma was pioneered by Japanese investigators who demonstrated that asymptomatic tumors could be detected in infants by measurement of urinary catecholamine metabolites. The implementation of infant screening for neuroblastoma resulted in a doubling of neuroblastoma incidence to 20.1 per million children,[5] and the tumors detected possessed favorable biological characteristics.[6] Although the outcome for the children with the detected tumors was excellent, these studies were not population based and did not demonstrate a resultant reduction in neuroblastoma mortality rates. The Quebec Neuroblastoma Screening Project and the German Neuroblastoma Screening Study were designed to identify whether screening a large cohort of infants for neuroblastoma at the ages of 3 weeks, 6 months, and 12 months could reduce the population-based incidence of advanced disease and mortality. These studies demonstrate that screening for neuroblastoma at or under the age of 1 year identifies tumors with a good prognosis and molecular pathology, doubles the incidence, and fails to detect the poor-prognosis disease that presents clinically at an older age.[7,8]

GENETIC PREDISPOSITION

Neuroblastoma can occur in patients affected with other neural crest disorders or malignancies, such as Hirschsprung disease, neurofibromatosis type 1, and congenital central hypoventilation syndrome.[9–11] Genomic linkage studies have not found evidence of a link between Hirschsprung disease and neuroblastoma development. The co-occurrence of neuroblastoma and von Recklinghausen disease is of interest because both disorders are deviations of normal neural-crest cell development in the embryo. An analysis of the reported coincidence of neuroblastoma and neurofibromatosis indicates that most of these cases can probably be accounted for by chance.[12] The *PHOX2B* gene is the major disease gene for the congenital central hypoventilation disorder, and constitutional *PHOX2B* mutations have been identified in familial neuroblastoma cases[13] and in 2.3% of patients who have sporadic neuroblastoma.[14]

Several cases of constitutional chromosome abnormalities have been reported in individuals who have neuroblastoma, but no consistent pattern has emerged.[12] Constitutional abnormalities involving the short arm of chromosome 1 have been reported for three neuroblastoma cases, possibly implicating chromosome 1 p loci in neuroblastoma predisposition. A report that familial neuroblastoma is not linked to 1p36 indicates that the predisposition locus for familial cases lies elsewhere.

Familial forms of neuroblastoma are rare, accounting for about 1% of all cases. There are few reported pedigrees of familial neuroblastoma.[15] In those families, the median age at diagnosis is 9 months, as opposed to 2 to 3 years in sporadic cases. An increased incidence of multiple primary tumors is also apparent. Analysis of the pedigree structures suggests a dominant mode of inheritance with low penetrance.[15] Germline mutations in the *ALK* oncogene are the main cause of familial susceptibility to neuroblastoma in otherwise healthy families. *ALK* is predicted to function as an oncogene in the pathogenesis of neuroblastoma. Disease-causing mutations are found almost exclusively within the tyrosine kinase domain of the *ALK* that lead to constitutive phosphorylation and activation of the *ALK* protein.[16–18a,b]

PATHOLOGY
Cell of Origin and Cancer Stem Cell Hypothesis

The peripheral neuroblastic tumors (pNTs), including neuroblastoma, belong to the "small blue round cell" neoplasms of childhood.[19] They are derived from progenitor cells of the sympathetic nervous system: the sympathogonia of the sympathoadrenal lineage. After migrating from the neural crest, these pluripotent sympathogonia form the sympathetic ganglia, the chromaffin cells of the adrenal medulla, and the paraganglia, reflecting the typical localizations of neuroblastic tumors.

The mechanisms causing persistence of embryonal cells that later give rise to pNTs are mainly unknown. Defects in embryonic genes controlling neural crest development are likely to underlie the unbalanced proliferation and disturbed differentiation of neuroblastoma.[13,14,20] These defects cause a disruption of the normal genetic differentiation program, resulting in an early or late differentiation block. The classic histopathologic pNT subtypes of neuroblastoma, ganglioneuroblastoma, and ganglioneuroma reflect a spectrum of maturation ranging from tumors with predominant undifferentiated neuroblasts to those largely consisting of fully differentiated neurons surrounded by a dense stroma of Schwann cells.

A hallmark of neuroblastoma is cellular heterogeneity. Although the presence of phenotypically diverse cells could be explained by ongoing mutagenesis, the cancer stem cell hypothesis has provided an intriguing alternative explanation for neuroblastoma heterogeneity. This hypothesis suggests that rare multipotent stem cells with indefinite potential for self-renewal drive the onset and growth of tumors. Although the existence of cancer stem cells in leukemia and some solid tumors has been established,[21–23] neuroblastoma stem cells have not been clearly identified. Developmental programs controlling self-renewal in neuronal stem cells, including the Notch, Sonic hedgehog, and Wnt/β-catenin pathways, have been implicated in embryonal tumorigenesis.[24–26] It is conceivable that neuroblastoma stem cells arise from normal neural crest stem cells, partly preserving and partly dysregulating these pathways. The identification and characterization of cancer stem cells in neuroblastoma should permit a targeted approach to more effective treatment.

Histopathologic Assessment

Primary, pretreatment tumor specimens obtained by open biopsy are optimal material for histologic examination and prognostic evaluation. The typical neuroblastoma is composed of small, uniformly sized cells containing dense hyperchromatic nuclei and scant cytoplasm. The Homer-Wright pseudorosette composed of neuroblasts surrounding areas of eosinophilic neuropil is seen in up to 50% of cases.[27] Distinguishing pNTs from other "small blue round cell" tumors often requires techniques beyond hematoxylin-eosin staining and light microscopy. In the immunohistochemical diagnosis of pNTs, positive staining for neural markers, including neuron-specific enolase, synaptophysin, neurofilament protein, ganglioside GD2, chromogranin A, and tyrosine hydroxylase, combined with negative staining for markers of other small-round-cell tumors should be considered. Electron microscopy typically demonstrates dense core, membrane-bound neurosecretory granules, microfilaments, and parallel arrays of microtubules within neuritic processes (neuropil).[19]

As early as 1963, Beckwith and Perrin suggested a natural history of pNTs that might include involution (regression) and maturation.[28] This hypothesis was based on their observation of "in situ neuroblastoma," an adrenal lesion of microscopic size that is cytologically identical to typical neuroblastoma and is detected in infants with a frequency of 50 times the expected incidence of primary adrenal neuroblastoma. The concept of Beckwith and Perrin has been adopted and incorporated in the International Neuroblastoma Pathology Classification (INPC).[29] The INPC was established in 1999 by adopting the original system proposed by Shimada in 1984.[30] The INPC was revised in 2003.[31] The INPC distinguishes a favorable histology group from an unfavorable histology group of pNTs by applying the concept of age-dependent normal ranges of morphologic features, such as Schwannian stromal development, grade of neuroblastic differentiation, and mitosis-karyorrhexis index (**Fig. 1**).

According to the INPC, the pNTs are assigned to one of the following four basic morphologic categories.

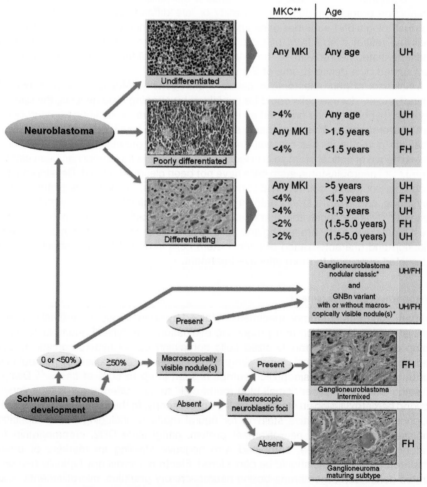

Fig. 1. International Neuroblastoma Pathology Classification.

Neuroblastoma (Schwannian-stroma poor)

A neuroblastoma is a tumor composed of neuroblastic cells forming groups or nests separated by stromal septa with none to limited Schwannian proliferation. This category consists of the three subtypes: (1) undifferentiated, (2) poorly differentiated (background of recognizable neuropil and <5% of cells showing differentiation), and (3) differentiating (abundant neuropil and >5% cells showing differentiation toward ganglion cells).

Ganglioneuroblastoma, intermixed (Schwannian stroma-rich)

An intermixed ganglioneuroblastoma is a tumor containing well-defined microscopic nests of neuroblastic cells intermixed or randomly distributed in the ganglioneuromatous stroma. The nests are composed of a mixture of neuroblastic cells in various stages of differentiation, usually dominated by differentiating neuroblasts and maturing ganglion cells in a background of neuropil.

Ganglioneuroblastoma, nodular (composite Schwannian stroma-rich/stroma dominant and stroma-poor)

A nodular ganglioneuroblastoma is characterized by the presence of grossly visible, usually hemorrhagic neuroblastic nodules (stoma-poor component, representing an aggressive clone) co-existing with ganglioneuroblastoma, intermixed (stroma-rich component) or with ganglioneuroma (stroma-dominant component), both representing a nonaggressive clone. The term "composite" implies that the tumor is composed of biologically different clones.

Ganglioneuroma (Schwannian-stroma-dominant)

This variant has two subtypes: maturing and mature. The maturing subtype is composed predominantly of ganglioneuromatous stroma with scattered collections of differentiating neuroblasts or maturing ganglion cells in addition to fully mature ganglion cells. The mature subtype is composed of mature Schwannian stroma and ganglion cells.

There is a significant correlation between morphologic features of the INPC and biological properties of the pNTS, such as *MYCN* amplification or *TrkA* Expression.

CLINICAL PRESENTATION, DIAGNOSIS, AND STAGING

Clinical presentation of neuroblastoma is dependent upon site of tumor origin, disease extent, and the presence of paraneoplastic syndromes. Neuroblastoma can arise anywhere along the sympathetic nervous system. The majority of tumors (65%) arise in the abdomen, with over half of these arising in the adrenal gland. Additional sites of origin include the neck, chest, and pelvis. There is a concordance with age and site of disease, with infants more likely to present with thoracic and cervical primary sites (**Fig. 2**). One percent of patients have no detectable primary tumor.

Approximately 50% of patients present with localized or regional disease, and approximately 35% of patients have regional lymph node spread at the time of diagnosis. Patients who have localized disease are often asymptomatic, with disease coincidently diagnosed after testing for unassociated medical conditions. Alternatively, mass or abdominal distension and pain are present. Patients who have localized cervical disease arising from the superior cervical ganglion may present with Horner syndrome. Epidural or intradural extension of tumor occurs in approximately 5% to 15% of patients diagnosed with neuroblastoma and may be accompanied by

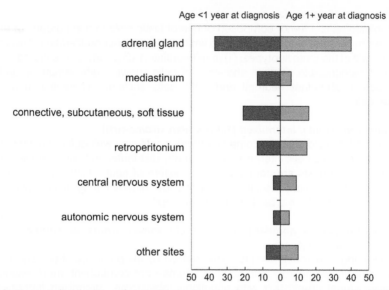

Fig. 2. Percent distribution of neuroblastomas by primary site and age; SEER 1975–1995. (*Data from* Ries LA, Smith MA, Gurney JG, et al. Cancer incidence and survival among children and adolescents: United States SEER Program 1975–1995. NIH Pub. No. 99-4649. Bethesda (MD): NIH; 1999.)

neurologic impairments.[32,33] Well-documented paraneoplastic or clinical syndromes can be present at diagnosis and are summarized in **Table 1**.

Disease dissemination occurs through lymphatic and hematogenous routes. Bone, bone marrow, and liver are the most common sites of hematogenous spread, with particular predilection for metaphyseal, skull, and orbital bone sites. In contrast to the frequent lack of symptoms with locoregional disease, patients who have widespread disease are often ill appearing with fever, pain, and irritability. A classic presentation of periorbital swelling and ecchymoses ("raccoon eyes") is seen in children who have disease spread to periorbital region. Rarely, infants can present with respiratory compromise secondary to diffuse tumor involvement in the liver and massive hepatomegaly.[34]

The current criteria for diagnosis and staging of neuroblastoma are based upon the International Neuroblastoma Staging System (INSS) criteria initially formulated in 1986 and revised in 1988.[35,36] Neuroblastoma diagnosis is defined by pathologic confirmation from tumor tissue or by pathologic confirmation of neuroblastoma tumor cells in a bone marrow sample in the setting of increased urine or serum catecholamines or catecholamine metabolites (dopamine, vanillylmandelic acid, and homovanillic acid). Initial diagnostic testing should include CT or MRI to evaluate primary tumor size and regional extent and to assess for distant spread to neck, thorax, abdomen, or pelvic sites. Brain imaging is recommended only if clinically indicated by examination or neurologic symptoms. Bilateral posterior iliac crest marrow aspirates and core biopsies are required to exclude marrow involvement. Metaiodobenzylguanidine, a norepinephrine analog, is concentrated selectively in sympathetic nervous tissue and, when labeled with radioactive iodine (I^{131} or I^{123}), is an integral component of neuroblastoma staging and response evaluation.[37] A technetium bone scan should be considered for detection of cortical bone disease, especially in patients who have a negative metaiodobenzylguanidine scan.

Table 1 Syndromes associated with neuroblastoma	
Eponym	**Syndrome Features**
Pepper syndrome	Massive involvement of the liver with metastatic disease with or without respiratory distress.
Horner syndrome	Unilateral ptosis, myosis, and anhydrosis associated with a thoracic or cervical primary tumor. Symptoms do not resolve with tumor resection.
Hutchinson syndrome	Limping and irritability in young child associated with bone and bone marrow metastases.
Opsoclonus Mycoclonus Ataxia syndrome	Myoclonic jerking and random eye movement with or without cerebellar ataxia. Often associated with a biologically favorable and differentiated tumor. The condition is likely immune mediated, may not resolve with tumor removal, and often exhibits progressive neuropsychologic sequelae.[119–121]
Kerner-Morrison syndrome	Intractable secretory diarrhea due to tumor secretion of vasointestinal peptides. Tumors are generally biologically favorable.[122–123]
Neurocristopathy syndrome	Neuroblastoma associated with other neural crest disorders, including congenital hypoventilation syndrome or Hirshprung disease. Germline mutations in the paired homeobox gene PHOX2B have been identified in a subset of such patients.[13,20]

Adapted from Castleberry RP. Biology and treatment of neuroblastoma. Pediatr Clin North Am 1997;44:919–37; with permission.

The INSS definitions for neuroblastoma stage are listed in **Table 2**. Resectability implies tumor removal without removal of vital organs, compromise of major vessels, or patient disfigurement. Completely resected tumors are classified as stage 1, and partially resected regional tumors with or without regional nodal involvement are classified as stages 2 and 3 dependent upon amount of tumor resection, local invasion, and regional lymph node involvement. Stage 4 disease is defined as distant nodal or hematogenous spread of disease. A unique pattern of dissemination limited to liver, skin, and minimal bone marrow involvement has been described in infants (stage 4s), which has a potential for spontaneous regression in marked contrast to the disseminated aggressive disease seen in the majority of patients greater than 18 months of age.[34]

TUMOR BIOLOGY AND PROGNOSIS

Numerous clinical and biologic factors have been shown to predict clinical behavior of neuroblastoma. There is international agreement that a combination of clinical and biologic factors best predicts clinical prognosis. The Children's Oncology Group stratifies patients into low-, intermediate-, or high-risk categories based upon age at diagnosis, INSS stage, tumor histopathology, DNA index (ploidy), and *MYCN* amplification status (**Table 3**), with each group displaying a unique risk for recurrence (**Fig. 3**). Similar strategies are used internationally; however, several factors outlined below suggest a potential for continued evolution of any classification algorithm.

Table 2	
International Neuroblastoma Staging System	
Stage 1	Localized tumor with complete gross excision with or without microscopic residual disease; representative ipsilateral lymph nodes negative for tumor microscopically (nodes attached to and removed with the primary tumor may be positive)
Stage 2A	Localized tumor with incomplete gross resection; representative ipsilateral nonadherent lymph nodes negative for tumor microscopically
Stage 2B	Localized tumor with or without complete gross excision with ipsilateral nonadherent lymph nodes positive for tumor; enlarged contralateral lymph nodes must be negative microscopically
Stage 3	Unresectable unilateral tumor infiltrating across the midline[a] with or without regional lymph node involvement, localized unilateral tumor with contralateral regional lymph node involvement, or midline tumor with bilateral extension by infiltration (unresectable) or by lymph node involvement[b]
Stage 4	Any primary tumor with dissemination to distant lymph nodes, bone, bone marrow, liver, skin, or other organs (except as defined for stage 4S)
Stage 4S	Localized primary tumor (as defined for stage 1, 2A, or 2B) with dissemination limited to skin, liver, or bone marrow[c] (limited to infants <1 yr of age)

Multifocal primary tumors (eg, bilateral adrenal primary tumors) should be staged according to the greatest extent of disease, as defined in the table, and followed by a subscript "M" (eg, 3_M).

[a] The midline is defined as the vertebral column. Tumors originating on one side and crossing the midline must infiltrate to or beyond the opposite side of the vertebral column.

[b] Proven malignant effusion within the thoracic cavity if it is bilateral or the abdominal cavity upstages the patient to INSS stage 3.

[c] Marrow involvement in stage 4S should be minimal (ie, <10% of total nucleated cells identified as malignant on bone marrow biopsy or marrow aspirate). More extensive marrow involvement would be considered to be stage 4. The metaiodobenzylguanidine scan (if performed) should be negative in the marrow.

Data from Brodeur GM, Pritchard J, Berthold F, et al. Revisions of the international criteria for neuroblastoma diagnosis, staging, and response to treatment. J Clin Oncol 1933;11(8):1466–77.

Stage and Age

Although the prognostic value of classifying patients according to the INSS has been confirmed,[38,39] an inherent bias toward complete resection exists. Variation in the surgical approach for resection of locoregional disease has the potential to dramatically alter INSS staging. Such variation has led to considerations of alternative staging approaches. In 1995, the European International Society of Pediatric Oncology Neuroblastoma group demonstrated that radiographic characteristics of the tumor, termed surgical risk factors, were useful in predicting the ability to resect the primary tumor and the risk of developing postoperative complications.[40] This led to proposing an International Risk Group imaging classification system that would use surgical risk factors to more uniformly define extent of disease/staging.[41a,b] The prognostic significance of the International Risk Group classification system will be prospectively validated in ongoing trials within the United States and Europe and, if validated, may replace the current INSS staging.

Age is an important clinical prognostic factor. Patients older than 1 to 2 years have a worse prognosis than those who are younger,[42,43] especially for patients who have disseminated disease at diagnosis. Until recently, an age of 365 days has been used as a surrogate for tumor behavior, although alternative ages have been explored. A review of over 3000 neuroblastoma cases confirmed age as a continuous prognostic

Table 3
Children's Oncology Group neuroblastoma risk stratification

Risk Group	Stage	Age	*MYCN* Amplification Status	Ploidy	Shimada
Low risk	1	Any	Any	Any	Any
Low risk	2a/2b	Any	Not amplified	Any	Any
High risk	2a/2b	Any	Amplified	Any	Any
Intermediate risk	3	<547 d	Not amplified	Any	any
Intermediate risk	3	≥547 d	Not amplified	Any	FH
High risk	3	Any	Amplified	Any	Any
High risk	3	≥547 d	Not amplified	Any	UH
High risk	4	<365 d	Amplified	Any	Any
Intermediate risk	4	<365 d	Not amp	Any	Any
High risk	4	365 to <547 d	Amplified	Any	Any
High Risk	4	365 to <547 d	Any	DI = 1	Any
High risk	4	365 to <547 d	Any	Any	UH
Intermediate risk	4	365 to <547 d	Not amplified	DI > 1	FH
High risk	4	≥547 d	Any	Any	Any
Low risk	4s	<365 d	Not amplified	DI > 1	FH
Intermediate risk	4s	<365 d	Not amplified	DI = 1	Any
Intermediate risk	4s	<365 d	Not amplified	Any	UH
High risk	4s	<365 d	Amplified	Any	Any

Abbreviations: DI, DNA index; FH, favorable histology; UH, unfavorable histology.
Courtesy of Children's Oncology Group.

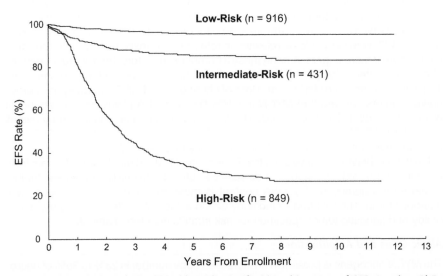

Fig. 3. Analysis of event free survival by risk stratification. (*Courtesy of* W.B. London, PhD, Children's Oncology Group Statistical Office.)

variable and identified 460 days as the most prognostic age cutoff.[44] Recent reviews demonstrated that patients up to 18 months of age who are diagnosed with biologically favorable INSS stage 3 and 4 neuroblastoma share the same excellent prognosis with those less than 1 year of age[45–47] and suggests that 18 months may be a more clinically relevant predictor of outcome. These outcomes were achieved with dose-intensive chemotherapy regimens, including myeloablative consolidation therapy as compared with the moderately dosed chemotherapy received by the more biologically favorable patient cohorts. The ability to treat children ages 12 to 18 months of age who have metastatic disease or locoregional disease using less aggressive therapy is under investigation.

Pathology

The pathologic characteristics of neuroblastoma have been used to further classify these tumors as outlined previously. Shimada initially proposed a histology-based classification of tumors into "favorable" and "unfavorable" by combining age with extent of tumor differentiation, presence of a Schwannian stromal components, and degree of mitosis and karyorrhexis.[30] The prognostic impacts of the original Shimada classification and the more recently revised INPC have been validated.[30,48] The inclusion of age, which is a strong independent prognostic variable, has led to consideration for examining cellular proliferation and extent of differentiation as independent variables in future multifactorial clinical and biological classification schemas.

Genetic Factors

Neuroblastoma can be divided into those with a near-diploid nuclear DNA content ($\approx 45\%$) and near-triploid tumors ($\approx 55\%$). Near-triploid neuroblastomas are characterized by whole chromosome gains and losses without structural genetic aberrations. Clinically, near-triploid tumors are more often localized and show a favorable outcome. Near-diploid neuroblastomas are characterized by the presence of genetic aberrations, such as *MYCN* amplification, 17q gain, and chromosomal losses (reviewed in references[12,49]). For many genetic, molecular, and clinical factors, a prognostic value has been reported. Recently, a systematic review of prognostic tumor markers in neuroblastoma has been published.[50] Riley and coworkers identified 3415 papers with a sensitive literature search for prognostic factors in neuroblastoma, of which 428 were judged to be relevant. In total, 31 prognostic factors were reported, each in five or more papers. Among these 31 prognostic factors, there were six genetic aberrations listed (ploidy, *MYCN* amplification, chromosome 1 p loss, chromosome 17q gain, chromosome 14q loss, and loss of chromosome 11q). Meta-analysis of prognostic markers showed that *MYCN* amplification and DNA ploidy had the strongest prognostic impact. The pooled hazard ratio for a bad outcome (measured by overall survival) for *MYCN* amplification was 5.48 (95% confidence interval, 4.30–6.97) and for DNA near-diploidy was 3.23 (95% confidence interval, 2.08–5.00).

Most neuroblastomas have a nuclear DNA content in the diploid range. Tumors from patients who have lower stages of disease can often be hyperdiploid or near-triploid (reviewed in references[12,49]). DNA content is most prognostic in infants who have neuroblastoma. The Children's Oncology Group is the only collaborative group using ploidy of diagnostic tumor specimen for risk stratification (see **Table 3**).

Allelic Gains and Amplifications

The *MYCN* oncogene is present in an increased copy number in 25% to 35% of neuroblastomas. *MYCN* amplification is found in 30% to 40% of stage 3 and 4 neuroblastomas and in only 5% of localized or stage 4s neuroblastomas. *MYCN*-amplified neuroblastomas are characterized by a highly aggressive behavior with unfavorable outcome (reviewed in[12,49]). Some discussion remains on the prognostic value of *MYCN* amplification in the rare cases of completely resected localized neuroblastoma. The unfavorable prognostic value also holds in the prognostically favorable group of infants who have stage 4s neuroblastoma. In *MYCN*-amplified neuroblastomas, loss of chromosome 1 p is almost invariably present.[49,51]

Allelic Gains

Gain of the entire chromosome 17 or gain of parts of chromosome 17q occur in greater than 60% of neuroblastomas. The partial 17q gain most often results from unbalanced translocation of 17q21–25 to another chromosome (eg, chromosome 1). Partial gain of 17q identifies unfavorable neuroblastoma.[52] Obvious candidate genes on 17q are the NM23 and the BIRC5 (survivin) gene.

Tumor Suppressor Genes

Loss of tumor suppressor regions is reported in neuroblastomas for many chromosomal regions. The most frequently affected regions are chromosome 1 p (30–40%), 4 p (20%), 1lq (25%), and 14q (25%).

Chromosome 1 p loss occurs more frequently in older children who have stage 3 and 4 neuroblastoma and is correlated with increased serum ferritin and serum lactate dehydrogenase. In almost all samples with *MYCN* amplification, concomitant 1 p loss is demonstrated, but loss of chromosome 1 p also occurs in *MYCN* single-copy cases.[53] Several studies have shown that 1 p loss is a strong predictor of outcome.[12,49,53] In the meta-analysis of Riley and colleagues,[50] *MYCN* amplification and ploidy were stronger predictors of outcome, indicating that 1 p loss might best be used to identify high-risk patients in *MYCN* single-copy tumors.

Chromosome 11q loss is demonstrated in approximately 40% of patients (reviewed in[12,49]). Chromosome 11q loss is inversely correlated with *MYCN* amplification and therefore identifies an additional high-risk subset of patients characterized by advanced stage, older age, and unfavorable pathology. It has recently become clear that "unbalanced" deletion of 11q (deletion of long-arm material with retention or gain of short-arm material) occurs in 15% to 20% of cases but is more clearly associated with high-risk biologic features.[54] Prospective evaluation of 1 p and 11q status is ongoing in several cooperative group trials and is especially aimed at risk stratification of intermediate-risk patients.

Molecular Factors

Despite extensive data correlating genomic alterations with disease outcome, no bona fide target genes have been identified for neuroblastoma, with the exception of *MYCN*.[55] A number of biological pathways regulating cancer seem to be disrupted or affected in neuroblastoma, including tumor differentiation, apoptosis, drug resistance, angiogenesis, and metastasis. Insight into the molecular regulation of these biological pathways will lead to the identification of novel drug targets.

Because neurotrophin signaling has a central role in normal neuronal development and may be involved in differentiation and regression of neuroblastoma there has been interest in alterations of these pathways. The clinical and biological roles of Trk receptors (*NTRK1*, *NTRK2*, and *NTRK3* encoding TrkA, TrkB, and TrkC, respectively) and their ligands (NGF, BDNF, and NT-3, respectively) have been extensively investigated. Trk-receptors have been identified as important prognostic factors in neuroblastoma.[56,57] High expression of TrkA is present in neuroblastomas, with favorable biological features and correlates with good outome.[58–61] By contrast, full-length TrkB is highly expressed in biologically unfavorable, *MYCN*-amplified, aggressive neuro-blastomas.[56,62] In neuroblastoma cell culture models, the biological effects of TrkA include neuronal differentiation or apoptosis, depending on the presence or absence of NGF and on inhibition of proliferation and angiogenesis.[63,64] TrkA signaling might also be related to Phox2B- or Delta-Notch–regulated differentiation programs. Depending on the microenvironment, NGF/TrkA signaling could provoke differentiation or regression in favorable neuroblastomas.[14,65] This would partly explain spontaneous regression as a delayed activation of developmentally programmed cell death resulting from the absence of NGF in the microenvironment.

Activation of TrkB by its ligand BDNF results in enhanced proliferation, migration, angiogenesis, and chemotherapy resistance of neuroblastoma cells.[66] Differential splicing of Trk receptors results in the expression of truncated receptors lacking the kinase domain,[67] which may function as dominant negative inhibitors or scavenger receptors sequestering the ligand.[68–70] Truncated TrkB seems to be preferentially expressed in more differentiated tumors.[62,71] Recently, a novel NGF-unresponsive TrkA splice variant has been identified, which is predominantly expressed in clinically aggressive neuroblastomas. This splice variant promotes cell survival, xenograft tumor growth, and angiogenesis.[72] Thus, the neurotrophins and their receptors govern numerous cellular functions in neuroblastoma, and the complexity of the signaling responses is reflected in the multiplicity of the pathways involved. More detailed insights into the mechanisms regulating differentiation might suggest new options for treatment.

Delayed activation or disruption of normal apoptotic pathways may be an important phenomenon involved in spontaneous regression and therapy resistance of neuro-blastoma. Major elements of the apoptotic signaling cascade with abnormal expression or activation patterns include the BCL2 family, survivin, and caspase-8.[73–76] The latter is mainly affected by inactivation due to epigenetic silencing. CpG-island hypermethylation of gene promoters is a frequent mechanism for functional inactivation of genes. In neuroblastoma, this mode of inactivation has been demonstrated not only for caspase-8 but also for the four TRAIL apoptosis receptors, the caspase-8 inhibitor FLIP, the RASSF1A tumor suppressor, p73, RB1, DAPK, CD44, p14ARF, and p16INK4a.[74,77] Because many of these genes are involved in apoptotic signaling and therapy responsiveness, gene hypermethylation might be a major event leading to resistance. Therefore, the antitumor effects of demethylating agents, including decitabine, are being investigated in preclinical studies.

Acquired resistance to chemotherapeutic agents may be conferred by enhanced drug efflux due to overexpression of classical multidrug resistance proteins, including multidrug resistance gene 1 and the gene for multidrug resistance-related protein. Their potential clinical significance in neuroblastoma has been addressed in several studies,[78–81] but their interaction with each other and the role of unknown cofactors remains to be elucidated. Several additional factors have been shown to contribute to treatment resistance in neuroblastoma, including expression of oncogenes such as MYCN, TrkB/BDNF signaling, or loss of p53 expression.[66,82,83]

Enhanced tumor angiogenesis and high expression of proangiogenic factors such as vascular endothelial growth factor and basic fibroblast growth factor are correlated with an aggressive phenotype in neuroblastoma,[64,84] making angiogenesis inhibitors an attractive treatment option that is being evaluated in preclinical studies. Despite the fact that approximately 50% of patients present with disseminated disease at the time of diagnosis, little is known about the biology of invasion and metastases in neuroblastoma. Major molecular players in the regulation of local invasiveness and metastases are metalloproteinases (mainly MMP9), activating matrix-degrading proteolytic enzymes, and molecules regulating tumor cell adhesion and migration, such as CD44 and NM23-H1.[85–88]

TREATMENT OVERVIEW

It is imperative that a multidisciplinary approach to diagnosis and therapy be undertaken for all patients. Tumor tissue obtained through surgical tumor biopsy is almost uniformly required to assess tumor genetic and histologic features. The improved understanding of neuroblastoma biology and its impact on prognosis has resulted in successful tailoring of therapy. The requirement for further surgical resection, chemotherapy, or radiotherapy is based upon a patient's risk stratification with general principles of therapy outlined below. When possible, exposure to chemotherapy is limited to patients who have regional or advanced-stage disease, whereas radiotherapy is limited to patients who have advanced disease and unfavorable biologic characteristics.

LOW-RISK NEUROBLASTOMA

Survival rates for patients who have INSS stage 1 disease, regardless of biologic factors, are excellent with surgery alone. Chemotherapy, when necessary, has been an effective salvage therapy for patients who have INSS stage 1 disease who relapse after surgery only.[89,90] Chemotherapy can be omitted for the majority of patients who have biologically favorable but incompletely resected localized tumors (INSS stage 2A and 2B), with a survival rate greater than 95%.[90–93] For patients who have INSS stage 1, 2A, or 2B disease, chemotherapy should be reserved for those who have localized neuroblastoma and experience life- or organ-threatening symptoms at diagnosis or for the minority of patients who experience recurrent or progressive disease.

Stage 4S neuroblastoma without *MYCN* amplification undergoes spontaneous regression in the majority of cases.[34,94] Chemotherapy or low-dose radiotherapy is reserved for patients who have large tumors or massive hepatomegaly causing mechanical obstruction, respiratory insufficiency, or liver dysfunction.[95,96]

INTERMEDIATE-RISK NEUROBLASTOMA

The intermediate-risk classification group encompasses a wide spectrum of disease. Surgical resection and moderate–dose, multiagent chemotherapy are the backbone of therapy. The prognosis for patients who have INSS stage 3 disease or infants who have INSS stage 4 disease is highly dependent upon the tumor's histologic and biologic features. Survival after surgical resection and moderate-dose chemotherapy, including cisplatin, doxorubicin, etoposide, and cyclophosphamide, is greater than 95% for children whose tumors exhibit favorable characteristics.[97,98] To reduce acute and long-term toxicity, international groups have successfully reduced the cumulative exposure to chemotherapy and substituted carboplatin for cisplatin while maintaining excellent survival.[99] These promising results have provided the basis for further reduction in therapy for patients who have intermediate-risk disease. Several small series have brought to question whether chemotherapy could be eliminated for patients who have regional disease and favorable biologic characteristics.[100,101] The challenge is to use more recently identified biologic features to identify patients within this heterogeneous intermediate risk group for whom therapy reduction may not be warranted. Prospective clinical trials in the United States and Europe will integrate additional molecular genetic variables (1 p and 11q allelic status) to further refine risk assessment within the intermediate-risk group.

HIGH-RISK NEUROBLASTOMA

High-risk neuroblastoma is largely chemotherapy responsive, but, despite improvements in complete response rates, only 30% to 40% of patients survive long term.[102] Standard therapy for patients who have high-risk neuroblastoma involves at least four components: induction, local control, consolidation, and treatment of minimal disease with biologic agents. The use of these four components has evolved over the last 20 years based upon work by the Pediatric Oncology Group, the Children's Cancer Group (CCG), international cooperative groups, and smaller cohort studies, with results summarized below.

Induction Therapy

There is a direct correlation between achieving complete tumor response after induction therapy and survival.[102] Standard induction chemotherapy consists of a combination of anthracyclines, alkylators, platinum compounds, and topoisomerase II inhibitors. Escalation in chemotherapy dose intensity may improve initial tumor response rates[103]; however, these results have not been reproduced in multicenter trials.[104,105] An alternative induction strategy is to add noncross-resistant cytotoxic agents into this multiagent chemotherapy backbone. The topoisomerase I inhibitor class of agents, including topotecan, has activity in recurrent neuroblastoma[106] and can be safely combined with multiagent induction chemotherapy.[107] The efficacy of this strategy is being studied in a phase III Children's Oncology Group trial for newly diagnosed neuroblastoma.

Local Control

Optimal local control is achieved with a combination of aggressive surgical resection and administration of external-beam radiotherapy to the primary tumor site regardless of response to induction chemotherapy. Resection of the primary tumor and bulky metastatic disease is usually necessary to achieve a chance of cure. Delayed surgical resection after initial induction chemotherapy improves resection of the primary tumor, may improve overall survival, and may minimize acute complications of surgical resection.[108]

Neuroblastoma is one of the most radiosensitive solid tumors of childhood.[109] Radiation doses of 2160 cGy in daily 180 cGy fractions administered to the primary tumor site, regardless of initial response to chemotherapy, seem to decrease the risk for local recurrence.[33,110,111] The presence of residual tumor at the time of radiation therapy affects risk for recurrence. A single-institution study suggests that patients undergoing an incomplete resection may benefit from a higher radiation dose.[112] Prospective studies are ongoing to assess whether higher-dose radiation to the volume of residual tumor improves local control rates.

Myeloablative Consolidation Therapy

Over the past decade, several clinical trials have assessed the efficacy of myeloablative consolidation chemotherapy. The CCG-3891 study demonstrated that myeloablative therapy with purged bone marrow transplant improved outcome for patients who had high-risk neuroblastoma.[102] Trials performed in Germany and Europe similarly demonstrate improved outcome after myeloablative therapy compared with maintenance chemotherapy[113] or observation.[114] Taken together, these data indicate that neuroblastoma is one of the few human cancers in which relapse rates are reduced by myeloablative consolidation in first remission and raise the possibility that further intensification of consolidation therapy may improve outcome. George and colleagues have recently published a 3-year, event-free survival of 55% after a rapid sequential tandem transplant consolidation therapy,[115] forming the basis for an ongoing randomized trial comparing single- versus tandem transplant consolidation for high-risk neuroblastoma.

Biologic Therapy

The CCG-3891 study demonstrated the efficacy of isotretinoin (cis-RA), a synthetic retinoid, in treating minimal residual neuroblastoma and established a standard for the use of noncytotoxic therapy for the treatment of minimal residual disease.[102] Although cis-RA is the standard of care for postremission induction maintenance therapy, monoclonal antibodies directed against neuroblastoma-specific antigens (gangliosidase, GD2) may provide an additional mechanism to kill residual neuroblastoma cells via antibody-dependant cellular cytotoxicity. Preclinical and clinical trials suggest that lymphocyte-, neutrophil-, or natural killer cell–mediated, antibody-dependent cellular cytotoxicity can be enhanced by coadministration of the cytokines granulocyte/macrophage colony-stimulating factor and interleukin-2.[116,117] The addition of anti-GD2 immunotherapy (chimeric 14.18 antibody) combined with cytokines granulocyte macrophage colony stimulating factor (GMCSF) and interleukin-2 (IL2) to standard cisRA significantly decreases risk for recurrence and improves overall survival for high risk neuroblastoma.[118] Clinical trials are underway to further analyze the efficacy of coadministration of soluble cytokines with anti-GD2 (gangliosidase) monoclonal antibodies or the development of fused anti-GD2/cytokine molecules in the setting of minimal residual disease. Alternative retinoid derivatives, including fenretinide, have been tested and show promising response rates in recurrent disease.

FUTURE DIRECTIONS

Neuroblastoma is a heterogenous tumor for which biology dictates clinical behavior. Further advances in our understanding of the molecular biology of neuroblastoma are supported by the use of high-throughput, array-based methods not only with the goal of patient-tailored prognostication but also to identify key targets that can efficiently be exploited therapeutically. We must continue to refine our ability to better identify the rare patients who have apparent low-risk or intermediate-risk disease who are destined to have a poor outcome. For the remaining patients who have low- and intermediate-risk disease, we must minimize the lasting effects of therapy, specifically avoiding organ damage or organ loss from surgery and organ dysfunction or risk for secondary malignancy after chemotherapy. Likewise, it is imperative that we use the mounting knowledge of neuroblastoma tumor biology toward the development of novel therapies for high-risk neuroblastoma. Several rationally chosen biologic agents are in ongoing clinical trials for recurrent neuroblastoma, including histone deacetylase inhibitors, Trk tyrosine kinase inhibitors, and anti-angiogenic agents. If effective, these agents will be moved into front-line therapy and may improve induction response. Alternatively, they may be used to optimize treatment of minimal residual disease.

REFERENCES

1. Stiller CA, Parkin DM. International variations in the incidence of neuroblastoma. Int J Cancer 1992;52(4):538–43.
2. Kushner BH, Gilbert F, Helson L. Familial neuroblastoma: case reports, literature review, and etiologic considerations. Cancer 1986;57(9):1887–93.

3. Belson M, Kingsley B, Holmes A. Risk factors for acute leukemia in children: a review. Environ Health Perspect 2007;115(1):138–45.

4. Connelly JM, Malkin MG. Environmental risk factors for brain tumors. Curr Neurol Neurosci Rep May 2007;7(3):208–14.

5. Yamamoto K, Hayashi Y, Hanada R, et al. Mass screening and age-specific incidence of neuroblastoma in Saitama Prefecture, Japan. J Clin Oncol 1995;13(8): 2033–8.

6. Kaneko Y, Kanda N, Maseki N, et al. Current urinary mass screening for catecholamine metabolites at 6 months of age may be detecting only a small portion of high-risk neuroblastomas: a chromosome and N-myc amplification study. J Clin Oncol 1990;8(12):2005–13.

7. Schilling FH, Spix C, Berthold F, et al. Neuroblastoma screening at one year of age. N Engl J Med 2002;346(14):1047–53.

8. Woods WG, Gao RN, Shuster JJ, et al. Screening of infants and mortality due to neuroblastoma. N Engl J Med 2002;346(14):1041–6.

9. Clausen N, Andersson P, Tommerup N. Familial occurrence of neuroblastoma, von Recklinghausen's neurofibromatosis, Hirschsprung's agangliosis and jaw-winking syndrome. Acta Paediatr Scand 1989;78(5):736–41.

10. Rohrer T, Trachsel D, Engelcke G, et al. Congenital central hypoventilation syndrome associated with Hirschsprung's disease and neuroblastoma: case of multiple neurocristopathies. Pediatr Pulmonol 2002;33(1):71–6.

11. Trochet D, O'Brien LM, Gozal D, et al. PHOX2B genotype allows for prediction of tumor risk in congenital central hypoventilation syndrome. Am J Hum Genet 2005;76(3):421–6.

12. Brodeur GM. Neuroblastoma: biological insights into a clinical enigma. Nat Rev Cancer 2003;3(3):203–16.

13. Trochet D, Bourdeaut F, Janoueix-Lerosey I, et al. Germline mutations of the paired-like homeobox 2B (PHOX2B) gene in neuroblastoma. Am J Hum Genet 2004;74(4):761–4.

14. van Limpt V, Schramm A, van Lakeman A, et al. The Phox2B homeobox gene is mutated in sporadic neuroblastomas. Oncogene 2004;23(57):9280–8.

15. Longo L, Panza E, Schena F, et al. Genetic predisposition to familial neuroblastoma: identification of two novel genomic regions at 2p and 12p. Hum Hered 2007;63(3–4):205–11.

16. Chen Y, Takita J, Choi YL, et al. Oncogenic mutations of ALK kinase in neuroblastoma. Nature 2008;455:971–4.

17. George RE, Sanda T, Hanna M, et al. Activating mutations in ALK provide a therapeutic target in neuroblastoma. Nature 2008;455:975–8.

18a. Janoueix-Lerosey I, Lequin D, Brugières L, et al. Somatic and germline activating mutations of the ALK kinase receptor in neuroblastoma. Nature 2008; 455:967–70.

18b. Mossé YP, Laudenslager M, Longo L, et al. Identification of ALK as a major familial neuroblastoma predisposition gene. Nature 2008;455:930–5.

19. Triche TJ. Neuroblastoma: biology confronts nosology. Arch Pathol Lab Med 1986;110(11):994–6.

20. Mosse YP, Laudenslager M, Khazi D, et al. Germline PHOX2B mutation in hereditary neuroblastoma. Am J Hum Genet 2004;75(4):727–30.

21. O'Brien CA, Pollett A, Gallinger S, et al. A human colon cancer cell capable of initiating tumour growth in immunodeficient mice. Nature 2007;445(7123):106–10.

22. Singh SK, Hawkins C, Clarke ID, et al. Identification of human brain tumour initiating cells. Nature 2004;432(7015):396–401.

23. Tirode F, Laud-Duval K, Prieur A, et al. Mesenchymal stem cell features of Ewing tumors. Cancer Cell 2007;11(5):421–9.

24. Allenspach EJ, Maillard I, Aster JC, et al. Notch signaling in cancer. Cancer Biol Ther 2002;1(5):466–76.

25. Blanc E, Goldschneider D, Douc-Rasy S, et al. Wnt-5a gene expression in malignant human neuroblasts. Cancer Letters 2005;228(1–2):117–23.

26. Taipale J, Beachy PA. The Hedgehog and Wnt signalling pathways in cancer. Nature 2001;411(6835):349–54.

27. Russell D, Rubinstein L. Pathology of tumours of the nervous system. London: Edward Arnold; 1989.

28. Beckwith J, Perrin E. In situ neuroblastomas: a contribution to the natural history of neural crest tumors. Am J Pathol 1963;43:1089–104.

29. Shimada H, Ambros IM, Dehner LP, et al. The International Neuroblastoma Pathology Classification (the Shimada system). Cancer 1999;86(2):364–72.

30. Shimada H, Chatten J, Newton W Jr, et al. Histophatologic prognostic factors in neuroblastic tumors: definition of subtypes of ganglineuroblastoma and an age-linked classification of neuroblastomas. J Natl Cancer Inst 1984;73:405–16.

31. Peuchmaur M, d'Amore ES, Joshi VV, et al. Revision of the international neuro-blastoma pathology classification: confirmation of favorable and unfavorable prognostic subsets in ganglioneuroblastoma, nodular. Cancer 2003;98(10): 2274–81.

32. de Bernardi B, Rogers D, Carli M, et al. Localized neuroblastoma: surgical and pathologic staging. Cancer 1987;60(5):1066–72.

33. Haas-Kogan DA, Swift PS, Selch M, et al. Impact of radiotherapy for high-risk neuroblastoma: a Children's Cancer Group study. Int J Radiat Oncol Biol Phys 2003;56(1):28–39.

34. Evans AE, Chatten J, D'Angio GJ, et al. A review of 17 IV-S neuroblastoma patients at the Children's Hospital of Philadelphia. Cancer 1980;45(5):833–9.

35. Brodeur GM, Pritchard J, Berthold F, et al. Revisions of the international criteria for neuroblastoma diagnosis, staging, and response to treatment. J Clin Oncol 1993;11(8):1466–77.

36. Brodeur GM, Seeger RC, Barrett A, et al. International criteria for diagnosis, staging, and response to treatment in patients with neuroblastoma. J Clin Oncol 1988;6(12):1874–81.

37. Messina JA, Cheng SC, Franc BL, et al. Evaluation of semi-quantitative scoring system for metaiodobenzylguanidine (mIBG) scans in patients with relapsed neuroblastoma. Pediatr Blood Cancer 2006;47(7):865–74.

38. Castleberry RP, Shuster JJ, Smith EI. The pediatric oncology group experience with the international staging system criteria for neuroblastoma. Member Institu-tions of the Pediatric Oncology Group. J Clin Oncol 1994;12(11):2378–81.

39. Haase GM, Atkinson JB, Stram DO, et al. Surgical management and outcome of locoregional neuroblastoma: comparison of the Childrens Cancer Group and the international staging systems. J Pediatr Surg 1995;30(2):289–94 [discus-sion: 295].

40. Cecchetto G, Mosseri V, De Bernardi B, et al. Surgical risk factors in primary surgery for localized neuroblastoma: the LNESG1 study of the European Inter-national Society of Pediatric Oncology Neuroblastoma Group. J Clin Oncol 2005;23(33):8483–9.

41a. Cohn SL, Pearson AD, London WB, et al. The international Neuroblastoma Risk Group (INRG) classification system: an INRG Task Force report. J Clin Oncol 2009;27:289–97.

41b. Monclair T, Brodeur GM, Ambros PF, et al. The International Neuroblastoma Risk Group (INRG) staging system: an INRG Task Force Report. J Clin Oncol 2009; 27:298–303.

42. Breslow N, McCann B. Statistical estimation of prognosis for children with neuroblastoma. Cancer Res 1971;31(12):2098–103.

43. Evans AE. Staging and treatment of neuroblastoma. Cancer 1980;45(Suppl 7): 1799–802.

44. London WB, Castleberry RP, Matthay KK, et al. Evidence for an age cutoff greater than 365 days for neuroblastoma risk group stratification in the Children's Oncology Group. J Clin Oncol 2005;23(27):6459–65.

45. George RE, London WB, Cohn SL, et al. Hyperdiploidy plus nonamplified MYCN confers a favorable prognosis in children 12 to 18 months old with disseminated neuroblastoma: a Pediatric Oncology Group study. J Clin Oncol 2005;23(27): 6466–73.

46. Schmidt ML, Lal A, Seeger RC, et al. Favorable prognosis for patients 12 to 18 months of age with stage 4 nonamplified MYCN neuroblastoma: a Children's Cancer Group Study. J Clin Oncol 2005;23(27):6474–80.

47. Park J, Villablanca J, Seeger R, et al. Favorable outcome of high risk (HR) stage 3 neuroblastoma (NB) with myeloablative therapy and 13-cis-retinoic acid. Presented at the 41st Annual Meeting of American Society of Oncology. Orlando, Florida, May 13–17, 2005.

48. Shimada H, Stram DO, Chatten J, et al. Identification of subsets of neuroblastomas by combined histopathologic and N-myc analysis. J Natl Cancer Inst 1995;87(19):1470–6.

49. Maris JM. The biologic basis for neuroblastoma heterogeneity and risk stratification. Curr Opin Pediatr 2005;17(1):7–13.

50. Riley RD, Heney D, Jones DR, et al. A systematic review of molecular and biological tumor markers in neuroblastoma. Clin Cancer Res 2004;10(1 Pt 1): 4–12.

51. Westermann F, Schwab M. Genetic parameters of neuroblastomas. Cancer Lett 2002;184(2):127–47.

52. Bown N, Cotterill S, Lastowska M, et al. Gain of chromosome arm 17q and adverse outcome in patients with neuroblastoma. N Engl J Med 1999;340(25):1954–61.

53. Caron H, van Sluis P, de Kraker J, et al. Allelic loss of chromosome 1p as a predictor of unfavorable outcome in patients with neuroblastoma. N Engl J Med 1996;334(4):225–30.

54. Attiyeh EF, London WB, Mosse YP, et al. Chromosome 1p and 11q deletions and outcome in neuroblastoma. N Engl J Med 2005;353(21):2243–53.

55. Maris JM, Hogarty MD, Bagatell R, et al. Neuroblastoma. Lancet 2007; 369(9579):2106–20.

56. Nakagawara A, Azar CG, Scavarda NJ, et al. Expression and function of Trk-B and BDNF in human neuroblastomas. Mol Cell Biol 1994;14:759–67.

57. Nakagawara A, Arima-Nakagawara M, Scavarda NJ, et al. Association between high levels of expression of the Trk gene and favorable outcome in human neuroblastomas. N Engl J Med 1993;328:847–54.

58. Combaret V, Gross N, Lasset C, et al. Clinical relevance of CD44 cell surface expression and MYCN gene amplification in neuroblastoma. Eur J Cancer 1997;33(12):2101–5.

59. Borrello MG, Bongarzone I, Pierotti MA, et al. TRK and RET protooncogene expression in human neuroblastoma specimens: high frequency of Trk expression in non-advanced stages. Int J Cancer 1993;54:540–5.

60. Kogner P, Barbany G, Dominici C, et al. Coexpression of messenger RNA for Trk protooncogene and low affinity nerve growth factor receptor in neuroblastomas with favorable prognosis. Cancer Res 1993;53:2044–50.
61. Suzuki T, Bogenmann E, Shimada H, et al. Lack of high affinity nerve growth factor receptors in aggressive neuroblastomas. J Natl Cancer Inst 1993;85: 377–84.
62. Aoyama M, Asai K, Shishikura T, et al. Human neuroblastomas with unfavorable biologies express high levels of brain-derived neurotrophic factor mRNA and a variety of its variants. Cancer Lett 2001;164(1):51–60.
63. Eggert A, Grotzer MA, Ikegaki N, et al. Expression of the neurotrophin receptor TrkA down-regulates expression and function of angiogenic stimulators in SH-SY5Y neuroblastoma cells. Cancer Res 2002;62(6):1802–8.
64. Eggert A, Ikegaki N, Kwiatkowski J, et al. High-level expression of angiogenic factors is associated with advanced tumor stage in human neuroblastomas. Clin Cancer Res 2000;6:1900–8.
65. van Limpt V, Chan A, Schramm A, et al. Phox2B mutations and the Delta-Notch pathway in neuroblastoma. Cancer Lett 2005;228(1–2):59–63.
66. Ho R, Eggert A, Hishiki T, et al. Resistance to chemotherapy mediated by TrkB in neuroblastomas. Cancer Res 2002;62(22):6462–6.
67. Barbacid M. The trk family of neurotrophin receptors. J Neurobiol 1994;25: 1386–403.
68. Biffo S, Offenhauser N, Carter BD, et al. Selective binding and internalisation by truncated receptors restrict the availability of BDNF during development. Development 1995;121(8):2461–70.
69. Eide FF, Vining ER, Eide BL, et al. Naturally occurring truncated trkB receptors have dominant inhibitory effects on brain-derived neurotrophic factor signaling. J Neurosci 1996;16(10):3123–9.
70. Haapasalo A, Koponen E, Hoppe E, et al. Truncated trkB.T1 is dominant negative inhibitor of trkB.TK+-mediated cell survival. Biochem Biophys Res Commun 2001;280(5):1352–8.
71. Brodeur GM, Nakagawara A, Yamashiro D, et al. Expression of TrkA, TrkB and TrkC in human neuroblastomas. J Neurooncol 1997;31:49–55.
72. Tacconelli A, Farina AR, Cappabianca L, et al. TrkA alternative splicing: a regulated tumor-promoting switch in human neuroblastoma. Cancer Cell 2004;6(4): 347–60.
73. Castle VP, Heidelberger KP, Bromberg J, et al. Expression of the apoptosis-suppressing protein bcl-2, in neuroblastoma is associated with unfavorable histology and N-myc amplification. Am J Pathol 1993;143(6):1543–50.
74. Eggert A, Grotzer MA, Zuzak TJ, et al. Resistance to tumor necrosis factor-related apoptosis-inducing ligand (TRAIL)-induced apoptosis in neuroblastoma cells correlates with a loss of caspase-8 expression. Cancer Res 2001;61(4): 1314–9.
75. Hopkins-Donaldson S, Bodmer JL, Bourloud KB, et al. Loss of caspase-8 expression in highly malignant human neuroblastoma cells correlates with resistance to tumor necrosis factor-related apoptosis-inducing ligand-induced apoptosis. Cancer Res 2000;60(16):4315–9.
76. Teitz T, Wei T, Valentine MB, et al. Caspase 8 is deleted or silenced preferentially in childhood neuroblastomas with amplification of MYCN. Nat Med 2000;6(5): 529–35.
77. van Noesel MM, van Bezouw S, Salomons GS, et al. Tumor-specific down-regulation of the tumor necrosis factor-related apoptosis-inducing ligand decoy

receptors DcR1 and DcR2 is associated with dense promoter hypermethylation. Cancer Res 2002;62(7):2157–61.

78. Chan HS, Haddad G, Thorner PS, et al. P-glycoprotein expression as a predictor of the outcome of therapy for neuroblastoma. N Engl J Med 1991;325(23): 1608–14.

79. Goldstein LJ, Fojo AT, Ueda K, et al. Expression of the multidrug resistance, MDR1, gene in neuroblastomas. J Clin Oncol 1990;8(1):128–36.

80. Haber M, Smith J, Bordow SB, et al. Association of high-level MRP1 expression with poor clinical outcome in a large prospective study of primary neuroblastoma. J Clin Oncol 2006;24(10):1546–53.

81. Norris MD, Bordow SB, Marshall GM, et al. Expression of the gene for multidrug-resistance-associated protein and outcome in patients with neuroblastoma. N Engl J Med 1996;334(4):231–8.

82. Jaboin J, Kim CJ, Kaplan DR, et al. Brain-derived neurotrophic factor activation of TrkB protects neuroblastoma cells from chemotherapy-induced apoptosis via phosphatidylinositol 3'-kinase pathway. Cancer Res 2002;62(22):6756–63.

83. Scala S, Wosikowski K, Giannakakou P, et al. Brain-derived neurotrophic factor protects neuroblastoma cells from vinblastine toxicity. Cancer Res 1996;56: 3737–42.

84. Meitar D, Crawford SE, Rademaker AW, et al. Tumor angiogenesis correlates with metastatic disease, N-myc amplification, and poor outcome in human neuroblastoma. J Clin Oncol 1996;14:405–14.

85. Almgren MA, Henriksson KC, Fujimoto J, et al. Nucleoside diphosphate kinase A/nm23-H1 promotes metastasis of NB69-derived human neuroblastoma. Mol Cancer Res 2004;2(7):387–94.

86. Chantrain CF, Shimada H, Jodele S, et al. Stromal matrix metalloproteinase-9 regulates the vascular architecture in neuroblastoma by promoting pericyte recruitment. Cancer Res 2004;64(5):1675–86.

87. Gross N, Balmas Bourloud K, Brognara CB. MYCN-related suppression of functional CD44 expression enhances tumorigenic properties of human neuroblastoma cells. Exp Cell Res 2000;260(2):396–403.

88. Jodele S, Chantrain CF, Blavier L, et al. The contribution of bone marrow-derived cells to the tumor vasculature in neuroblastoma is matrix metalloproteinase-9 dependent. Cancer Res 2005;65(8):3200–8.

89. Alvarado CS, London WB, Look AT, et al. Natural history and biology of stage A neuroblastoma: a Pediatric Oncology Group Study. J Pediatr Hematol Oncol 2000;22(3):197–205.

90. Perez CA, Matthay KK, Atkinson JB, et al. Biologic variables in the outcome of stages I and II neuroblastoma treated with surgery as primary therapy: a children's cancer group study. J Clin Oncol 2000;18(1):18–26.

91. Simon T, Spitz R, Faldum A, et al. New definition of low-risk neuroblastoma using stage, age, and 1p and MYCN status. J Pediatr Hematol Oncol 2004;26(12):791–6.

92. Simon T, Spitz R, Hero B, et al. Risk estimation in localized unresectable single copy MYCN neuroblastoma by the status of chromosomes 1p and 11q. Cancer Lett 2006;237(2):215–22.

93. Strother DR, London W, Schmidt ML, et al. Surgery alone or followed by chemotherapy for patients with stages 2A and 2B neuroblastoma: results of Children's Oncology Group Study P9641. Presented at the 12th meeting of Advances in Neuroblastoma Research. Los Angeles, May 18–20, 2006.

94. D'Angio GJ, Evans AE, Koop CE. Special pattern of widespread neuroblastoma with a favourable prognosis. Lancet 1971;1(7708):1046–9.

95. Nickerson HJ, Matthay KK, Seeger RC, et al. Favorable biology and outcome of stage IV-S neuroblastoma with supportive care or minimal therapy: a Children's Cancer Group study. J Clin Oncol 2000;18(3):477–86.

96. Katzenstein HM, Bowman LC, Brodeur GM, et al. Prognostic significance of age, MYCN oncogene amplification, tumor cell ploidy, and histology in 110 infants with stage D(S) neuroblastoma: the pediatric oncology group experience–a pediatric oncology group study. J Clin Oncol 1998;16(6):2007–17.

97. Matthay KK, Perez C, Seeger RC, et al. Successful treatment of stage III neuroblastoma based on prospective biologic staging: a Children's Cancer Group study. J Clin Oncol 1998;16(4):1256–64.

98. Schmidt ML, Lukens JN, Seeger RC, et al. Biologic factors determine prognosis in infants with stage IV neuroblastoma: a prospective Children's Cancer Group study. J Clin Oncol Mar 2000;18(6):1260–8.

99. Baker DL, Schmidt ML, Cohn SL, et al. A phase III trial of biologically-based therapy reduction for intermediate risk neuroblastoma. Presented at the 43rd Annual meeting of the American Society of Clinical Oncology. Chicago, June 2–6, 2007.

100. Kushner BH, Cheung NK, LaQuaglia MP, et al. Survival from locally invasive or widespread neuroblastoma without cytotoxic therapy. J Clin Oncol 1996;14(2):373–81.

101. Hero B, Thorsten S, Benz-Bohm G, et al. Is a "wait and see" strategy justified in localised neuroblastoma in infancy? Presented at the 12th meeting of Advances in Neuroblastoma Research. Los Angeles, May 18–20, 2006.

102. Matthay KK, Villablanca JG, Seeger RC, et al. Treatment of high-risk neuroblastoma with intensive chemotherapy, radiotherapy, autologous bone marrow transplantation, and 13-cis-retinoic acid. Children's Cancer Group. N Engl J Med 1999;341(16):1165–73.

103. Kushner BH, LaQuaglia MP, Bonilla MA, et al. Highly effective induction therapy for stage 4 neuroblastoma in children over 1 year of age. J Clin Oncol 1994; 12(12):2607–13.

104. Valteau-Couanet D, Michon J, Boneu A, et al. Results of induction chemotherapy in children older than 1 year with a stage 4 neuroblastoma treated with the NB 97 French Society of Pediatric Oncology (SFOP) protocol. J Clin Oncol 2005; 23(3):532–40.

105. Kreissman SG, Villablanca JG, Diller L, et al. Response and toxicity to a dose-intensive multi-agent chemotherapy induction regimen for high risk neuroblastoma: a Children's Oncology Group study. Presented at the 43rd Annual meeting of the American Society of Clinical Oncology. Chicago, June 2–6, 2007.

106. Frantz CN, London WB, Diller L, et al. Recurrent neuroblastoma: randomized treatment with topotecan + cyclophosphamide (T + C) vs. topotecan alone(T). A POG/CCG Intergroup Study. J Clin Oncol 2004;22(14S):8512.

107. Park JR, Stewart CF, London W, et al. Targeted topotecan during induction therapy of high risk neuroblastoma: a Children's Oncology Group pilot study. Presented at the 42nd annual meeting of the American Society of Clinical Oncology. Atlanta, Georgia, June 2–6, 2006.

108. Adkins ES, Sawin R, Gerbing RB, et al. Efficacy of complete resection for high-risk neuroblastoma: a Children's Cancer Group study. J Pediatr Surg 2004; 39(6):931–6.

109. Brodeur GM, Maris JM. Neuroblastoma. 4th edition. Philadelphia: Lippincott; 2002.

110. Kushner BH, Wolden S, LaQuaglia MP, et al. Hyperfractionated low-dose radiotherapy for high-risk neuroblastoma after intensive chemotherapy and surgery. J Clin Oncol 2001;19(11):2821–8.

111. Bradfield SM, Douglas JG, Hawkins DS, et al. Fractionated low-dose radio-therapy after myeloablative stem cell transplantation for local control in patients with high-risk neuroblastoma. Cancer 2004;100(6):1268–75.

112. Simon T, Bongartz R, Hero B, et al. Intensified external beam radiation therapy improves the outcome of stage 4 neuroblastoma in children >1 year with residual local disease. [abstract: 314]. Advances in Neuroblastoma Research 2006.

113. Berthold F, Boos J, Burdach S, et al. Myeloablative megatherapy with autologous stem-cell rescue versus oral maintenance chemotherapy as consolidation treatment in patients with high-risk neuroblastoma: a randomised controlled trial. Lancet Oncol 2005;6(9):649–58.

114. Pritchard J, Cotterill SJ, Germond SM, et al. High dose melphalan in the treatment of advanced neuroblastoma: results of a randomised trial (ENSG-1) by the European Neuroblastoma Study Group. Pediatr Blood Cancer 2005;44(4):348–57.

115. George RE, Li S, Medeiros-Nancarrow C, et al. High-risk neuroblastoma treated with tandem autologous peripheral-blood stem cell-supported transplantation: long-term survival update. J Clin Oncol 2006;24(18):2891–6.

116. Albertini MR, Gan J, Jaeger P, et al. Systemic interleukin-2 modulates the anti-idiotypic response to chimeric anti-GD2 antibody in patients with melanoma. J Immunother Emphasis Tumor Immunol 1996;19(4):278–95.

117. Hank JA, Surfus J, Gan J, et al. Treatment of neuroblastoma patients with anti-ganglioside GD2 antibody plus interleukin-2 induces antibody-dependent cellular cytotoxicity against neuroblastoma detected in vitro. J Immunother 1994;15(1):29–37.

118. Yu AL, Gilman AL, Ozkaynak MF, et al. A phase III randomized trial of the chimeric anti-GD2 antibody ch14.18 with GM-CSF and IL2 as immunotherapy following does intensive chemotherapy for high-risk neuroblastoma: Children's Oncology Group (COG) study ANBL0032 [abstract]. J Clin Oncol 2009;27: 10067z.

119. Roberts KB. Cerebellar ataxia and "occult neuroblastoma" without opsoclonus. Pediatrics 1975;56(3):464–5.

120. Altman AJ, Baehner RL. Favorable prognosis for survival in children with coincident opso-myoclonus and neuroblastoma. Cancer 1976;37(2):846–52.

121. Matthay KK, Blaes F, Hero B, et al. Opsoclonus myoclonus syndrome in neuroblastoma: a report from a workshop on the dancing eyes syndrome at the advances in neuroblastoma meeting in Genoa, Italy. Cancer Lett 2005; 228(1–2):275–82.

122. Scheibel E, Rechnitzer C, Fahrenkrug J, et al. Vasoactive intestinal polypeptide (VIP) in children with neural crest tumours. Acta Paediatr Scand 1982;71(5): 721–5.

123. El Shafie M, Samuel D, Klippel CH, et al. Intractable diarrhea in children with VIP-secreting ganglioneuroblastomas. J Pediatr Surg 1983;18(1):34–6.

Central Nervous System Tumors

Roger J. Packer, MD[a,b,c,d,]*, Tobey MacDonald, MD[c,d,e],
Gilbert Vezina, MD[c,d,f]

KEYWORDS

• Brain tumors • Medulloblastoma • Pediatric brain tumors

Central nervous system (CNS) tumors comprise 15% to 20% of all malignancies occurring in childhood and adolescence.[1] Despite being relatively common, they only occur in between 2500 to 3500 children in the United States each year and may present in a myriad of ways, often delaying diagnosis. Symptoms and signs depend on the growth rate of the tumor, its location in the central nervous system (CNS), and the age of the child. Childhood brain tumors demonstrate greater histological variation, are more likely to be disseminated at the time of diagnosis, and more frequently are embryonal than those arising in adults.[1]

The etiology for most childhood brain and spinal cord tumors is unknown. Specific syndromes are associated with a higher incidence of tumors.[2] Patients who have neurofibromatosis type 1 (NF-1) have a higher incidence of low-grade gliomas, including visual pathway gliomas and other types of CNS tumors.[3] Children who have tuberous sclerosis are prone to harbor giant-cell astrocytomas,[4] and those who have the Li-Fraumeni syndrome have an increased predisposition to various different tumors including gliomas.[5] Rarer conditions, such as the autosomally dominant inherited nevoid basal cell carcinoma syndrome (Gorlin syndrome) and the

A version of this article was previously published in the *Pediatric Clinics of North America*, 55:1.

[a] Center for Neuroscience and Behavioral Medicine, Children's National Medical Center, 111 Michigan Avenue, Washington, DC 20010, USA

[b] Division of Neurology, Children's National Medical Center, 111 Michigan Avenue, Washington, DC 20010, USA

[c] The Brain Tumor Institute, Children's National Medical Center, 111 Michigan Avenue, Washington, DC 20010, USA

[d] The George Washington University School of Medicine and Health Sciences, Washington, DC, USA

[e] Division of Oncology, Center for Cancer and Blood Disorders, Center for Cancer and Immunology Research, Children's National Medical Center, 111 Michigan Avenue NW, Washington, DC 20010, USA

[f] Department of Radiology, Children's National Medical Center, 111 Michigan Avenue NW, Washington, DC 20010, USA

* Corresponding author. Department of Neurology, Children's National Medical Center, 111 Michigan Avenue, NW, Washington, DC 20010.

E-mail address: rpacker@cnmc.org (R.J. Packer).

Hematol Oncol Clin N Am 24 (2010) 87–108
doi:10.1016/j.hoc.2009.11.012
0889-8588/10/$ – see front matter © 2010 Elsevier Inc. All rights reserved.

recessively inherited Turcot's syndrome (germ line mutation of the adenomatosis polyposis coli gene) are associated with an increased incidence of medulloblastoma.[6,7] Exposure to radiation therapy has been the only environmental factor consistently related to the development of brain tumors.[8]

PRESENTATION

Approximately one-half of all childhood brain tumors arise in the posterior fossa (**Table 1**).[1] The five major tumor types that arise subtentorially may present with focal neurologic deficits, but those filling the fourth ventricle are as likely to come to clinical attention because of obstruction of cerebrospinal fluid with associated hydrocephalus. The classical triad associated with increased intracranial pressure of morning headaches, nausea, and vomiting, may occur, but nonspecific headaches are more frequent. In infants, cerebrospinal fluid obstruction with dilatation of the third ventricle and the resultant tectal pressure causes paresis of upgaze may result in downward deviation of the eyes, the setting sun sign.

The suprasellar and pineal regions are relatively frequent sites for supratentorial childhood brain tumors.[1,9] Tumors in the suprasellar region, primarily craniopharyngiomas, visual pathway gliomas, and germinomas, may present with complex visual findings including unilateral or bilateral decreased visual acuity and hard to characterize visual field loss, as well as hormonal dysfunction. In the pineal region, various different tumor types may occur in the pediatric years, including germinomas, mixed germ cell tumors, pineoblastomas, and lower-grade pineocytomas. Pineal region lesions characteristically cause compression or destruction of the tectal region of the brain stem, and result in Parinaud's syndrome, manifested by paralysis or paresis of upgaze, retraction or convergence nystagmus, pupils that react better to accommodation than light, and lid retraction. Most cortical childhood tumors are gliomas, usually low-grade, but they are anaplastic in approximately 20% of cases. Other tumor types (supratentorial primitive neuroectodermal tumors and ependymomas) may occur. Unlike the situation in adulthood, pediatric low-grade gliomas do not mutate frequently to higher-grade gliomas during childhood. In younger children, large benign supratentorial lesions, such as diffuse infantile gangliogliomas/gliomas and dysembryoplastic neuroepithelial tumors may be misdiagnosed as more aggressive lesions.

DIAGNOSIS

The diagnosis of pediatric brain and spinal cord tumors has been simplified by advances in neuroimaging.[10] Because of the speed and availability of CT, it is often the first imaging technique obtained for children with suspected intracranial pathology and, if properly done, CT will detect 95% or more of brain tumors. Because of the superior image contrast of MRI, however, it is essential in the diagnosis of brain tumors, and its multiplanar capabilities offer far superior tumor localization. Based on clinical and neuroradiographic findings, brain tumors have characteristic presentations, especially those arising in the posterior fossa (**Fig. 1**). Other MRI techniques such as magnetic resonance spectroscopy, which supplements anatomic findings with biochemical data and possibly, in the future, diffusion tensor imaging, especially tractography, may aid in characterizing the type of tumor and its anatomic interrelationships.

For the diagnosis of spinal cord tumors or determination of leptomeningeal dissemination of tumors, spinal MRI has supplanted all other techniques, including myelography or CT studies. In attempts to avoid postoperative artifacts, an MRI of the

Table 1
Posterior-Fossa tumors of childhood

Tumor	Relative Incidence	Presentation	Diagnosis	Prognosis
Medulloblastoma	35% to 40%	2–3 months of headaches, vomiting, truncal ataxia	Heterogeneous or homogeneously enhancing fourth ventricular mass; may be disseminated	65% to 85% survival; dependent on stage/type; poorer (20% to 70%) in infants
Cerebellar astrocytoma	35% to 40%	3–6 months of limb ataxia; secondary headaches, vomiting	Cerebellar hemisphere mass, usually with cystic and solid (mural nodule) components	90% to 100% in totally resected pilocytic type
Brain stem glioma	10% to 15%	1–4 months of double vision, unsteadiness, weakness, and other cranial nerve deficits, facial weakness, swallowing deficits, and other deficits	Diffusely expanded, minimally or partially enhancing mass in 80%; 20% more focal tectal or cervicomedullary lesion	90% + 18-month mortality in diffuse tumors; better in localized
Ependymoma	10% to 15%	2–5 months of unsteadiness, headaches, double vision, and facial asymmetry	Usually enhancing, fourth ventricular mass with cerebellopontine predilection	75% + survival in totally resected lesions
Atypical Teratoid/Rhabdoid	>5 (10% to 15% of infantile malignant tumors)	As in medulloblastoma, but primarily in infants; often associated facial weakness and strabismus	As in medulloblastoma, but often more laterally extended	10% to 20% (or less) survival in infants

Ages 0-14 (n=4,214)   Ages 15-19 (n=1,241)

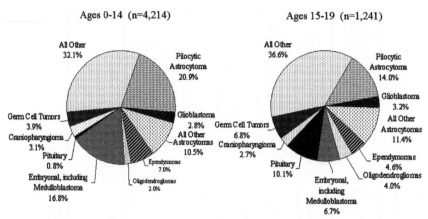

Fig. 1. Distribution of childhood primary brain and other central nervous system tumors by histology from the Central Brain Tumor Registry of the United States (CBTRUS) 1998–2002.

entire neurospinal axis often is undertaken before surgery in patients who have presumed malignant tumors.

In selected cases, positron emission tomography (PET) scanning may provide additional information, but it is usually most useful in supplying baseline diagnostic information, as a means to follow the tumor over time. PET is most helpful in the determination of transformation of a lower-grade tumor (primarily glial) to a higher-grade neoplasm and the separation of post-therapy, especially postradiation, treatment effects from tumor progression.

CLASSIFICATION

Because of the histologic variability of childhood brain and spinal cord tumors, classification is often difficult and, at times, subjective.[11] In most cases, diagnosis continues to be made predominantly upon light microscopy findings. In selective situations, such as in embryonal tumors, especially atypically teratoid/rhabdoid lesions, immunohistochemistry has aided diagnosis greatly. Although the molecular underpinnings of childhood brain tumors increasingly have been unraveled, molecular techniques have not been incorporated extensively into most classification systems. Evaluation of the mitotic activity of the tumor, assessed by mitotic indices, usually does not change classification, but may be helpful, in selected situations, in determining prognosis and approach to therapy.

SPECIFIC TUMOR TYPES

Discussions of the biology of the tumor, its growth pattern, management, and prognosis are discussed best within individual tumor types. For most tumors, the same modalities of treatment are used (ie, surgery, radiation, and in an increasing number of patients chemotherapy), but the use of each of these types of treatment is not only dependent on the type of tumor present, but also on its location in the CNS tumor and the age of the child. Biologic therapies are just being introduced into management, and to date, have been reserved primarily for those patients who fail initial treatment.

Medulloblastoma

Medulloblastoma, which by definition arises in the posterior fossa, is the most common malignant brain tumor of childhood (**Fig. 2**A). Medulloblastomas usually are diagnosed in children less than 15 years of age, and they have a bimodal distribution, peaking at 3 to 4 years of age and then again between 8 and 9 years of age.[12] For unknown reasons, there is a male predominance.[12] Ten percent to 15% of patients are diagnosed in infancy. The classical, or undifferentiated, type of medulloblastoma, comprising 70% or more of medulloblastomas, is composed of densely packed cells with hyperchromatic, round, oval, or carrot-shaped nuclei and minimal cytoplasm.[11] The large-cell, or anaplastic variant, which has pleomorphic nuclei, prominent nucleoli

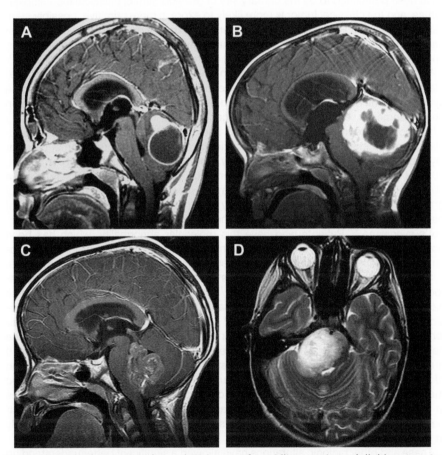

Fig. 2. (*A*) Sagittal contrast-enhanced T1 image of a midline, cystic medulloblastoma. An enhancing solid nodule is seen superiorly within the vermis; the cystic component (with a thin enhancing wall) is inferior. (*B*) Sagittal contrast-enhanced T1 image of a midline, mixed solid–cystic pilocytic astrocytoma. A large enhancing mass occupies the upper half of the vermis. Central, nonenhancing cystic/microcystic elements are evident. Severe hydrocephalus is caused by compression of the fourth ventricle. (*C*) Sagittal contrast-enhanced T1 image of a fourth ventricular ependymoma. A lobulated mass expands the fourth ventricle and shows irregular moderate enhancement. (*D*) Axial T2 weighted image of an infiltrative brainstem (pontine) glioma. An intrinsic T2 bright mass replaces most of the pons and infiltrates the right middle cerebellar peduncle.

and more abundant cytoplasm, as well as possibly higher mitotic and apoptotic indices, increasingly has been recognized and may carry a poorer prognosis.[13] By contrast, the desmoplastic, at times nodular, medulloblastoma variant seems more responsive to therapy and may have a better prognosis.[14]

BIOLOGY

Medulloblastoma is thought to originate from a primitive cell type in the cerebellum, arising from one of the two cerebellar germinal zones, the ventricular zone that forms the innermost boundary of the cerebellum or the external germinal layer that lines the outside of the cerebellum.[15] The multipotent progenitor cells of the ventricular zone have been postulated to be the primary site of development of classical medulloblastomas, and the classical tumor is more likely to express more primitive, possibly stem cell markers. Medulloblastomas arising from the external granular layer on the other hand are believed to originate from a more neuronally restricted granular cell precursor, and are more likely to be desmoplastic and express markers of granular cell lineage.

Various genes and signaling pathways have been identified as active in medulloblastoma and support progenitor cell theories. The nevoid basal cell carcinoma syndrome, which is caused by an inherited germ line mutation of the PTCH gene on chromosome 22, encodes the sonic hedgehog (SHH) receptor PATCHED1 (PTC1), which normally represses SHH signaling.[15] Somatic mutation of PTC1 has been associated predominantly with the desmoplastic variant, possibly from external granular layer precursors, and this pathway is likely a potential therapeutic target for 10% to 20% of medulloblastomas.[13,16] Classical medulloblastomas are less likely to have abnormalities in the SHH pathway and may be more likely to arise from the internal granular layer. Another signaling pathway that has been identified in a subset of patients with medulloblastoma has been the WNT pathway, which is aberrant in Turcot's syndrome.[17] Patients who have this molecular abnormality, which has been noted in as many as 15% of patients and may affect growth and survival of multipotential cerebellar progenitor cells, have been demonstrated to have better prognosis.

Specific molecular genetic abnormalities have been associated with medulloblastoma and variably correlated with survival.[13,18] Amplification of the MYCC oncogene has been associated with the large-cell variant and poorer outcome. Similarly, expression of the tyrosine kinase receptor ERBB2 has been demonstrated in 40% of medulloblastomas and is also predictive of poor outcome.[19] Increased expression of the neurotrophin-3 receptor (TRKC), which regulates proliferation, differentiation, and granular layer cell death, has been associated with better survival.[20,21] Amplification of the OXT2 homeobox gene, a retinoid target, has been identified in the anaplastic medulloblastoma variant.[22] Gene expression profiling has demonstrated differences in metastatic and nonmetastatic tumors, as platelet-derived growth factor receptor beta and members of the RAS-MAP kinase pathway are up-regulated significantly in metastatic tumors.[23]

These and other biologic alterations have allowed a significant better understanding of medulloblastoma. In time, it is likely that they will be incorporated into staging schema for medulloblastoma and also will act as therapeutic targets.[24,25] To date, however, medulloblastomas predominantly are staged and treated based on clinical parameters.

MANAGEMENT

In most patients who have medulloblastomas, the initial step in treatment is surgical resection. Total or near-total resection of the primary tumor site has been correlated with better survival, predominantly in nondisseminated patients.[26] Such resections will result in avoidance of permanent ventriculoperitoneal cerebrospinal drainage in over 60% of patients. Significant postoperative complications may occur, including both septic and aseptic meningitis, postoperative cerebrospinal fluid leaks, and increased neurologic morbidity caused by direct cerebellar or brain stem damage. The cerebellar mutism syndrome has been identified in up to 25% of patients following resection of midline cerebellar tumors.[27] This syndrome presents as the late (delayed) onset of mutism associated with a variable constellation of nystagmus, truncal hypotonia, dysmetria, dysphagia, other supranuclear cranial nerve palsies, and marked emotional lability. The neurophysiologic mechanism underlying this syndrome is unclear, but it is believed to be related to vermian damage and possibly impaired dentatorubrothalamic connections to the supplementary motor cortex. Symptoms may persist from weeks to months and approximately 50% of those affected will have significant sequelae 1 year after surgery. Neurosurgery-related complications have not been related clearly to more aggressive surgery.

Following surgery, patients usually are stratified into one of two risk groups, based on extent of surgical resection and disease extent at the time of diagnosis (**Table 2**). Neuroradiographic staging, although critical, remains problematic, as central review of international studies has demonstrated inadequate spinal neuroimaging or misinterpreted studies in nearly 25% of patients.[12,25] Adequate staging requires meticulous, multiplanar neuro-axis imaging and lumbar cerebrospinal fluid analysis. In time, as these risk groups are modified by the inclusion of other factors, including histological features and molecular genetic parameters, an intermediate risk group of patients may become more apparent (see **Table 2**).

Patients greater than 3 years of age with average-risk disease are treated conventionally with craniospinal (2400 cGy) and local boost radiotherapy (5580 cGy), supplemented with adjuvant chemotherapy.[28] The dose of craniospinal radiation therapy for children who have nondisseminated disease has been decreased by one-third (from 3600 cGy) with maintained efficacy, as long as chemotherapy is given during and after radiotherapy. Studies are underway attempting to determine if a further reduction of the dose of craniospinal radiotherapy from 2340 cGy to 1800 cGy will result in equivalent survival figures and better neurocognitive outcome.

Different chemotherapeutic regimens have shown benefit in medulloblastoma. Probably the best tested is the use of vincristine during radiotherapy and the combination of CCNU, cisplatin and vincristine, or cyclophosphamide, cisplatin, and vincristine following radiotherapy.[28,29] Another approach, demonstrating similar survival, has used essentially the same agents in a truncated, higher-dose fashion supported by peripheral stem cell rescue.[30] With such combination approaches used during and after radiotherapy, over 80% of children with average-risk medulloblastoma are alive and free of disease five years following diagnosis, most of whom are apparently cured

Table 2
Staging of medulloblastoma in children older than 3 years of age

	Average-Risk	High-Risk
Tumor extent	Localized	Disseminated
Tumor resection	Total; near total	Subtotal; biopsy
Histology	Classical; desmoplastic/nodular	Anaplastic/large cell
Biologic parameters	Neurotrophin-3 receptor expression; sonic hedgehog lineage markers	↑ MYCC amplification; ↑ ERBB2 expression; OXT2 amplification

from their disease. The use of preradiotherapy chemotherapy has resulted in inferior survival.[28–32]

Children older than 3 years who have high-risk medulloblastoma have approximately a 50% to 60% 5-year disease-free survival after treatment with higher doses of craniospinal radiation therapy (3600 cGy) and similar doses of local radiotherapy, as used for children with average-risk disease, and chemotherapy during and after radiation therapy.[30] Recent trials have included the use of carboplatin as a radiosensitizer during radiation therapy and the delivery of higher-dose chemotherapy, essentially an intensified cisplatin, cyclophosphamide, vincristine, and etoposide regimen, supported by peripheral stem cell rescue, following radiotherapy, with possibly better results.[30] The added efficacy of biologic therapy, such as retinoic acid and tyrosine kinase inhibitors, is being explored in this subset of patients.

Treatment of children younger than 3 years of who have medulloblastoma is problematic. Because of the immaturity of the brain and the resultant deleterious effects of whole brain irradiation on the very young child, there is significant reluctance to use craniospinal radiation therapy. Management of infants is complicated further by the increased likelihood of dissemination at the time of diagnosis in younger patients, because as many as 40% of children younger than 3 years who have medulloblastoma will have disseminated disease at diagnosis.[12] Although various chemotherapeutic approaches have been used, and others are under active study, the most important predictor of outcome is likely not the type of regimen employed, but rather the biology of the tumor.[33–35] Infants who have desmoplastic/nodular tumors are quite responsive to chemotherapy, and 75% or greater of patients harboring this histologic variant may be cured by chemotherapy alone. Outcome is less favorable in infants who have classical, undifferentiated medulloblastoma, especially in those who have disseminated disease at the time of diagnosis. More intensive chemotherapeutic regimens using peripheral stem cell support or regimens that have been supplemented with high-dose, intravenous, and intrathecal methotrexate have shown possible increased efficacy.[34,35] The safety and efficacy of focal radiation therapy to the primary tumor site also is being explored in this age group.

Children of all ages with medulloblastoma who survive are at risk for significant long-term sequelae. The whole brain portion of craniospinal radiation therapy has been implicated as the primary cause of long-term neurocognitive deficits. Other factors, however, may play a significant role in sequelae encountered. These include: the tumor's location extent and the presence of hydrocephalus at diagnosis, postsurgical complications, the age of the patient, the potential deleterious effects of concomitant chemotherapy, and the additive toxicity of local radiotherapy.[36,37] Neurocognitive difficulties are the most common sequelae seen, and even after reduction of whole-brain radiotherapy from 3600 cGy to 2340 cGy, most children, especially those younger than 7 years of age, will have significant intellectual difficulties.[36,37] Deficits include demonstrable post-treatment drop in overall intelligence, as well as deficits in perceptual motor ability, memory tasks, verbal learning, and executive function. Moderate-to-severe learning difficulties are common.

Neuroendocrine sequelae are also relatively common, but these seem to be somewhat less frequent in those children who have been treated with reduced doses of craniospinal radiation therapy.[12] Of the endocrinologic sequelae, growth hormone insufficiency is the most common, occurring in almost all prepubertal children who have received 3600 cGy of craniospinal radiation and probably 50% or more of those children receiving 2340 cGy of whole-brain irradiation therapy.[12,38] Thyroid dysfunction also occurs frequently and is caused not only by the dose of radiotherapy delivered to the hypothalamic region, but also by scatter radiation to the thyroid gland.

Permanent neurologic sequelae, including motor difficulties, sensory dysfunction, hearing impairments caused by the tumor, chemotherapy (especially cisplatinum), or radiation therapy, and visual abnormalities increasingly have been recognized in long-term survivors.[39] Late-onset cerebrovascular damage resulting in stroke-like episodes is not uncommon, and can cause devastating long-term complications.[39] Survivors are at risk for small vessel microangiopathy and more subtle vascular-related sequelae, such as seizures. Secondary tumors are another long-term complication of medulloblastoma and may be related to the underlying genetic predisposition of these patients to tumors and/or to the radiotherapy employed. Both meningiomas and gliomas can occur at any time following successful treatment, and, in general, high-grade gliomas tend to predominate in the first 5 to 10 years following therapy, while the risk of meningiomas continues to increase over time.[40]

Supratentorial Primitive Neuroectodermal Tumors

Supratentorial primitive neuroectodermal tumors are characterized by undifferentiated or poorly differentiated neuroepithelial cells that may show some degree of differentiation. Although similar histologically, they are biologically different from medulloblastomas.[21] Various different names, including cerebral neuroblastomas, have been used for these tumors, which, by definition, must occur above the tentorium, primarily in the cerebral cortex and less frequently in the diencephalic region. They are infrequent, comprising 2.5% of all childhood brain tumors. The tumors are staged based predominantly on tumor extent at diagnosis, although approximately 20% or less of lesions have evidence of dissemination.

The degree of surgical resection has been related variably to outcome.[41–44] Postsurgical management has been similar to that employed for high-risk medulloblastoma patients, with most children being treated with craniospinal and local boost radiotherapy and aggressive adjuvant chemotherapy. The need for craniospinal radiation therapy has never been demonstrated clearly, although it is used frequently. Reported 5-year progression-free survival rates have ranged from 30% to 60%, with most series finding that approximately 50% of affected patients survive.[41–44]

Pineoblastomas

Although pineoblastomas are classified as pineal parenchymal tumors, they are conceptualized most commonly as a subvariant of embryonal tumors and are managed similarly to high-risk medulloblastomas. They represent approximately 25% of tumors that occur in the pineal region. Dissemination at the time of diagnosis is present in 20% to 30% of patients.[41–44]

Total resections before the initiation of adjuvant treatment are uncommon because of tumor location. Survival figures after treatment with craniospinal plus local boost radiation therapy and adjuvant chemotherapy, similar to that being used for high-risk medulloblastoma patients, have been quite variable, with some studies reporting relatively optimistic 5-year progression-free survival rates of as high as 60%.[41–44] Other series have reported much less favorable outcomes, especially in very young children who are not treated with craniospinal radiotherapy.

Atypical Teratoid/Rhabdoid Tumors

Atypical teratoid/rhabdoid tumors (AT/RTs) first were recognized as a discreet entity in the late 1980s.[45] These lesions, which predominantly occur in children younger than 3 years, but may be first diagnosed in older children and adolescents, histologically are characterized by rhabdoid cells intermixed with a variable component of primitive neuroectodermal, mesenchymal, and epithelial cells. The rhabdoid cell is a medium-sized round-to-oval cell with distinct borders, an eccentric nucleus, and a prominent nucleolus. The primitive neuroectodermal component of AT/RTs is indistinguishable from that found in other forms of primitive neuroectodermal tumors. Immunohistochemical studies demonstrated that AT/RTs were different from medulloblastomas, because the rhabdoid component of the tumor characteristically stained positive for epithelial membrane antigen, vimentin, cytokeratin, glial fibrillary acidic protein, and, at times, smooth muscle actin and neurofilament protein. Molecular genetic studies have demonstrated that AT/RTs are distinct from other embryonal tumors and are characterized by deletions or mutations of the tumor suppressor gene hSNF5/INI1 located in the chromosomal region 22q11.2.[46]

Management of AT/RTs has been extremely problematic. The tumor arises equally in the posterior fossa or supratentorium.[47] Dissemination has been reported in approximately 25% of patients at diagnosis. Outcome after treatment of infants on protocols used for children younger than 3 years with medulloblastoma, including high-dose chemotherapy protocols, has been disappointing, with prolonged survival occurring in less than 20% of patients who had nondisseminated tumors, primarily in those who had undergone a total or near-total resection. Various different chemotherapeutic approaches are under study, including adding methotrexate to the drug regimen or using protocols that are hybrids of the infant medulloblastoma and sarcoma treatment regimens. Survival seems more favorable in patients older than 3 years at diagnosis treated with extensive resections, craniospinal and local boost radiotherapy, and chemotherapy.

Gliomas

High-grade gliomas

These tumors present most frequently between 5 and 10 years of age.[48] Patients may present with headaches, motor weakness, personality changes and seizures; however, seizures are more typical of low-grade cortical lesions.[49] On CT and MRI, high-grade gliomas (HGG) typically appear as irregularly shaped lesions with partial contrast enhancement and peritumoral edema with or without mass effect.[49]

Radical (greater than 90%) surgical resection is the most powerful predictor of favorable outcome in HGG when followed by irradiation.[50,51] Only 49% of tumors in the superficial hemisphere and 8% of tumors in the midline or deep cerebrum are amenable to radical resection, however. Local or wide-field irradiation to 5000 cGy to 6000 cGy is the mainstay of therapy. The addition of radiation therapy has improved 5-year survival rates (10% to 30%) compared with surgery alone (0%).[50] Although initial reports demonstrated a benefit of adjuvant chemotherapy with prednisone, CCNU, and vincristine (pCV) compared with radiotherapy alone (46% versus 18%), a subsequent trial comparing pCV with the eight-in-one regimen failed to show the same benefit (26%).[52,53] A review of the histology from the original trial with pCV suggested that a significant portion of patients (69/250) actually did not meet the central consensus definition of HGG. Most recently, temozolamide and concurrent radiation followed by maintenance temozolomide therapy has been used; however this regimen has shown no improvement in survival. To date, no large randomized clinical trial has demonstrated a benefit of chemotherapy clearly. High-dose chemotherapy for HGG has shown effective responses, and despite significant associated toxicity, may warrant further investigation.[54,55]

Biologic therapy, such as drugs that target angiogenesis, is being investigated as an alternative approach. Specific biologic therapeutic targets have not been defined well for childhood HGG. For example, although 80% of pediatric HGG overexpress the EGFR protein, amplification of the EGFR gene is rare compared with EGFR amplification in one-third of adult glioblastomas.[56–58] A more recent expression profiling study of childhood HGG revealed increased expression of the EGFR/HIF/ IGFBP2 pathway.[57] The TP53 gene is mutated in 34% of HGG in children younger than 3 years and only 12% of HGG in children older than 3 years, while the 5-year progression-free survival in those with low expression of p53 protein is 44% compared with 17% in those with high expression.[59,60] Deletions for p16INK4a and p14ARF of the Rb pathway are observed in only 10% of pediatric HGG.[61] These data indicate that the development of pediatric HGG may follow different pathways from the primary or secondary paradigm of adult glioblastomas and as such may require differently tailored biologic therapy than is being employed for adults with HGG.

Low-grade gliomas

Most low-grade cortical gliomas in children are juvenile pilocytic astrocytoma (JPA) or diffuse fibrillary astrocytoma. Other forms, such as oligodendroglioma, oligoastrocytoma and mixed glioma are much less common.[62] Low-grade cortical gliomas (LGG) most commonly present with headache and seizure. On CT, diffuse astrocytomas appear as ill-defined, homogeneous masses of low density without contrast enhancement. MRI usually shows a mass that is hypodense on T1 weighted and hyperintense on T2 weighted images with little enhancement. Imaging of JPA lesions is similar to the cerebellar counterpart.[63]

Complete surgical resection is curative for most, and even with incomplete excision, long-term progression-free survival is common.[64] If subsequent progression occurs, then re-resection generally is undertaken. For patients who have progressive disease not amenable to resection, irradiation with 5000 cGy to 5500 cGy is warranted. Chemotherapy is reserved for very young children and infants and most commonly includes carboplatin and vincristine.

Overall 5-year survival is 95%, while progression-free survival is 88%. Less favorable results have been seen in patients who have nonpilocytic astrocytoma.[65]

Chiasmatic gliomas

Gliomas of the visual pathway, which also may extend to the hypothalamus and thalamus, comprise a relatively common form of childhood glioma. Tumors of the optic chiasm are usually low-grade. Twenty percent of children who have (NF-1) will develop visual pathway tumors, predominantly JPA, during childhood.[66] Visual pathway tumors may cause visual loss, strabismus, proptosis and/or nystagmus. Extension to the hypothalamus may present with endocrinologic disturbances, including precocious puberty. Imaging demonstrates similar characteristics of low-grade gliomas that present elsewhere (**Fig. 3**). Optic pathway lesions have limited capacity to spread, as they are confined to migrate between the optic nerve and chiasm.[66]

Radiation therapy with 5000 cGy to 5500 cGy generally is reserved for older children who have progressive or symptomatic tumors. Therapy with carboplatin and vincristine has demonstrated tumor shrinkage and/or stabilization in over 90% of children younger than 5 years of age.[67,68] In children who have NF-1, tumor biopsy for histologic confirmation is not necessary because of the highly characteristic appearance on MRI. In these children, lesions may be detected by routine screening before the onset of symptoms, and treatment is often withheld until there is clear radiographic or clinical progression.

Brain stem gliomas

Brain stem gliomas (BSGs) comprise 10% to 15% of all pediatric CNS tumors and are generally uncommon in the adult population. Peak incidence is between 5 and 9 years of age, but may occur anytime during childhood.[62] BSGs most commonly arise in the

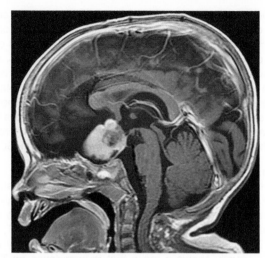

Fig. 3. Sagittal contrast-enhanced T1 image a of a chiasmatic glioma. A large, enhancing suprasellar mass is evident, which replaces the chiasm. Nonenhancing cystic/microcystic components are evident posteriorly.

pons (diffuse intrinsic), in which location they typically resemble adult glioblastomas multiforme (GBM) and have an almost uniformly dismal prognosis (see **Fig. 2**). In contrast, those arising from midbrain or medulla are likely to be low-grade lesions that have a more indolent course and better outcome. BSGs commonly present with multiple cranial nerve deficits, especially sixth and seventh nerve palsies, long track signs, and cerebellar deficits.[69] Diffuse pontine gliomas show CT and MRI characteristics similar to HGG within an enlarged pons. Low-grade BSGs are relatively discrete, often exophytic, and contrast, enhancing with cyst formation.[11]

Treatment is local irradiation with 5500 cGy to 6000 cGy. Over 90% of patients who have diffuse intrinsic lesions transiently respond, but ultimately succumb to disease progression within 18 months of diagnosis. Neither hyperfractionated radiotherapy nor chemotherapy has been shown to add benefit.[70] Low-grade lesions are treated with similar irradiation doses but overall respond less favorably than their counterparts in other locations.[69,71]

Cerebellar gliomas

Cerebellar glioma is found almost exclusively in children, occurring most frequently between ages 4 and 9. JPA is the most common subtype, accounting for 85% of cerebellar gliomas.[72] Diffuse astrocytoma is the next most common, while malignant astrocytoma is rare in this location. Children typically present with headache, vomiting, papilledema. and gait disturbance. CT and MRI reveal either a large solid (20%) or mixed solid and cystic (80%) circumscribed mass that enhances with contrast (see **Fig. 2**B).[73,74] Pilocytic tumors are circumscribed well and characterized by a biphasic pattern with varying proportion of bipolar cells with Rosenthal fibers and loose multipolar cells with microcysts.[11]

Total surgical resection is curative in 95% to 100% of cases.[73,74] JPAs may stabilize for long periods of time or even spontaneously regress. however, the behavior of cerebellar gliomas in children who have NF-1 may be more aggressive. Those children whose lesions are inoperable because of brain stem involvement may require additional therapy, although residual tumor may remain quiescent for years. Thus irra-diation and/or chemotherapy should be reserved for tumors that demonstrate clear growth or symptomatic change.[73,74] Rare malignant cerebellar astrocytomas have a poor outcome and require aggressive treatment similar to supratentorial HGG.

Ependymomas

Ependymomas comprise 5% to 10% of all childhood brain tumors.[75,76] Most (70% to 80%) arise in the posterior fossa and, because of a relative predilection for the cere-bellopontine angle and lateral portion of the lower brainstem, often cause multiple cranial nerve deficits including sixth and seventh nerve palsies, hearing loss, and swal-lowing difficulties. Ependymomas tend to present more insidiously than medulloblas-tomas and at the time of diagnosis, despite their lateral posterior fossa location, frequently cause obstructive hydrocephalous (see **Fig. 2**C). Various histological subtypes of ependymoma are recognized; however, clinically, the most important distinction is between anaplastic lesions and somewhat lower grade, usually cellular tumors.[77] The myxopapillary ependymoma, which occurs predominantly in the conus and cauda equina region of the spinal cord, is likely a biologically different subtype of tumor with an even more indolent natural history.

Although probably no greater than 5% of ependymomas are disseminated at the time of diagnosis, staging for extent of disease usually is undertaken either before or after surgery.[78] The degree of surgical resection is a critical determinant of outcome for children who have ependymomas, as those who have total or near-total resections have the highest likelihood of long-term disease control.[79] Infratentorial tumors noto-riously extend along the upper cervical cord, making total resection and radiotherapy planning difficult. Such contiguous extension has been related to poorer disease control, especially if radiation planning does not take into consideration the tendency of these tumors to contiguously spread.

The need for radiotherapy in totally resected nonanaplastic ependymomas is some-what controversial. Small series have suggested that totally resected supratentorial lesions can be treated with surgery alone. most patients with completely resected in-fratentorial tumors have received radiotherapy, with resultant 5-year progression-free survival rates of 75% to 80%.[79] Local radiotherapy, using conformal treatment plan-ning and doses ranging between 5500 cGy and 5960 cGy, is as effective as craniospi-nal and local boost radiotherapy. Patients who have anaplastic tumors may fare less well. Patients who have subtotally resected ependymomas, after local radiotherapy, have 5-year progression-free survival rates of probably no higher than 50%. Combina-tion therapy with radiation and chemotherapy has been reserved predominantly for children older than 3 years and those patients who have subtotally resected and/or anaplastic tumors.[80,81] Randomized studies, using chemotherapy as an adjuvant after radiotherapy, have not demonstrated significant improvements in survival, although more recent preirradiation phase 2 investigations suggest there may be a role for adju-vant, predominantly cisplatin-based combination drug regimens.

Because of the apparent crucial role of extensive surgery in patients with ependy-momas, studies are underway evaluating the feasibility, safety, and utility of second-look surgery after chemotherapy before radiation. Postsurgical neurologic complications due to the location of the tumor and its involvement of multiple lower cranial nerves are a major risk, however, and the need for total resection has to be counterbalanced by the risk of surgically induced long-term neurologic impairment.

Ependymomas are relatively common in younger patients, as they comprise 20% or more of infantile infratentorial tumors. Chemotherapy usually is used in attempts to delay the need for radiotherapy, although there has been renewed interest in using local radiotherapy in children as young as 1 year who have infratentorial tumors, especially for patients who have tumors not amenable to total surgical resection.[82]

Craniopharyngiomas

Craniopharyngiomas account for 5% to 10% of all childhood brain tumors and are believed to arise from embryonic remnants of Rathke's pouch in the sellar region.[83] Clinical presentation is variable, and symptoms may be secondary to blockage of cerebrospinal fluid and resultant increased intracranial pressure or direct chiasmatic or hypothalamic damage from the solid tumor and associated cyst. Visual symptoms are variable and may include decreased visual acuity in one or both eyes and visual field deficits. Endocrinologic abnormalities at the time of diagnosis are common and may include failure of growth, delayed sexual maturation, weight gain, and, in a significant minority of patients, diabetes insipidus. Craniopharyngiomas peak at 6 to 10 years and then later at 11 to 15 years. They are notoriously large at the time of diagnosis and are often multilobulated heterogeneous masses with cystic and solid components and significant amounts of calcification (**Fig. 4**).

The tumor's size and its proximity to the hypothalamus, visual pathway, and carotid vessels, as well as craniopharyngioma's tendency to be quite gritty and adherent to these critical brain structures and the undersurface of the frontal lobes, make surgical removal difficult.[83,84] Despite decades of clinical experience, controversy exists over optimal management. Complete tumor removal results in an 80% to 95% 10-year progression-free survival rate and cure, but this also may be associated with significant behavioral and neurocognitive difficulties and, in most patients, permanent hormonal deficits.[83] After total removal, most patients will require growth, thyroid, and cortisol supplementation; chronic DDAVP replacement to correct diabetes insipidus will be needed in up to 75% of patients. The degree of neurocognitive/ psychological damage, manifested by severe memory loss, behavioral difficulties, and associated obesity secondary subfrontal and hypothalamic damage can be severe and, in the cases of severe obesity, can be life-threatening.[85] Alternative approaches, which include partial tumor resection and/or cyst aspiration followed

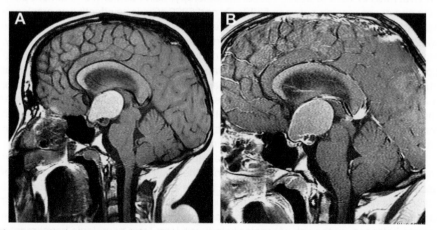

Fig. 4. Sagittal precontrast (*A*) and postcontrast (*B*) T1 images of a cystic suprasellar craniopharyngioma. The proteinaceous contents of the dominant, superior cyst are very bright on the precontrast image (*A*); following contrast (*B*), the capsule surrounding the large cyst and a more solid nodule (inferior) enhance and become hyperintense to the cyst contents.

by radiotherapy, may be nearly as effective in controlling disease and result in less morbidity.[86] Intercavitary brachytherapy using p[32] or y[90], repeated cyst aspiration, or the use of intracyst bleomycin may be useful in selected situations.[87,88] Even after less aggressive surgery and other means of treatment, sequelae may occur. Hormonal deficits are less likely if the pituitary stalk is preserved.[89]

Germ Cell Tumors

Germ cell tumors, which comprise approximately 2% to 5% of all childhood brain tumors, arise predominantly in the pineal and suprasellar region, but may occur throughout the brain.[90] Despite their relatively rapid growth rate, they may present insidiously and delays of 6 months to 1 year between initial onset of symptoms, which may include school difficulties, polyuria, and behavioral problems, occurs in up to one-third of patients. Germinomas and mixed germ cell tumors account for approximately 60% of all pineal region masses. Germinomas may present in both the pineal region and the suprasellar region in 10% to 20% of patients. Those patients with pineal region symptomatology, which is classically manifested by symptoms of hydrocephalus and/or direct tectal damage (Parinaud's syndrome), with associated diabetes insipidus or other hormonal deficits, are considered to have both pineal and suprasellar involvement, even in the case of equivocal neuroradiographic findings. Tumors in the thalamic region and those disseminated throughout the brain and spinal cord may be more difficult to diagnose neuroradiographically and may not show characteristic enhancement.

Histological confirmation is usually, but not always, required for the diagnosis of germinomas and distinction from other pineal region tumors such as pineoblastomas, pineocytomas, and teratomas.[90,91] Elevated cerebrospinal fluid and, in selected cases, blood levels of alpha-feta protein and β-HCG can be used to confirm a mixed germ cell tumor. Highly elevated levels of beta-human chorionic gonadotrophin (β-HCG) alone are diagnostic of a choriocarcinoma. A subvariety of germinoma, the syncytiotrophoblastic variant, secretes moderate levels of β-HCG into the cerebrospinal fluid. Surgery for patients who have presumed germ cell tumors usually is preserved for those patients for whom a diagnosis cannot be made by cerebrospinal fluid markers or when the tumor is very large and requires debulking.

Radiation therapy has been the primary modality of therapy for patients who have pure germinomas, and craniospinal plus local boost radiotherapy can result in cure in 95% or more of patients, including those with disseminated disease at the time of diagnosis.[92,93] Germinomas, however, are also chemosensitive, and treatment with preradiation chemotherapy followed by more localized radiotherapy, usually whole ventricular therapy, may be as effective and result in somewhat less sequelae because of the avoidance of whole-brain radiation.[94–96] In contradistinction, patients with mixed germ cell tumors have only a 40% to 60% likelihood of long-term disease control after treatment with radiotherapy alone. In these patients, multidrug chemotherapeutic regimens, either given before or after radiotherapy, have seemed to result in improved survival rates.[97]

Choroid Plexus Tumors

Tumors of the choroid plexus are relatively uncommon, contributing 1% to 5% of all pediatric tumors.[98–100] Choroid plexus papillomas, because of their intraventricular location and associated cerebrospinal fluid overproduction, and blockage of cerebrospinal fluid reabsorbtion pathways, predominantly result in hydrocephalus. Papillomas notoriously occur in very young infants and result in massive hydrocephalus. They increasingly are being diagnosed during prenatal ultrasound evaluations. Unlike the situation in older patients and adults, where the tumor more commonly arises in the fourth ventricle, infantile tumors classically arise in the lateral ventricles and may be bilateral. The treatment of choice for choroid plexus papillomas is surgical removal. Because of the marked vascularity of these tumors, the massive hydrocephalus often present, and the age of the patient, however, there may be considerable surgical mortality.

Choroid plexus carcinomas are much more likely to invade the contiguous brain parenchyma than papillomas. Despite their histological aggressivity, gross total resections alone can result in long-term disease control. Optimal treatment for subtotally resected choroid plexus carcinomas is unclear. Although adjuvant chemotherapy and radiotherapy have been used and may result in tumor response, the long-term efficacy of such approaches has been difficult to demonstrate.[98–100]

Spinal Cord Tumors

Spinal cord tumors may be extremely difficult to diagnose in young children who may present with delays in walking and, in older patients, who develop difficult-to-characterize gait disturbances.[101,102] Back pain is frequent but often nonspecific and initially nonlocalizing, and sensory abnormalities are often hard to characterize in children. Tumors in the conus region result in early bowel and bladder difficulties. In total, spinal cord tumors account for less than 10% of all CNS neoplasms. The most common primary central nervous system lesions are gliomas and ependymomas. Patients who have NF-1 are prone to develop intramedullary astrocytomas, and are at high risk for extrinsic cord compression by neurofibromas. Children who have neurofibromatosis type 2 are more likely to harbor intramedulllary ependymomas, which are often indolent lesions requiring little therapy for many years.

In patients who have low-grade gliomas, MRI usually reveals an enlarged hypointense cord, at times associated with a thin syrinx. There may be focal enhancement, especially in pilocytic tumors. In general, ependymomas are somewhat more circumscribed than astrocytomas.

Low-grade spinal astrocytomas can be treated effectively by extensive surgical resections or by partial resections followed by radiotherapy, or possibly, in very young children, chemotherapy.[103,104] The outcome for patients who have ependymomas is somewhat more variable, although long-term control after resection and usually adjuvant radiotherapy is possible. High-grade lesions may be very difficult to resect, and even after treatment with radiation therapy, most patients will suffer tumor relapse within 3to 5 years of diagnosis, often associated with neuro-axis dissemination.[103]

REFERENCES

1. CBTRUS 2005. Statistical report: primary brain tumors in the United States, 1995–1999. Published by the Central Brain Tumor Registry of the United States.
2. Lindor NM, Greene MH. Mayo Familial Cancer Program. The concise handbook of family cancer syndromes. J Natl Cancer Inst 1998;90:1039–71.
3. McGaughran JM, Harris DL, Donnai E, et al. A clinical study of type 1 neurofibromatosis in northwest England. J Med Genet 1999;36:197–203.
4. Webb DW, Fryer AE, Osborne JP. Morbidity associated with tuberous sclerosis: a population study. Dev Med Child Neurol 1996;38:146–55.
5. Varley JM, Evans DGR, Birch JM. Li-Fraumeni syndrome—a molecular and clinical review. Br J Cancer 1997;76:1–14.

6. Cowan R, Hoban P, Kelsey A, et al. The gene for the nevoid basal cell carcinoma syndrome acts as a tumour suppressor gene in medulloblastoma. Br J Cancer 1997;76:141–5.
7. Paraf F, Jothy S, van Meir EG. Brain tumor polyposis syndrome: two genetic diseases? J Clin Oncol 1997;15:2744–58.
8. Ron E, Modan B, Boice JD, et al. Tumors of the brain and nervous system after radiotherapy in childhood. N Engl J Med 1988;319:1033–9.
9. Pollack IF. Brain tumors in children. N Engl J Med 1994;331:1500–7.
10. Vézina L-G. Neuroradiology of childhood brain tumors: new challenges. J Neuro-Oncol 2005;75:243–52.
11. Kleihues P, Cavenee WK. Survival and prognostic factors following radiation therapy and chemotherapy for ependymoma in children: a report of the Children's Cancer Group. Lyon, France: IARC Press; 2000.
12. Packer RJ, Cogen P, Vézina G, et al. Medulloblastoma: clinical and biologic aspects. Neuro Oncol 1999;1:232–50.
13. Eberhart CG, Kratz J, Wang Y, et al. Histopathological and molecular prognostic markers in medulloblastoma: c-myc, N-myc, TrkC, and anaplasia. J Neuropathol Exp Neurol 2004;63(5):4441–9.
14. Giangaspero F, Rigobello L, Badiali M, et al. Large-cell medulloblastomas. a distinct variant with highly aggressive behavior. Am J Surg Pathol 1992; 16(7):687–93.
15. Read T-A, Hegedus B, Wechsler-Reya R, et al. The neurobiology of neuro-oncology. Ann Neurol 2006;6:3–11.
16. Raffel C, Jenkins RB, Frederick L, et al. Sporadic medulloblastomas contain PTCH mutation. Cancer Res 1997;57:842–5.
17. Ellison DW, Onilude OE, Lindsey JC, et al. Beta-catenin status predicts a favorable outcome in childhood medulloblastoma: the United Kingdom Children's Cancer Study Group brain tumour committee. J Clin Oncol 2005;23: 7951–7.
18. Grotzer MA, Hogarty MD, Janss AJ, et al. MYC messenger RNA expression predicts survival outcome in childhood primitive neuroectodermal tumor/medulloblastoma. Clin Cancer Res 2001;7:2425–33.
19. Gilbertson S, Wickramasinghe C, Hernan R, et al. Clinical and molecular stratification of disease risk in medulloblastoma. Br J Cancer 2001;85:705–12.
20. Grotzer MA, Janss AJ, Fung K, et al. TrkC expression predicts good clinical outcome in primitive neuroectodermal brain tumors. J Clin Oncol 18:1027–1035.
21. Pomeroy S, Tamayo P, Gaasenbeek M, et al. Prediction of central nervous system embryonal tumour outcome based on gene expression. Nature 2002; 415(6870):436–42.
22. MacDonald TJ, Rood B, Santi MR, et al. Advances in the diagnosis, molecular genetics, and treatment of pediatric embryonal CNS tumors. Oncologist 2003; 8:174–86.
23. MacDonald TJ, Brown KM, LaFleur B, et al. Expression profiling of medulloblastoma: PDGFRA and the RAS/MAPK pathway as therapeutic targets for metastatic disease. Nat Genet 2001;29:143–52.
24. Gajjar A, Hernan R, Kocak M, et al. Clinical, histopathologic, and molecular markers of prognosis: toward a new disease risk stratification system for medulloblastoma. J Clin Oncol 2004;22(6):984–93.
25. Ray A, Ho M, Ma J, et al. A clinicobiological model predicting survival in medulloblastoma. Clin Cancer Res 2004;10:7613–20.

26. Albright AL, Sposto R, Holmes E, et al. Correlation of neurosurgical subspecialization with outcomes in children with malignant brain tumors. Neurosurgery 2000;47:879–87.
27. Robertson PL, Muraszko KM, Holmes EJ, et al. Incidence and severity of postoperative cerebellar mutism syndrome in children with medulloblastoma: a prospective study by the Children's Oncology Group. J Neurosurg 2006; 105(S6 Pediatrics):444–51.
28. Packer RJ, Gajjar A, Vézina G, et al. Phase III study of craniospinal radiation therapy followed by adjuvant chemotherapy for newly diagnosed average-risk medulloblastoma. J Clin Oncol 2006;24(25):4202–8.
29. Packer RJ, Sutton LN, Elterman R, et al. Outcome for children with medulloblastoma treated with radiation and cisplatin, CCNU, and vincristine chemotherapy. J Neurosurg 81(5): 690–8.
30. Gajjar A, Chintagumpala M, Ashley D, et al. Risk-adapted craniospinal radiotherapy followed by high-dose chemotherapy and stem cell rescue in children with newly diagnosed medulloblastoma (St Jude Medulloblastoma-96): longterm results from a prospective, multicentre trial. Lancet 2006;7:813–20.
31. Taylor RE, Bailey CC, Robinson K, et al. Results of a randomized study of preradiation chemotherapy versus radiotherapy alone for nonmetastatic medulloblastoma: The International Society of Paediatric Oncology/United Kingdom Children's Cancer Study Group PNET-3 Study. J Clin Oncol 2003;21(8):1582–91.
32. Kuhl J, Muller HL, Berthold F, et al. Preradiation chemotherapy of children and young adults with malignant brain tumors: results of the German pilot trial HIT '88/'89. Klin Padiatr 1998;210(4):227–33.
33. Duffner PK, Horowitz ME, Krischer JP, et al. Postoperative chemotherapy and delayed radiation in children less than three years of age with malignant brain tumors. N Engl J Med 1993;328(24):1725–31.
34. Rutkowski S, Bode U, Deinlein F, et al. Treatment of early childhood medulloblastoma by postoperative chemotherapy alone. N Engl J Med 2005;352(10):978–86.
35. Geyer JR, Jennings M, Sposto, et al. Multiagent chemotherapy and deferred radiotherapy in infants with malignant brain tumors: a report from the Children's Cancer Group. J Clin Oncol 2005;23:7621–31.
36. Ris MD, Packer R, Goldwein J, et al. Intellectual outcome after reduced-dose radiation therapy plus adjuvant chemotherapy for medulloblastoma: a Children's Cancer Group study. J Clin Oncol 2001;19:3470–6.
37. Mulhern RK, Kepner JL, Thomas PR, et al. Neuropsychologic functioning of survivors of childhood medulloblastoma randomized to receive conventional or reduced-dose craniospinal irradiation: a Pediatric Oncology Group study. J Clin Oncol 1889;16:1723–8.
38. Gurney JG, Kadan-Lottick NS, Packer RJ, et al. Endocrine and cardiovascular late effects among adult survivors of childhood brain tumors: Childhood Cancer Survivor Study. Cancer 2003;47:663–73.
39. Packer RJ, Gurney JG, Punyko JA, et al. Longterm neurologic and neurosensory sequelae in adult survivors of a childhood brain tumor: Childhood Cancer Survivor Study. J Clin Oncol 2003;21:3255–61.
40. Neglia JP, Robison LL, Stovall M, et al. New primary neoplasms of the central nervous system in survivors of childhood cancer: a report from the Childhood Cancer Survivor Study. J Natl Cancer Inst 2006;98:1528–37.
41. Reddy AT, Janss AJ, Phillips PC, et al. Outcome for children with supratentorial primitive neuroectodermal tumors treated with surgery, radiation, and chemotherapy. Cancer 2000;88(9):2189–93.

42. Massimino M, Gandola L, Spreafico F, et al. Supratentorial primitive neuroecto-dermal tumors (S-PNEET) in children: a prospective experience with adjuvant intensive chemotherapy and hyperfractionated accelerated radiotherapy. Int J Radiat Oncol Biol Phys 2006;64:1031–7.

43. Jakacki R, Zeltzer PM, Boyett JM, et al. Survival and prognostic factors following radiation and/or chemotherapy for primitive neuroectodermal tumors of the pineal region in infants and children: a report of the Children's Cancer Group. J Clin Oncol 1995;13(6):1377–83.

44. Timmermann B, Kortmann RD, Kuhl J, et al. Role of radiotherapy in the treatment of supratentorial primitive neuroectodermal tumors in childhood: results of the prospective German brain tumor trials HIT 88/89 and 91. J Clin Oncol 2002;20: 842–9.

45. Rorke LB, Packer RJ, Biegel JA. Central nervous system atypical teratoid/rhab-doid tumors of infancy and childhood: definition of an entity. J Neurosurg 1996; 85:56–65.

46. Biegel JA, Zhou J-Y, Rorke LB, et al. Germ-line and acquired mutations of INI1 in atypical teratoid and rhabdoid tumours. Cancer Res 1999;59:74–9.

47. Packer RJ, Biegel JA, Blaney S, et al. Atypical teratoid/rhabdoid tumor of the central nervous system: report on workshop. J Ped Hem/Onc 2002;24(5):337–42.

48. Ciurea AV, Vasilescu G, Nuteanu L, et al. Neurosurgical management of cerebral astrocytomas in children. Ann N Y Acad Sci 1997;824:237–40.

49. Marchese MJ, Chang CH. Malignant astrocytic gliomas in children. Cancer 1990;65:2771–8.

50. Wolff JE, Gnekow AK, Kortmann RD, et al. Preradiation chemotherapy for pedi-atric patients with high-grade glioma. Cancer 2002;94:264–71.

51. Wisoff JH, Boyett JM, Berger MS, et al. Current neurosurgical management and the impact of the extent of resection in the treatment of malignant gliomas of childhood: a report of the Children's Cancer Group trial no CCG-945. J Neuro-surg 1998;89:52–9.

52. Sposto R, Ertel IJ, Jenkin RD, et al. The effectiveness of chemotherapy for treat-ment of high-grade astrocytoma in children: results of a randomized trial. A report from the Children's Cancer Study Group. J Neurooncol 1989;7:165–77.

53. Finlay JL, Boyett JM, Yates AJ, et al. Randomized phase III trial in childhood high-grade astrocytoma comparing vincristine, lomustine, and prednisone with the eight drugs- in 1 day regimen. Children's Cancer Group. J Clin Oncol 1995;13:112–23.

54. MacDonald TJ, Arenson E, Sposto R, et al. Phase II study of high-dose chemo-therapy before radiation in children with newly diagnosed high-grade astrocy-toma: final analysis of Children's Cancer Group study 9933. Cancer 2005;104: 2862–71.

55. Coppes MJ, Lau R, Ingram LC, et al. Open-label comparison of the antiemetic efficacy of single intravenous doses of dolasetron mesylate in pediatric cancer patients receiving moderately to highly emetogenic chemotherapy. Med Pediatr Oncol 1999;33:99–105.

56. Sung T, Miller DC, Hayes RL, et al. Preferential inactivation of the p53 tumor suppressor pathway and lack of EGFR amplification distinguish de novo high-grade pediatric astrocytomas from de novo adult astrocytomas. Brain Pathol 2000;10:249–59.

57. Khatua S, Peterson KM, Brown KM, et al. Overexpression of the EGFR/FKBP12/ HIF-2alpha pathway identified in childhood astrocytomas by angiogenesis gene profiling. Cancer Res 2003;63:1865–70.

58. Bredel M, Pollack IF, Hamilton RL, et al. Epidermal growth factor receptor expression and gene amplification in high-grade nonbrainstem gliomas of childhood. Clin Cancer Res 1999;5:1786–92.
59. Pollack IF, Finkelstein SD, Burnham J, et al. Age and TP53 mutation frequency in childhood malignant gliomas: results in a multi-institutional cohort. Cancer Res 2001;61:7404–7.
60. Pollack IF, Finkelstein SD, Woods J, et al. Expression of p53 and prognosis in children with malignant gliomas. N Engl J Med 2002;346:420–7.
61. Newcomb EW, Alonso M, Sung T, et al. Incidence of p14ARF gene deletion in high-grade adult and pediatric astrocytomas. Hum Pathol 2000;31:115–9.
62. Gurney JG, Bunin GR. CNS and miscellaneous intracranial and intraspinal neoplasms. In: Ries LAG, S M, Gurney JG, et al, editors. Cancer incidence and survival among children and adolescents: United States SEER Program 1975–1995. NIH Pub No 99–4649. Bethesda (MD): National Cancer Institute SEER program; 1999. p. 51–63.
63. Finizio FS. CT and MRI aspects of supratentorial hemispheric tumors of childhood and adolescence. Childs Nerv Syst 1995;11:559–67.
64. Pollack IF. The role of surgery in pediatric gliomas. J Neurooncol 1999;42: 271–88.
65. Pollack IF, Claassen D, al-Shboul Q, et al. Low-grade gliomas of the cerebral hemispheres in children: an analysis of 71 cases. J Neurosurg 1995;82: 536–47.
66. Burger PC, Cohen KJ, Rosenblum MK, et al. Pathology of diencephalic astrocytomas. Pediatr Neurosurg 2000;32:214–9.
67. Gropman AL, Packer RJ, Nicholson HS, et al. Treatment of diencephalic syndrome with chemotherapy: growth, tumor response, and long-term control. Cancer 1998;83:166–72.
68. Packer RJ. Chemotherapy: low-grade gliomas of the hypothalamus and thalamus. Pediatr Neurosurg 2000;32:259–63.
69. Farmer JP, Montes JL, Freeman CR, et al. Brainstem gliomas. a 10-year institutional review. Pediatr Neurosurg 2001;34:206–14.
70. Mandell LR, Kadota R, Freeman C, et al. There is no role for hyperfractionated radiotherapy in the management of children with newly diagnosed diffuse intrinsic brainstem tumors: results of a pediatric oncology group phase III trial comparing conventional vs. hyperfractionated radiotherapy. Int J Radiat Oncol Biol Phys 1999;43:959–64.
71. Rubin G, Michowitz S, Horev G, et al. Pediatric brain stem gliomas: an update. Childs Nerv Syst 1998;14:167–73.
72. Rickert CH, Paulus W. Epidemiology of central nervous system tumors in childhood and adolescence based on the new WHO classification. Childs Nerv Syst 2001;17:503–11.
73. Undjian S, Marinov M, Georgiev K. Long-term follow-up after surgical treatment of cerebellar astrocytomas in 100 children. Childs Nerv Syst 1989;5:99–101.
74. Kayama T, Tominaga T, Yoshimoto T. Management of pilocytic astrocytoma. Neurosurg Rev 1996;19:217–20.
75. Robertson PL, Zeltzer PM, Boyett JM, et al. Survival and prognostic factors following radiation therapy and chemotherapy for ependymoma in children: a report of the Children's Cancer Group. J of Neurosurg 1998;88:695–703.
76. Horn B, Heideman R, Geyer R, et al. A multi-institutional retrospective study of intracranial ependymoma in children: identification of risk factors. J Pediatr Hematol Oncol 1999;21:203–11.

77. Merchant TE, Jenkins JJ, Burger PC, et al. Influence of tumor grade on time to progression after irradiation for localized ependymoma in children. Int J Radiat Oncol Biol Phys 2002;53:52–7.
78. Bouffet E, Perilongo G, Canete A, et al. Intracranial ependymomas in children: a critical review of prognostic factors and a plea for cooperation. Med Pediatr Oncol 1998;30:319–29.
79. Pollack IF, Gerszten PC, Martinez AJ, et al. Intracranial ependymomas of childhood: long-term outcome and prognostic factors. Neurosurgery 1995;37: 655–66.
80. Merchant TE, Mulhern RK, Krasin MJ, et al. Preliminary results from a phase II trial of conformal radiation therapy and evaluation of radiation-related CNS effects for pediatric patients with localized ependymoma. J Clin Oncol 2004; 22:3156–62.
81. Needle MN, Goldwein JW, Grass J, et al. Adjuvant chemotherapy for the treatment of intracranial ependymoma of childhood. Cancer 1997;80:341–7.
82. Massimino M, Giangaspero F, Garre ML, et al. Salvage treatment for childhood ependymoma after surgery only: pitfalls of omitting at once adjuvant treatment. Int J Radiat Oncol Biol Phys 2006;65(4):1440–5.
83. Grill J, Le Lelay Mc, Gambarell D, et al. Postoperative chemotherapy without irradiation for ependymoma in children under 5 years of age: a multicenter trial of the French Society of Pediatric Oncology. J Clin Oncol 2001;19:1288–96.
84. Müller HL, Albanese A, Calaminus G, et al. Consensus and perspectives on treatment strategies in childhood craniopharyngioma: results of a meeting of the craniopharyngioma study group (SIOP), Genova, 2004. J Pediatr Endocrinol Metab 2006;19:453–4.
85. Puget S, Garnett M, Wray A, et al. Pediatric craniopharyngiomas: classification and treatment according to the degree of hypothalamic involvement. J Neurosurg 2007;106(Peds 1):3–12.
86. Sands SA, Milner JS, Goldberg J, et al. Quality of life and behavioral follow-up study of pediatric survivors of craniopharyngioma. J Neurosurg 2005;103(Peds 4):302–11.
87. Merchant TE, Kiehna EN, Kun LE, et al. Phase II trial of conformal radiation therapy for pediatric patients with craniopharyngioma and correlation of surgical factors and radiation dosimetry with change in cognitive function. J Neurosurg 2006;104(Peds 2):94–102.
88. Kobayashi T, Kida Y, Mori Y, et al. Long-term results of gamma knife surgery for the treatment of craniopharyngioma in 98 consecutive cases. J Neurosurg 2005; 102(Peds 6):428–88.
89. Cáceres A. Intracavitary therapeutic options in the management of cystic craniopharyngioma. Childs Nerv Syst 2005;21:705–18.
90. Müller HL, Bruhnken G, Emser A, et al. Longitudinal study on quality of life in 102 survivors of childhood craniopharyngioma. Childs Nerv Syst 2005;21:975–80.
91. Balmaceda C, Modak S, Finlay J. Central nervous system germ cell tumors. Semin Oncol 1998;25(2):243–50.
92. Packer RJ, Cohen BH, Cooney K. Intracranial germ cell tumors. Oncologist 2000;5:312–20.
93. Legido A, Packer RJ, Sutton LN, et al. Suprasellar germinomas in childhood. A reappraisal. Cancer 1989;63:340–4.
94. Bamberg M, Kortmann RD, Calaminus G, et al. Radiation therapy for intracranial germinoma: results of the German cooperative prospective trials MAKEI 83/86/ 89. J Clin Oncol 1999;17:2585–92.

95. Bouffet E, Baranzelli MC, Patte C, et al. Combined treatment modality for intracranial germinomas: results of a multicentre SFOP experience. Sociéét Francaise d'Oncologie Pédiatrique. Br J Cancer 1999;79:1199–204.

96. Balmaceda C, heller G, Rosenblum M, et al. Chemotherapy without irradiation—a novel approach for newly diagnosed CNS germ cell tumors: results of an international cooperative trial. The First International Central Nervous System Germ Cell Tumor Study. J Clin Oncol 1996;14:2908–15.

97. Yoshida J, Sugita K, Kobayashi T. Treatment of intracranial germ cell tumors: effectiveness of chemotherapy with cisplatin and etoposide (CDDP and VP16). Acta Neurochir (Wien) 1993;120:111–7.

98. Berger C, Thiesse P, Lellouch-Tubiana A, et al. Choroid plexus carcinoma in childhood: clinical features and prognostic factors. Neurosurgery 1998;42:470–5.

99. Pencalet P, Sainte-Rose C, Lellouch-tubiana A, et al. Papillomas and carcinomas of the choroid plexus in children. J Neurosurg 1998;88:521–8.

100. McEvoy AW, Harding BN, Phipps KP, et al. Management of choroid plexus tumours in children: 20 years experience at a single neurosurgical center. Pediatr Neurosurg 2000;32:192–9.

101. Merchant TE, Kiehna EN, Thompson SJ, et al. Pediatric low-grade and ependymal spinal cord tumors. Pediatr Neurosurg 2000;32:30–6.

102. Epstein F, Constantini S. Spinal cord tumors of childhood. In: Pang D, editor. Disorders of the pediatric spine. New York: Raven Press; 1995. p. 55–76.

103. Constantini S, Miller DC, Allen JC, et al. Radical excision of intramedullary spinal cord tumors: surgical morbidity and long-term follow-up evaluation in 164 children and young adults. J Neurosurg 2000;93:183–93.

104. Bouffet E, Pierre-Kahn A, Marchal JC, et al. Prognostic factors in pediatric spinal cord astrocytoma. Cancer 1998;83:2391–9.

Cancer Immunotherapy: Will Expanding Knowledge Lead to Success in Pediatric Oncology?

Terry J. Fry, MD[a],*, Arjan C. Lankester, MD, PhD[b]

KEYWORDS

- Cancer vaccines • Adoptive cell transfer • T cells • NK cells
- B cells • Tumor immunity

The initial use of immunotherapy for cancer occurred in the early 1900s when Coley[1] used bacterial products to treat patients who had Ewing sarcoma based on the observation that postoperative infections seemed to diminish the likelihood of tumor recurrence. A number of patients were treated with these bacterial products, resulting in regression in a few.[2] James Ewing was simultaneously testing radiation as a means to treat these sarcomas, and controversy as to which approach was superior ensued. The consistency in response seen with radiation led to this treatment being more widely accepted, and the field of immunotherapy would need to wait approximately 50 years until it was explored further. The past 25 years have seen an increase in our understanding of immunology and further expansion in the clinical use of immunotherapeutic modalities. How immunotherapy will be integrated with chemotherapy, radiation, and surgery remains to be established. Although there have been successes in the field of immunotherapy, they have been inconsistent, and it is hoped that increased understanding of the basic principles of immunology will improve the consistency of beneficial effects. In this article, we briefly provide a general overview of our current understanding of the immune system, with a focus on concepts in tumor immunology, followed by a discussion of how these concepts are being used in the

A version of this article was previously published in the *Pediatric Clinics of North America*, 55:1.
[a] Division, Blood/Marrow Transplantation and Immunology, Center for Cancer and Blood Disorders, Children's National Medical Center, 111 Michigan Avenue, NW, Washington, DC 10010, USA
[b] Department of Pediatrics, BMT-Unit, Leiden University Medical Center, Leiden, the Netherlands
* Corresponding author.
E-mail address: tfry@cnmc.org (T.J. Fry).

Hematol Oncol Clin N Am 24 (2010) 109–127
doi:10.1016/j.hoc.2009.11.010
0889-8588/10/$ – see front matter © 2010 Elsevier Inc. All rights reserved.

clinic. Although this overview illustrates the highly integrated nature of the immune system, we divide the clinical section into specific arms of the immune response. It is likely that, as with the natural immune response, immunotherapy is most effective when the components of the immune armamentarium are used in combination.

PRINCIPLES OF THE IMMUNE RESPONSE

The immune system evolved to protect the host from invading pathogens. These processes can effectively clear aberrant self-antigens, including malignant cells.[3] A complete description of the immune response is beyond the scope of this article, but we highlight areas relevant to cancer immunotherapy. In general, the immune system can be divided into the innate response, which allows rapid, nonspecific protection, and the adaptive response, which develops more slowly but provides specific recognition of antigens via expression of carefully rearranged receptors. **Fig. 1** illustrates the various components of the immune response. Although the innate system is an essential part of successful immune clearance, this article focuses on adaptive immunity.

The adaptive immune system contains millions of potential specificities requiring amplification upon initial antigen encounter, which results in delayed onset but allows for a memory effect such that subsequent exposures to antigen result in a more rapid

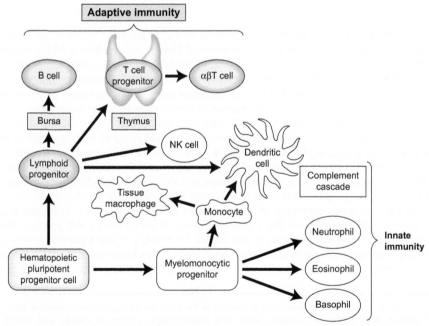

Fig. 1. The immune response can be divided into innate and adaptive components. The innate system provides rapid and relatively nonspecific protection, whereas the adaptive response is delayed but more specific. Innate and adaptive responses are critical for effective immunity, although each plays more or less prominent roles depending on the nature of the immune response (viral, bacterial, etc). Monocytes/macrophages, neutrophils, basophils, and eosinophils serve as the primary players in innate immunity. B cells and αβ T cells represent the central components of adaptive immunity. NK cells are generally considered a member of the innate response, although there is some specificity to NK cell recognition.

clearance. One potential danger of this type of system is the recognition of self-antigens resulting in autoimmunity. To prevent this, a number of strategies have evolved, including central deletion of specificities directed against self-antigens (in the thymus for T cells); the development of a complex network of regulatory cell types that maintain tolerance to self-antigens in the periphery (outside the thymus); and the requirement for professional antigen-presenting cells, such as dendritic cells (DCs), to effectively initiate the adaptive immune response. DCs are capable of sensing, filtering, and interpreting signals for the adaptive immune cells, providing an important link between the innate and adaptive immune response.[4]

T Cells and B Cells

Developing T cells and B cells rearrange germline DNA to generate receptors that are maintained throughout subsequent progeny and are capable of recognizing specific antigens. For B cells, gene rearrangement initially occurs in the bone marrow, with further rearrangements possible in the germinal center of the lymph node during maturation of the immune response after antigen encounter. For T cells, this process occurs in the thymus, where specificities are selected on the basis of recognition of self–human leukocyte antigens (HLAs) followed by deletion of T cells with high affinity for self-antigens. Although this process is complex and results in loss of greater than 95% of all rearranged T cells in the thymus, it allows for sufficient repertoire to protect throughout the lifespan of the host without causing autoimmunity in most individuals. Naive T cells and B cells circulate in a resting state until they encounter an antigen that binds to the specific receptor expressed on the surface of a responding cell. For T cells, this antigen is presented in the context of self HLA molecules on specialized antigen-presenting cells (APCs), such as DCs. CD4+ T cells recognize antigen in the context of HLA class II molecules, and for CD8+ T cells this recognition occurs on HLA class I molecules. Effective stimulation of the immune response also requires a second costimulatory signal provided by the APCs. The nature of a costimulatory signal (positive, negative, and how strong) is modulated by factors sensed by the APCs, such as bacterial products or inflammatory substances produced during the innate immune response (also referred to as "danger signals".[4]) An important group of receptors known as toll-like receptors (TLRs) recognizes these products and modulates the capacity for the APCs to stimulate a T-cell response, thus demonstrating one important link between innate and adaptive immunity.[5] Once activated, T and B lymphocytes undergo rapid clonal expansion, providing large numbers of effectors. T cells mediate an immune response via direct cytotoxicity of the target cell (perforin, granzyme, fas/fasL) or by secretion of effector cytokines, such as interferons, whereas B cells differentiate into antibody-secreting plasma cells. T and B lymphocytes also "talk" to other immune cells (innate and adaptive) by secretion of cytokines or through expression of surface molecules, resulting in further refinement in the immune response. Cytokines such as interleukin (IL)-2, IL-7, or IL-15 have been administered in clinical and preclinical studies to enhance antitumor immune responses.[6–8] In addition, agents that interfere with regulatory signals generated by surface receptors on responding immune cells, such as CTLA-4 (a negative regulator of T-cell immunity), have been used in patients who have cancer and who have demonstrated clinical activity.[9] **Fig. 2** demonstrates a schematic of the immune response.

An important subset of T cells generated in the thymus acquires a regulatory phenotype before export into the periphery, providing further protection against autoimmunity.[10] These naturally occurring regulatory T cells (Tregs) can be identified by expression of CD4 and CD25 (a component of the IL-2 receptor), low or absent expression of the IL-7 receptor, and the FoxP3 transcription factor. There is a subset

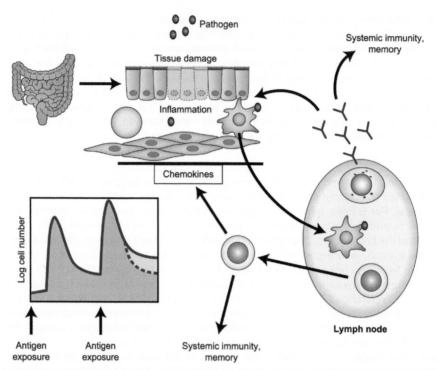

Fig. 2. Representation of the immune response to a gut pathogen. Initial pathogen-induced tissue damage results in invasion of submucosa by the pathogen and the generation of inflammation mediated, in part by the initial innate response. DCs resident in the gut acquire pathogen-derived antigens and signals from the inflammatory environment, resulting in further activation. The loaded and activated DCs migrate to the lymph node and initiate antigen-specific B-cell activation. B cells secrete antibodies directed against pathogen-derived antigens and activated T cells with pathogen specificity traffic to the gut directed, in part, by chemokines. Inset: Graphical representation of sequential adaptive immune responses to the same antigen. The response to the initial encounter is delayed, followed by a rapid amplification and subsequent contraction. The response does not return to initial baseline, instead remaining at a higher-level reflective of memory, which allows for a more rapid response upon subsequent encounter. One principal of vaccination against infections or tumors is that repeated boosting results in greater and greater amplification and a larger memory pool. Responses to tumors likely follow a similar pattern, although there is the added complexity of immune evasion as described in the section on immune escape.

of Tregs that can be induced during an immune response that may express the CD4 or CD8 co-receptor.[10] Our growing understanding of Tregs has led to the recognition that these cells may be detrimental to an effective antitumor immune response, particularly when the antigens targeted are self-antigens for which these regulatory networks are well developed.[11] Current immunotherapeutic protocols are exploring depletion or the modulation of Tregs as a means to enhance adaptive immune responses.[12]

Natural Killer Cells

Natural killer (NK) cells are bone-marrow–derived lymphocytes that do not bear clonally rearranged antigen-specific receptors. In humans, NK cells are phenotypically defined as CD3$^-$/CD56$^+$ lymphocytes, which can be divided into CD56^{dim} (CD16$^+$) cytotoxic and CD56^{bright} immunoregulatory NK-cell subsets.[13] NK cells have the potential to recognize and eliminate a wide range of tumors and virally infected cells. Besides acting as cytotoxic effector cells in immune responses, evidence is accumulating that NK cells play a crucial role in the translation of signals from innate toward adaptive immunity via bidirectional interaction with DCs.[14] Recent evidence indicates that type I interferon (IFN)-experienced DCs prime NK cells in an IL-15–dependent manner.[15] Primed NK cells can promote maturation of DCs in an IFN-γ–dependent manner, thereby facilitating further induction of T$_{H1}$ (cellular) T-cell responses.[16,17] Therefore, NK cells may exert a dual function in antitumor responses by acting as direct effector cells and as initiators of T-cell–mediated antitumor responses.[18]

The functional status of NK cells is regulated by the balance of inhibitory and activating NK-cell ligands on the target cells. Inhibitory signals are provided by classical and nonclassical HLA class I molecules, which bind to killer immunoglobulin- like receptors (KIRs) or NKG2A/CD94 on NK cells.[19] Within the human population, there is a wide variation in the repertoire of KIR genes. Together with the clonal distribution within the NK repertoire, this results in a wide diversity of expression profiles between and within individuals.

The inhibitory signals can be decreased in patients who have solid tumors caused by a down-regulation of HLA class I on the tumor cells (see "Immune escape"). Lack of HLA-dependent inhibitory signals may permit recognition and elimination of tumor cells by NK cells according to mechanism of "missing self" recognition.[20] In addition, interaction between NK-cell–activating receptors and their specific ligands on target cells seems necessary for adequate NK cell stimulation.[21] NK cells can be triggered by stress-induced ligands that are expressed by the tumor itself, such as the MIC (MICA/B) and ULBP (ULBP1-4) family of proteins. The expression of these molecules on tumors can be induced by DNA damage. The activating receptor NKG2D on the NK cell can bind to these ligands and lead to an activating signal.[22] Other activating NK cell receptors include the DNAX accessory molecule-1, which is activated by the CD112 (Nectin-2) and CD155 (PVR) molecules.[23] A third group of activating receptors is represented by the natural cytotoxicity receptors NKp30, NKp44, and NKp46. Their physiologic ligands remain to be identified.[14]

Many preclinical studies have provided evidence that a broad spectrum of human and murine tumor cell lines are susceptible to NK-cell cytotoxicity, albeit with different efficacy. The variation in NK-cell susceptibility seems related to differences in expression levels of the aforementioned activating and inhibitory ligands on tumor cells.[24,25] In addition to tumor cell lines, NK cells have been shown to have the potential to eliminate or prevent outgrowth of murine tumors in in vivo models.[26] In humans, the clinical significance of NK cells in the control of solid tumors is unresolved and is the subject of many studies.

NK-cell activation and cytolytic potential can be increased upon stimulation with various cytokines (eg, IL-2, IL-12, and IL-15) and type I IFN.[27] In various clinical trials, in vivo administration of some of these agents has been used to induce NK-cell–mediated antitumor responses with limited clinical efficacy.[28] Further insight in the role of these agents in NK cell regulation will provide tools to manipulate NK-cell function and will be of benefit in future adoptive transfer studies.

Another dimension of NK tumor target recognition may be seen in an allogeneic setting where a KIR–HLA mismatch between donor and patient may result in the absence of tumor cells of ligands for inhibitory KIR on donor NK cells. In this setting of "missing self-recognition," the available alloreactive donor NK-cell repertoire may be exploited to eliminate recipient tumor cells. Combined with the preferential expression of activating NK-cell ligands on malignant cells, this might result in a selective elimination of these targets without the risk of inducing concurrent graft-versus-host disease (GvHD). The first evidence for the clinical implication of this model has been reported by Ruggeri and colleagues in patients who have acute myeloid leukemia undergoing haploidentical stem cell transplantation.[29] In their experience, KIR-HLA mismatch was associated with a better clinical outcome, lower relapse rate, and reduced frequency of GvHD.[30] In subsequent studies, conflicting results have been reported on the advantage of KIR-HLA that may be related to the level of T-cell depletion and the repertoire of alloreactive donor NK cells.[31] Further insight into reconstitution, regulation, and functional properties of the (alloreactive) NK-cell repertoire after allogeneic stem cell transplantation (SCT) is needed to optimize exploitation of its potential. Altogether, the mode of action of NK cells indicates that they have the potential to exert potent antitumor immunity and may act complementary to and in synergy with T cells.

Immune Escape

As first proposed by Burnett,[32] tumors are not passive targets for cellular immune responses and are capable of escaping from and disabling the host immune system.[3,15] Changes in tumor phenotype not only permit tumor escape from normal immunologic surveillance but may also negatively influence the susceptibility and response to antitumor immunotherapy. In the setting of clinically established tumors, initial immune surveillance has failed to eliminate tumor cells. Immune pressure may have resulted in the generation of immune escape variants via the mechanism of immuno-editing.[33,34] General mechanisms of immune escape include interference with specific recognition of tumors by the immune system, reduced susceptibility of tumors to the apoptosis-inducing capacity of cytotoxic effector cells, and immunosuppressive potential of the tumor. These mechanisms have been described in detail elsewhere[35,36] and are therefore only be briefly discussed here.

Immune Cell Recognition of Tumors

Appropriate expression of HLA/peptide complexes on tumor cells plays a crucial role in the effector phase of cellular immunotherapy because they present antigenic epitopes to CTLs. A commonly known mechanism of immune escape involves impaired antigen processing or presentation. Total or selective loss of HLA I expression has been reported in a large variety of human tumors, including sarcomas, carcinomas, and lymphomas. The clinical relevance has been demonstrated by the observation that a lack of HLA expression often relates to metastatic disease and an unfavorable outcome.[37] The basis of aberrant HLA expression has been reported to be genetic, regulatory, or epigenetic in origin. Lack of HLA expression in tumors may be caused by loss of heterozygosity, mutations, or deletions in individual HLA genes and in genes encoding β2 microglobulin and components of the antigen-processing machinery, including peptide transporters TAP1 and TAP2, tapasin, and the proteosomal subunits LMP-2 and LMP-7.[38] The aberrant HLA expression pattern in tumors at diagnosis, which may be heterogeneous within individual tumors, indicates that a process of selection pressure has occurred. Evidence that immune surveillance and immune pressure may result in selective outgrowth of tumor variants has come from observations in clinical trials in which progressive disease after cellular immunotherapy revealed total or allelic loss of HLA expression.[39–41]

Recently, a unique category of CTLs has been identified in mice bearing TAP-deficient tumors. These tumors were found to express peptides derived from self-antigens in the context of classical and nonclassical MHC class I molecules, named T-cell epitopes, associated with impaired peptide processing, which may serve as alternative tumor-specific CTL targets.[42] Together with conventional tumor-specific T cells, T cell epitopes associated with impaired peptide processing (TEIPP)-specific CTLs might be considered in future studies to prevent outgrowth of or treat TAP-deficient tumors.

In addition to genetic causes, aberrant HLA expression may be the result of transcriptional regulation. During normal immune responses, HLA class I and II expression is strictly orchestrated and mediated by several immune regulators, including IFN-γ and TNF-α,[43] that have the potential to increase HLA expression in a variety of HLA-deficient tumor cell lines. Another possible mechanism responsible for transcriptional regulation of HLA expression is represented by epigenetic modifications, including histone acetylation and DNA methylation. Treatment with histone deacetylase inhibitors and methyltransferase inhibitors has been demonstrated to restore HLA expression in a variety of tumors and hematologic malignancies.[44] Whether this category of agents, which has been used as anticancer therapy in clinical trials, may be beneficial in future clinical immunotherapy studies remains to be resolved.

Tumors may specifically down-regulate expression of CTL tumor target antigens, which result in antigenic loss variants.[45] The clinical significance of this mechanism has been clearly observed in immunotherapy trials with patients who have melanoma in whom metastases occurring after treatment were found to selectively lack expression of CTL target antigens.[46] This illustrates the biological mechanism that selective pressure has the potential to generate immune escape variants. In addition, it shows that antigen-specific therapies, although elegant, may be vulnerable to the process of immune editing, especially in cases where tumor target antigens are used that are not essential for tumor biology and survival. Another potential hurdle for antigen-specific therapy is the often heterogeneous expression of target antigens, such as cancer-testis antigens, within individual tumors. Epigenetic regulation has been found to play a significant role in the expression of these genes, and treatment with the aforementioned hypomethylating agents has the potential to restore or increase expression, which may be beneficial in future immunotherapy studies.[47]

Although partial or complete loss of HLA/peptide complex expression impairs T-cell–mediated recognition, it may increase susceptibility to NK cells, which may be inhibited by self-HLA (see section on NK cells). Aberrant expression on the tumor of the ligands for NK-cell–activating receptors or expression of HLA-surrogate molecules can protect tumor cells from NK-cell–mediated recognition and killing. Several mechanisms leading to this so-called "NK-cell tolerance" have been described. First, sustained expression of its ligand induced down-regulation of NKG2D in a murine tumor model,[48] resulting in increased tumorigenesis. This process seemed to be reversible by stimulating innate immunity through TLRs. Similarly, expression of natural cytotoxicity receptors was found to be reduced in patients who have acute myelogenous leukemia (AML) compared with healthy control subjects, which was in part reversible by cytokine stimulation.[49] Second, NKG2D expression and consequent NK-cell (but also T-cell) function may be blocked and thus impaired by tumor-derived soluble ligands, as reported for soluble MICA in various human tumors.[50] Third, expression of the nonclassical HLA-E and G molecules on tumors has the potential to inhibit NK-cell function via interaction with their respective receptors.[51,52] A fourth potential mechanism is the aberrant expression of NK co-receptors and (soluble) adhesion molecules, which may prevent a functional interaction.[38]

Tumor Susceptibility to Immune Cell-mediated Killing

Interference with the induction of apoptosis is a frequently observed phenomenon in tumors and may be caused by a variety of mechanisms. This article focuses on the mechanisms directly related to the mode of action used by cytotoxic effector lympho-cytes and particularly those reported in human tumors. Tumor cells may interfere with the cytolytic pathways used by NK and T cells by overexpression of antiapoptotic genes or by down-regulation of proapoptotic molecules.

Overexpression of serine protease-inhibitor 9 has been shown to irreversibly inacti-vate GrB, resulting in defective apoptosis in tumor cell lines via the granule exocytosis pathway. The clinical significance has been suggested by the correlation between protease inhibitor–9 overexpression and clinical outcome in lymphomas and the outcome after tumor vaccination in patients who have melanoma.[53,54] Escape from death receptor (DR)-mediated apoptosis by overexpression of cellular FLICE inhibitory protein, which is a catalytic inactive homolog of procaspase 8, has been demon-strated in various types of tumors in vitro and in vivo.[27,28] Negatively affecting the same pathway, lack of caspase 8 expression has been reported to interfere with DR-mediated apoptosis in several human tumors and to favor formation of metastases.[55,56]

Other possible mechanisms to escape from DR pathway–mediated apoptosis include the expression of soluble (eg, soluble CD95[57]); and decoy receptors (eg, DcR 3[58]); and the presence of mutations in proteins involved in the DR cascade that may interfere with DR-mediated apoptosis.[59] Although the presence of these mecha-nisms was found to be correlated with clinical outcome of various tumors, their direct involvement in escape from immune pressure in vivo is remains to be resolved.

Tumor-induced Immune Suppression

It has been extensively reported that cancer patients are often characterized by a general state of decreased immune competence by mechanisms that are only partially understood. These mechanisms have been described in detail in several recent reviews.[15,60] Therefore, only a selection of mechanisms actively induced by the tumor is mentioned here. First, tumors may actively secrete immune suppressive cytokines (eg, IL-10, TGF-β and Indolamine 2,3-Dioxygenase [IDO]) that are able to interfere in various ways with innate and adaptive immune responses. Second, an increased frequency of circulating Tregs and their migration to the tumor environment has been reported in cancer patients.[11] The influx of Tregs in tissue or the surrounding stroma varied among different tumor types and between individuals. An association between Tregs numbers and clinical behavior (progressive disease) was first described in ovarian cancer patients.[61] The immunosuppressive effect induced by Tregs involves several potential mechanisms mediated via soluble factors and direct cell–cell contact as described in the previous sections on T-cell–mediated responses. Third, tumors have the potential to attract myeloid suppressor cells that may exert multiple inhibitory functions, including suppression of tumor infiltrated lymphocytes.[62] Fourth, down-regulation of T-cell receptor signaling molecules that may be reversible upon removal of the tumor has been reported in cancer patients.[63]

Lymphocyte Migration

For cellular immunotherapy to be effective, migration of effector T or NK cells to the tumor site, extravasation, and invasion into the tumor are pivotal. The presence of and variability in the amount of tumor-infiltrating lymphocytes (TILs) have been re-ported in many human tumors. In some studies, the presence of these TILs was re-ported to be correlated with the pattern of HLA expression. Recent studies in colorectal, ovarian, and cervical tumors have shown that the phenotypical profile of the TIL at diagnosis was a strong predictor of clinical outcome.[64–66] Particularly, the CD8/Treg ratio was found to be positively correlated with a favorable prognosis. These findings illustrate that insight into the molecular mechanisms involved in tumor site–directed migration are important to the understanding of the quantitative and qualitative differences in the naturally occurring TIL responses. This provides knowledge required to develop strategies to manipulate the natural immune response and to support (adoptive) immunotherapy interventions.

Site-directed migration of T/NK cells is a nonrandom process induced by inflammatory and other pathogenic stimuli. In lymphoid and in inflamed nonlymphoid tissues, lymphocyte adherence and tissue influx are facilitated by specialized high-endothelial venules (HEVs). HEVs express various adhesion molecules (eg, VCAM-1 and ICAM-1) and chemokines (eg, CCL21, CXCL9, and CXCL25), which create a highly regulated interface between lymphocytes and endothelial cells.[67] In contrast, intratumoral vessels are characterized by squamous endothelial cells with low expression of these molecules.[68] Generally, lymphocyte extravasation at the tumor site is limited. Significant differences have been reported between intratumoral- (low) and peritumoral- (dense) vessel lymphocyte extravasation. The molecular basis for these differences remains to be resolved, but a regulatory role has been suggested for pro- and antiangiogenic factors (eg, vascular endothelial growth factor), anti-inflammatory cytokines (eg, TGF-β), and the tumor cells themselves.[69] Transformation of squamous "nonattractive" tumor vessel endothelium into endothelial cells with a HEV-like appearance could have a beneficial effect on lymphocyte migration at the tumor site. Potential approaches include stimulation with inflammatory mediators (eg, TLR ligands), ionizing irradiation, and transgenic expression of recruiting cytokines.[70]

Chemokines are a superfamily of small molecules that regulate this selective process of migration. Directional migration of T/NK cells expressing the appropriate chemokine receptor(s) occurs along a chemical gradient of ligand(s).[71] In cancer, chemokines produced by the tumor may play a role in the pattern of leukocyte infiltration.[72] Several recent studies on human tumors have provided evidence for the significance of tumor-secreted chemokines on TIL responses and clinical outcome. Immune stimulatory and inhibitory effects have been proposed depending on the extent and by which cells the chemokines are produced in the tumor environment.[71,72] Identification of the relevant chemokines involved in the attraction of cytotoxic effector T or NK cells and Tregs combined with insight in the patterns of expression and regulation of these chemokines in human tumors may provide tools to manipulate the attractive capacity of the tumor and thereby improve the process of tumor-site–directed migration during T/NK-cell–mediated immunotherapy studies.

CLINICAL EXPERIENCE WITH IMMUNE-BASED THERAPIES FOR CANCER
T-cell Therapy

A number of strategies have been developed to use T cells as immunotherapeutic tools against tumors. Adoptive therapies involve the infusion of large numbers of T cells into patients (autologous or allogeneic). Vaccine therapy attempts to expand T cells, recognizing tumor associated antigens in vivo. Finally, cytokines have been used alone or combined with other strategies to expand or enhance the function of antitumor T cells.

Autologous

The use of autologous T cells to target malignancy can involve the infusion of manipulated or unmanipulated T cells or the administration of vaccines to expand tumor-reactive T cells in vivo. The existence of tumor-specific or tumor-associated antigens that can be targeted using these approaches has been clearly demonstrated.[73] The majority of these antigens are self-antigens expressed during a restricted period of development or in restricted tissues. Therefore, the process of inducing effective anti-tumor T-cell immunity requires that the self-tolerance mechanisms previously described be overcome.[10,74] This has presented one of the major obstacles to effective T-cell–based therapies.

For adoptive T-cell therapies, the source can be peripheral blood T cells or tumor-infiltrating T cells, which can then be harvested and reinfused into patients. T cells reactive against tumor antigens are present but infrequent in the blood of cancer patients. Although these T cells may be present at higher frequency in tumor infiltrates, the total number of cells that can be harvested is insufficient. Thus, effective adoptive immunotherapy requires manipulation and expansion in vitro to increase the frequency of T-cell–recognizing tumor antigens in the infused product. This approach has been used in the clinic and has resulted in regression in patients who have melanoma. A number of other clinical trials using adoptive immunotherapy have been undertaken, some demonstrating clinical benefit.[75] The experience of Dudley and colleagues[76] suggested that regression required that extremely high doses of T cells be infused such that a high percentage of circulating T cells recognized the tumor (~20–30%). These important findings indicate proof of the principle that, at least for melanoma, adoptive T-cell therapies represent a promising immunotherapeutic modality.[77,78] An alternative method to overcome the low frequency of tumor reactive T cells in autologous products that is being explored is gene transfer of T-cell receptors known to recognize tumor antigens into cells with cytotoxic potential, such as T cells or NK cells.[79–81] Although there has been much progress in the area of autologous adoptive immunotherapy for cancer in adults, there are limited data in pediatric patients.[82]

Another approach that can be used alone or in combination with adoptive T-cell therapy is the use of vaccines to expand tumor-reactive T cells. The types of vaccines used include whole tumor cells, peptides derived from known tumor antigens, replication-deficient viruses expressing tumor antigens, and DCs loaded with tumor antigens.[83] A large and growing number of clinical trials have been undertaken using each of these vaccine strategies resulting in vaccine responses and some evidence of clinical response, but the potency and consistency of these responses has been poor.[84,85] Most of these trials have been undertaken in the setting of bulky tumors where immune-based therapies may be less effective due to the tumor suppressive mechanisms discussed previously. Furthermore, the magnitude of the immune response generated by vaccines alone suggests that combining vaccines with adoptive therapies or T-cell–active cytokines may be necessary. Another strategy is the use of adjuvants to amplify weak vaccine-induced T-cell responses. There is the most clinical experience with Freund's adjuvant, but newer agents are being explored that specifically target innate immune cells via TLRs.[86,87] It is likely that effective vaccination protocols will need to incorporate multiple strategies to generate sufficient immune responses to induce clinically meaningful responses.[88] As with adoptive immunotherapy, experience in pediatrics is limited, but there has been one promising clinical response in pediatric sarcoma.[89–92]

Allogeneic

Perhaps the most potent form of immune-based therapy is the graft-versus-tumor reaction that occurs after allogeneic transplantation.[93] T cells and NK cells contribute to this response. The T-cell contribution is evident from the increased risk of relapse that occurs after transplantation of stem cell products that are depleted of T lymphocytes and when patients are treated with T-cell immunosuppressants. For chronic myeloid leukemia (CML) that recurs after transplant, remissions can be induced in up 50% or more of patients by stopping immunosupression or infusing donor lympho-cytes (DLI).[94] For AML, responses to donor lymphocyte infusions occur, but the frequency of responses is substantially lower than for CML ($\sim$20–30%). For pediatric acute lymphocytic leukemia, 5-year disease-free survival after allogeneic transplanta-tion ranges from approximately 40% to 80%, depending on risk status and type of donor used.[95] If relapse occurs, the poor response to immune manipulation suggests that the graft-versus-leukemia effect is far less potent than for AML or CML, although the reasons for this are not clear. Acute lymphocytic leukemia blasts are inferior at initi-ating immune responses but are susceptible to autologous T-cell–mediated immune responses.[96] Thus, for the most common form of pediatric leukemia, strategies to enhance the graft-versus-leukemia response are needed if outcomes are to be improved.

The effectiveness of the graft-versus-malignancy response is, to a large extent, due to the ability to target minor histocompatibility antigens that are disparate between the donor and recipient because these antigens do not require the immune response to overcome tolerance to self-antigens.[97] Another advantage of allogeneic transplant is the availability of donor-immune cells that have not been depleted or exposed to cytotoxic therapy and are not contaminated by tumor cells. Finally, it is possible that tumor restricted immune responses induced in the allogeneic transplant environ-ment may be more potent than similar responses induced using the autologous envi-ronment. Thus, there are a number of potential benefits in considering allogeneic transplantation as a platform for immune-based therapies.

The main hurdle to overcome when using allogeneic transplantation as immuno-therapy is the induction of GvHD. Most of the available approaches to enhance graft-versus-tumor reactions are nonspecific, such that the antitumor reaction is closely linked to GvHD. The use of strategies such as vaccines[98,99] or adoptive therapy with antitumor T-cell–enriched donor lymphocytes may be potential mecha-nisms to overcome this hurdle. An alternative would be to develop strategies to selec-tively modulate alloresponses against GvHD target organs. For example, selective depletion of alloreactive T cells in vitro before infusion of stem cells has been explored in preclincical and clinical settings.[100–102] The ability to manipulate the post-transplant environment to enhance the graft-versus-malignancy reaction would result in less reli-ance on pretransplant conditioning for cure, potentially allowing the use of reduced-intensity conditioning regimens, which have been used successfully for pediatric nonmalignant diseases and adult malignancies. Given the long-term morbidity associated with myeloablative transplantation for pediatric patients, this would be a desirable scenario.

Natural Killer Cell Therapy

Autologous
The first studies in this field were performed in the 1980s by the Rosenberg team.[103] Autologous IL-2/lymphokine-activated killer cells, combined with high-dose IL-2 in vivo, were used to treat cancer patients who had refractory disease, including melanoma and renal cell carcinoma.

In subsequent years, many more patients were included in similar studies receiving lymphokine activated killer cells combined with IL-2 or IL-2 alone, resulting in a response rate of 10% to 20%.[104] The limited efficacy and substantial toxicity of this approach together with the identification of tumor antigens as targets has shifted attention to T-cell–mediated strategies. Progress in our understanding of NK-cell biology and the aforementioned implications of KIR-HLA (mis)matching in allogeneic

SCT have resulted in renewed attention for the clinical application of allogeneic NK-cell–mediated immunotherapy strategies.

Allogeneic

The use of haploidentical NK cells in a nontransplant setting was first explored by Miller and colleagues[105] in patients who had refractory hematologic malignancies and solid tumors. For this purpose, NK-cell preparations were obtained from leukapheresis products using immunomagnetic CD3 depletion followed by overnight IL-2 stimulation. From this and subsequent studies, they concluded that a high-dose cyclophosphamide/fludarabine regimen was required to obtain long-term survival and expansion of the infused cells. In addition, NK-cell expansion was found to be correlated with endogenous IL-15 levels, which is in agreement with its role in survival and homeostatic proliferation. Infusion of the NK-cell products did not result in GvHD or other toxicity events. Clinical efficacy was demonstrated by achievement of a CR in a subgroup of patients who had AML. This was only observed in the patients receiving high-dose NK-cell treatment and was correlated with KIR–ligand mismatch in the GvHD direction. This and other pilot studies have provided evidence for the safety and feasibility of allogeneic NK-cell infusions.[106] Further studies are required to investigate the antitumor efficacy in vivo and to unravel the relevant mechanisms involved. In addition to primary NK cells, adoptive transfer studies have been performed using the NK cell line NK-92, expressing activating receptors and lacking inhibitory receptors. The use of these cells was found to be safe, and antitumor responses have been observed.[107]

Several important issues remain unresolved and require further study to optimize the clinical use of allogeneic NK-cell preparations.[108] One of these issues includes the technical approach used to obtain a defined number of NK cells from leukapheresis products and to reduce the amount of contaminating alloreactive T cells. Several procedures, including negative (ie, T and B cells) and positive (ie, CD56) selection steps, which are available under clinical grade conditions, are being investigated by several groups. Second, the absolute number and functional status of NK cells required for efficacy needs to be established. Little is known about dose-response ratios and the in vivo behavior of infused NK cells, but it is likely that this is influenced by multiple factors. Miller and colleagues[105] have demonstrated that a leuko/lymphopenia-inducing preparative regimen seems required to permit engraftment and expansion of adoptively transferred NK cells. Substantial evidence obtained from in vitro and in vivo studies indicates that the functional properties and survival of NK-cell populations, including responses toward tumor cells, can be increased after cytokine stimulation. This seems to justify the preferential use of ex vivo–stimulated NK-cell populations. Endogenous production of cytokines that influence NK-cell activation and survival (eg, IL-15) could play a significant role and is probably dependent on the preparative regimen, timing of NK-cell infusion, and postinfusion therapeutic regimens. By definition, the NK-cell repertoire is phenotypically and functionally heterogeneous, implying that significant interindividual differences will probably be encountered when these cells are used in adoptive transfer studies. In the allogeneic KIR-ligand mismatched setting, the interindividual variability in the amount of alloreactive NK cells is an additional factor that may influence outcome.[30] The challenge is to obtain further insight in the impact of all these parameters on clinical immune and antitumor responses in the scheduled and ongoing clinical trials. Given the reported favorable outcome of KIR-ligand mismatched haploidentical SCT in patients who have refractory AML and the apparent safety profile of allogeneic NK-cell infusions, it seems interesting to investigate exploitation of the NK-cell effect in patients who have NK-cell–permissive solid tumors in a similar haploidentical setting.

B Cells

Antibody therapy

Although this review has emphasized cellular therapies, the use of monoclonal antibodies targeting malignancy is rapidly expanding. Although the majority of these antibodies has been developed for adult cancers, some have demonstrated utility in pediatric malignancy.[109] For example, anti-CD20 has been used in pediatric lymphomas. Although this agent may theoretically target CD20-expressing pediatric B-cell leukemias, responses in this setting have been less promising. One difficulty with monoclonal antibodies alone is that, unless they interfere with receptor signaling on which the tumor is dependant, they require a mechanism such as antibody-dependant cytotoxicity to clear tumor cells. To overcome this, a newer generation of antibodies has been conjugated to radioisotopes or toxins to deliver these directly to the tumor.[110,111] A number of these antibodies are in clinical trials in pediatric malignancies.

SUMMARY

Although the immune system has long been recognized as providing a strategy to treat cancer, the full potential of immune-based therapies for malignancy has not been realized. Rapid increases in our understanding of basic immunologic principles and mechanisms by which tumors evade the immune response have served as a basis for improving on these approaches. Current strategies have used numerous arms of the adaptive and innate immune response. It will likely require a multipronged approach incorporating combination therapy to maximize the potential of the immune response against cancer. In addition, it will be important to establish how immunotherapy is to be best integrated into the standard armamentarium of chemotherapy therapy, radiation therapy, and surgery. This will be particularly true for pediatric cancers, where remissions can be induced using standard treatments in the majority of patients and preventing relapse presents the major obstacle to cure. Immunotherapy may ultimately prove most effective in this setting.

REFERENCES

1. Coley WB. Sarcoma of the long bones: the diagnosis, treatment and prognosis, with a report of sixty-nine cases. Ann Surg 1907;45(3):321–68.
2. Brunschwig A. The efficacy of "Coley's Toxin" in the treatment of sarcoma: an experimental study. Ann Surg 1939;109(1):109–13.
3. Dunn GP, Old LJ, Schreiber RD. The immunobiology of cancer immunosurveillance and immunoediting. Immunity 2004;21(2):137–48.
4. Matzinger P. An innate sense of danger. Ann N Y Acad Sci 2002;961:341–2.
5. Iwasaki A, Medzhitov R. Toll-like receptor control of the adaptive immune responses. Nat Immunol 2004;5(10):987–95.
6. Waldmann TA. The biology of interleukin-2 and interleukin-15: implications for cancer therapy and vaccine design. Nat Rev Immunol 2006;6(8):595–601.
7. Fry TJ, Mackall CL. The many faces of IL-7: from lymphopoiesis to peripheral T cell maintenance. J Immunol 2005;174(11):6571–6.
8. Rosenberg SA, Sportes C, Ahmadzadeh M, et al. IL-7 administration to humans leads to expansion of CD8+ and CD4+ cells but a relative decrease of CD4+ T-regulatory cells. J Immunother (1997) 2006;29(3):313–9.

9. Langer LF, Clay TM, Morse MA. Update on anti-CTLA-4 antibodies in clinical trials. Expert Opin Biol Ther 2007;7(8):1245–56.

10. Zou W. Regulatory T cells, tumour immunity and immunotherapy. Nat Rev Immunol 2006;6(4):295–307.

11. Beyer M, Schultze JL. Regulatory T cells in cancer. Blood 2006;108(3):804–11.

12. Banham AH, Powrie FM, Suri-Payer E. FOXP3+ regulatory T cells: current controversies and future perspectives. Eur J Immunol 2006;36(11):2832–6.

13. Cooper MA, Fehniger TA, Caligiuri MA. The biology of human natural killer-cell subsets. Trends Immunol 2001;22(11):633–40.

14. Moretta L, Ferlazzo G, Bottino C, et al. Effector and regulatory events during natural killer-dendritic cell interactions. Immunol Rev 2006;214:219–28.

15. Whiteside TL. Immune suppression in cancer: effects on immune cells, mechanisms and future therapeutic intervention. Semin Cancer Biol 2006;16(1):3–15.

16. Lucas M, Schachterle W, Oberle K, et al. Dendritic cells prime natural killer cells by trans-presenting interleukin 15. Immunity 2007;26(4):503–17.

17. Degli-Esposti MA, Smyth MJ. Close encounters of different kinds: dendritic cells and NK cells take centre stage. Nat Rev Immunol 2005;5(2):112–24.

18. Raulet DH. Interplay of natural killer cells and their receptors with the adaptive immune response. Nat Immunol 2004;5(10):996–1002.

19. Parham P. MHC class I molecules and KIRs in human history, health and survival. Nat Rev Immunol 2005;5(3):201–14.

20. Ljunggren HG, Karre K. In search of the 'missing self': MHC molecules and NK cell recognition. Immunol Today 1990;11(7):237–44.

21. Bryceson YT, March ME, Ljunggren HG, et al. Activation, coactivation, and costimulation of resting human natural killer cells. Immunol Rev 2006;214:73–91.

22. Hayakawa Y, Smyth MJ. NKG2D and cytotoxic effector function in tumor immune surveillance. Semin Immunol 2006;18(3):176–85.

23. Pende D, Bottino C, Castriconi R, et al. PVR (CD155) and Nectin-2 (CD112) as ligands of the human DNAM-1 (CD226) activating receptor: involvement in tumor cell lysis. Mol Immunol 2005;42(4):463–9.

24. Castriconi R, Dondero A, Corrias MV, et al. Natural killer cell-mediated killing of freshly isolated neuroblastoma cells: critical role of DNAX accessory molecule-1-poliovirus receptor interaction. Cancer Res 2004;64(24):9180–4.

25. Pende D, Spaggiari GM, Marcenaro S, et al. Analysis of the receptor-ligand interactions in the natural killer-mediated lysis of freshly isolated myeloid or lymphoblastic leukemias: evidence for the involvement of the Poliovirus receptor (CD155) and Nectin-2 (CD112). Blood 2005;105(5):2066–73.

26. Wu J, Lanier LL. Natural killer cells and cancer. Adv Cancer Res 2003;90: 127–56.

27. Becknell B, Caligiuri MA. Interleukin-2, interleukin-15, and their roles in human natural killer cells. Adv Immunol 2005;86:209–39.

28. Smyth MJ, Cretney E, Kershaw MH, et al. Cytokines in cancer immunity and immunotherapy. Immunol Rev 2004;202:275–93.

29. Ruggeri L, Capanni M, Urbani E, et al. Effectiveness of donor natural killer cell alloreactivity in mismatched hematopoietic transplants. Science 2002; 295(5562):2097–100.

30. Ruggeri L, Mancusi A, Capanni M, et al. Donor natural killer cell allorecognition of missing self in haploidentical hematopoietic transplantation for acute myeloid leukemia: challenging its predictive value. Blood 2007;110(1):433–40.

31. Farag SS, Bacigalupo A, Eapen M, et al. The effect of KIR ligand incompatibility on the outcome of unrelated donor transplantation: a report from the center for

international blood and marrow transplant research, the European blood and marrow transplant registry, and the Dutch registry. Biol Blood Marrow Transplant 2006;12(8):876–84.

32. Burnett FM. The concept of immunological surveillance. Prog Exp Tumor Res 1970;13:1–27.

33. Khong HT, Restifo NP. Natural selection of tumor variants in the generation of "tumor escape" phenotypes. Nat Immunol 2002;3(11):999–1005.

34. Zitvogel L, Tesniere A, Kroemer G. Cancer despite immunosurveillance: immunoselection and immunosubversion. Nat Rev Immunol 2006;6(10):715–27.

35. Malmberg KJ, Ljunggren HG. Escape from immune- and nonimmune-mediated tumor surveillance. Semin Cancer Biol 2006;16(1):16–31.

36. Kim R, Emi M, Tanabe K. Cancer immunoediting from immune surveillance to immune escape. Immunology 2007;121(1):1–14.

37. Algarra I, Garcia-Lora A, Cabrera T, et al. The selection of tumor variants with altered expression of classical and nonclassical MHC class I molecules: implications for tumor immune escape. Cancer Immunol Immunother 2004;53(10):904–10.

38. Chang CC, Ferrone S. Immune selective pressure and HLA class I antigen defects in malignant lesions. Cancer Immunol Immunother 2007;56(2):227–36.

39. Lehmann F, Marchand M, Hainaut P, et al. Differences in the antigens recognized by cytolytic T cells on two successive metastases of a melanoma patient are consistent with immune selection. Eur J Immunol 1995;25(2):340–7.

40. Restifo NP, Marincola FM, Kawakami Y, et al. Loss of functional beta 2-microglobulin in metastatic melanomas from five patients receiving immunotherapy. J Natl Cancer Inst 1996;88(2):100–8.

41. Seliger B, Cabrera T, Garrido F, et al. HLA class I antigen abnormalities and immune escape by malignant cells. Semin Cancer Biol 2002;12(1):3–13.

42. van Hall T, Wolpert EZ, van Veelen P, et al. Selective cytotoxic T-lymphocyte targeting of tumor immune escape variants. Nat Med 2006;12(4):417–24.

43. van den Elsen PJ, Gobin SJ, van Eggermond MC, et al. Regulation of MHC class I and II gene transcription: differences and similarities. Immunogenetics 1998;48(3):208–21.

44. van den Elsen PJ, Holling TM, van der Stoep N, et al. DNA methylation and expression of major histocompatibility complex class I and class II transactivator genes in human developmental tumor cells and in T cell malignancies. Clin Immunol 2003;109(1):46–52.

45. Ohnmacht GA, Marincola FM. Heterogeneity in expression of human leukocyte antigens and melanoma-associated antigens in advanced melanoma. J Cell Physiol 2000;182(3):332–8.

46. Yee C, Thompson JA, Byrd D, et al. Adoptive T cell therapy using antigen-specific CD8+ T cell clones for the treatment of patients with metastatic melanoma: in vivo persistence, migration, and antitumor effect of transferred T cells. Proc Natl Acad Sci U S A 2002;99(25):16168–73.

47. Meklat F, Li Z, Wang Z, et al. Cancer-testis antigens in haematological malignancies. Br J Haematol 2007;136(6):769–76.

48. Oppenheim DE, Roberts SJ, Clarke SL, et al. Sustained localized expression of ligand for the activating NKG2D receptor impairs natural cytotoxicity in vivo and reduces tumor immunosurveillance. Nat Immunol 2005;6(9):928–37.

49. Fauriat C, Just-Landi S, Mallet F, et al. Deficient expression of NCR in NK cells from acute myeloid leukemia: evolution during leukemia treatment and impact of leukemia cells in NCRdull phenotype induction. Blood 2007;109(1):323–30.

50. Gonzalez S, Groh V, Spies T. Immunobiology of human NKG2D and its ligands. Curr Top Microbiol Immunol 2006;298:121–38.
51. Menier C, Riteau B, Carosella ED, et al. MICA triggering signal for NK cell tumor lysis is counteracted by HLA-G1-mediated inhibitory signal. Int J Cancer 2002; 100(1):63–70.
52. Malmberg KJ, Levitsky V, Norell H, et al. IFN-gamma protects short-term ovarian carcinoma cell lines from CTL lysis via a CD94/NKG2A-dependent mechanism. J Clin Invest 2002;110(10):1515–23.
53. Bladergroen BA, Meijer CJ, ten Berge RL, et al. Expression of the granzyme B inhibitor, protease inhibitor 9, by tumor cells in patients with non-Hodgkin and Hodgkin lymphoma: a novel protective mechanism for tumor cells to circumvent the immune system? Blood 2002;99(1):232–7.
54. van Houdt IS, Oudejans JJ, van den Eertwegh AJ, et al. Expression of the apoptosis inhibitor protease inhibitor 9 predicts clinical outcome in vaccinated patients with stage III and IV melanoma. Clin Cancer Res 2005;11(17):6400–7.
55. Harada K, Toyooka S, Shivapurkar N, et al. Deregulation of caspase 8 and 10 expression in pediatric tumors and cell lines. Cancer Res 2002;62(20): 5897–901.
56. Stupack DG, Teitz T, Potter MD, et al. Potentiation of neuroblastoma metastasis by loss of caspase-8. Nature 2006;439(7072):95–9.
57. Ugurel S, Rappl G, Tilgen W, et al. Increased soluble CD95 (sFas/CD95) serum level correlates with poor prognosis in melanoma patients. Clin Cancer Res 2001;7(5):1282–6.
58. Roth W, Isenmann S, Nakamura M, et al. Soluble decoy receptor 3 is expressed by malignant gliomas and suppresses CD95 ligand-induced apoptosis and chemotaxis. Cancer Res 2001;61(6):2759–65.
59. Gronbaek K, Straten PT, Ralfkiaer E, et al. Somatic Fas mutations in non-Hodgkin's lymphoma: association with extranodal disease and autoimmunity. Blood 1998;92(9):3018–24.
60. Ben-Baruch A. Inflammation-associated immune suppression in cancer: the roles played by cytokines, chemokines and additional mediators. Semin Cancer Biol 2006;16(1):38–52.
61. Curiel TJ, Coukos G, Zou L, et al. Specific recruitment of regulatory T cells in ovarian carcinoma fosters immune privilege and predicts reduced survival. Nat Med 2004;10(9):942–9.
62. Serafini P, Borrello I, Bronte V. Myeloid suppressor cells in cancer: recruitment, phenotype, properties, and mechanisms of immune suppression. Semin Cancer Biol 2006;16(1):53–65.
63. Baniyash M. TCR zeta-chain downregulation: curtailing an excessive inflammatory immune response. Nat Rev Immunol 2004;4(9):675–87.
64. Galon J, Costes A, Sanchez-Cabo F, et al. Type, density, and location of immune cells within human colorectal tumors predict clinical outcome. Science 2006; 313(5795):1960–4.
65. Sato E, Olson SH, Ahn J, et al. Intraepithelial CD8+ tumor-infiltrating lymphocytes and a high CD8+/regulatory T cell ratio are associated with favorable prognosis in ovarian cancer. Proc Natl Acad Sci U S A 2005;102(51): 18538–43.
66. Piersma SJ, Jordanova ES, van Poelgeest MI, et al. High number of intraepithelial CD8+ tumor-infiltrating lymphocytes is associated with the absence of lymph node metastases in patients with large early-stage cervical cancer. Cancer Res 2007;67(1):354–61.

67. von Andrian UH, Mempel TR. Homing and cellular traffic in lymph nodes. Nat Rev Immunol 2003;3(11):867–78.
68. Chen Q, Wang WC, Evans SS. Tumor microvasculature as a barrier to antitumor immunity. Cancer Immunol Immunother 2003;52(11):670–9.
69. Carriere V, Colisson R, Jiguet-Jiglaire C, et al. Cancer cells regulate lymphocyte recruitment and leukocyte-endothelium interactions in the tumor-draining lymph node. Cancer Res 2005;65(24):11639–48.
70. Fisher DT, Chen Q, Appenheimer MM, et al. Hurdles to lymphocyte trafficking in the tumor microenvironment: implications for effective immunotherapy. Immunol Invest 2006;35(3–4):251–77.
71. Zlotnik A, Yoshie O. Chemokines: a new classification system and their role in immunity. Immunity 2000;12(2):121–7.
72. Balkwill F. Cancer and the chemokine network. Nat Rev Cancer 2004;4(7): 540–50.
73. Dunn GP, Old LJ, Schreiber RD. The three Es of cancer immunoediting. Annu Rev Immunol 2004;22:329–60.
74. Mapara MY, Sykes M. Tolerance and cancer: mechanisms of tumor evasion and strategies for breaking tolerance. J Clin Oncol 2004;22(6):1136–51.
75. June CH. Adoptive T cell therapy for cancer in the clinic. J Clin Invest 2007; 117(6):1466–76.
76. Dudley ME, Wunderlich JR, Robbins PF, et al. Cancer regression and autoimmunity in patients after clonal repopulation with antitumor lymphocytes. Science 2002;298(5594):850–4.
77. Gattinoni L, Powell DJ Jr, Rosenberg SA, et al. Adoptive immunotherapy for cancer: building on success. Nat Rev Immunol 2006;6(5):383–93.
78. June CH. Principles of adoptive T cell cancer therapy. J Clin Invest 2007;117(5): 1204–12.
79. Berger C, Berger M, Feng J, et al. Genetic modification of T cells for immunotherapy. Expert Opin Biol Ther 2007;7(8):1167–82.
80. Morgan RA, Dudley ME, Wunderlich JR, et al. Cancer regression in patients after transfer of genetically engineered lymphocytes. Science 2006;314(5796): 126–9.
81. Dotti G, Heslop HE. Current status of genetic modification of T cells for cancer treatment. Cytotherapy 2005;7(3):262–72.
82. Savoldo B, Goss JA, Hammer MM, et al. Treatment of solid organ transplant recipients with autologous Epstein Barr virus-specific cytotoxic T lymphocytes (CTLs). Blood 2006;108(9):2942–9.
83. Banchereau J, Palucka AK. Dendritic cells as therapeutic vaccines against cancer. Nat Rev Immunol 2005;5(4):296–306.
84. Figdor CG, de Vries IJ, Lesterhuis WJ, et al. Dendritic cell immunotherapy: mapping the way. Nat Med 2004;10(5):475–80.
85. Rosenberg SA, Yang JC, Restifo NP. Cancer immunotherapy: moving beyond current vaccines. Nat Med 2004;10(9):909–15.
86. Paulos CM, Kaiser A, Wrzesinski C, et al. Toll-like receptors in tumor immunotherapy. Clin Cancer Res 2007;13(18):5280–9.
87. Krieg AM. Development of TLR9 agonists for cancer therapy. J Clin Invest 2007; 117(5):1184–94.
88. Schlom J, Arlen PM, Gulley JL. Cancer vaccines: moving beyond current paradigms. Clin Cancer Res 2007;13(13):3776–82.
89. Dagher R, Long LM, Read EJ, et al. Pilot trial of tumor-specific peptide vaccination and continuous infusion interleukin-2 in patients with recurrent Ewing

sarcoma and alveolar rhabdomyosarcoma: an inter-institute NIH study. Med Pediatr Oncol 2002;38(3):158–64.

90. Geiger JD, Hutchinson RJ, Hohenkirk LF, et al. Vaccination of pediatric solid tumor patients with tumor lysate-pulsed dendritic cells can expand specific T cells and mediate tumor regression. Cancer Res 2001;61(23):8513–9.

91. Rousseau RF, Brenner MK. Vaccine therapies for pediatric malignancies. Cancer J 2005;11(4):331–9.

92. Rousseau RF, Haight AE, Hirschmann-Jax C, et al. Local and systemic effects of an allogeneic tumor cell vaccine combining transgenic human lymphotactin with interleukin-2 in patients with advanced or refractory neuroblastoma. Blood 2003; 101(5):1718–26.

93. Nash RA, Storb R. Graft-versus-host effect after allogeneic hematopoietic stem cell transplantation: GVHD and GVL. Curr Opin Immunol 1996;8(5):674–80.

94. Gilleece MH, Dazzi F. Donor lymphocyte infusions for patients who relapse after allogeneic stem cell transplantation for chronic myeloid leukaemia. Leuk Lymphoma 2003;44(1):23–8.

95. Hahn T, Wall D, Camitta B, et al. The role of cytotoxic therapy with hematopoietic stem cell transplantation in the therapy of acute lymphoblastic leukemia in children: an evidence-based review. Biol Blood Marrow Transplant 2005;11(11):823–61.

96. Cardoso AA, Schultze JL, Boussiotis VA, et al. Pre-B acute lymphoblastic leukemia cells may induce T-cell anergy to alloantigen. Blood 1996;88(1):41–8.

97. Bleakley M, Riddell SR. Molecules and mechanisms of the graft-versus-leukaemia effect. Nat Rev Cancer 2004;4(5):371–80.

98. Molldrem JJ. Vaccinating transplant recipients. Nat Med 2005;11(11):1162–3.

99. Rousseau RF, Biagi E, Dutour A, et al. Immunotherapy of high-risk acute leukemia with a recipient (autologous) vaccine expressing transgenic human CD40L and IL-2 after chemotherapy and allogeneic stem cell transplantation. Blood 2006;107(4):1332–41.

100. Amrolia PJ, Muccioli-Casadei G, Yvon E, et al. Selective depletion of donor alloreactive T cells without loss of antiviral or antileukemic responses. Blood 2003;102(6):2292–9.

101. Solomon SR, Mielke S, Savani BN, et al. Selective depletion of alloreactive donor lymphocytes: a novel method to reduce the severity of graft-versus-host disease in older patients undergoing matched sibling donor stem cell transplantation. Blood 2005;106(3):1123–9.

102. Mielke S, Nunes R, Rezvani K, et al. A clinical scale selective allodepletion approach for the treatment of HLA-mismatched and matched donor-recipient pairs using expanded T lymphocytes as antigen-presenting cells and a TH9402-based photodepletion technique. Blood 2007 [epub ahead of print].

103. Rosenberg SA, Lotze MT, Muul LM, et al. Observations on the systemic administration of autologous lymphokine-activated killer cells and recombinant interleukin-2 to patients with metastatic cancer. N Engl J Med 1985;313(23):1485–92.

104. Atkins MB, Lotze MT, Dutcher JP, et al. High-dose recombinant interleukin 2 therapy for patients with metastatic melanoma: analysis of 270 patients treated between 1985 and 1993. J Clin Oncol 1999;17(7):2105–16.

105. Miller JS, Soignier Y, Panoskaltsis-Mortari A, et al. Successful adoptive transfer and in vivo expansion of human haploidentical NK cells in patients with cancer. Blood 2005;105(8):3051–7.

106. Passweg JR, Koehl U, Uharek L, et al. Natural-killer-cell-based treatment in haematopoietic stem-cell transplantation. Best Pract Res Clin Haematol 2006;19(4):811–24.

107. Klingemann HG. Natural killer cell-based immunotherapeutic strategies. Cytotherapy 2005;7(1):16–22.
108. Ljunggren HG, Malmberg KJ. Prospects for the use of NK cells in immunotherapy of human cancer. Nat Rev Immunol 2007;7(5):329–39.
109. Wayne AS, Kreitman RJ, Pastan I. Monoclonal antibodies and immunotoxins as new therapeutic agents for childhood acute lymphoblastic leukemia. American Society of Clinical Oncology 2007 Educational Book. Alexandria (VA): ASCO; 2007. p. 596–601.
110. Pastan I, Hassan R, Fitzgerald DJ, et al. Immunotoxin therapy of cancer. Nat Rev Cancer 2006;6(7):559–65.
111. Boerman OC, Koppe MJ, Postema EJ, et al. Radionuclide therapy of cancer with radiolabeled antibodies. Anticancer Agents Med Chem 2007;7(3):335–43.

Challenges After Curative Treatment for Childhood Cancer and Long-Term Follow up of Survivors

Kevin C. Oeffinger, MD[a],*, Paul C. Nathan, MD, MSc[b],
Leontien C.M. Kremer, MD, PhD[c]

KEYWORDS

- Childhood cancer • Survivor • Late effects

Cancer in childhood or adolescence is rare. Each year, for every 100,000 persons under the age of 21 years, 16 are diagnosed with cancer. Today, more than 80% of those diagnosed with a childhood cancer will become a long-term survivor.[1] Many cancer survivors will develop serious morbidity, die at a young age from noncancer causes, and experience diminished health status. Among children treated in the 1970s to 1990s, about 75% will develop a chronic disease by 40 years of age, and over 40% will develop a serious health problem.[2,3] The absolute excess risk of premature death from a second cancer, cardiovascular disease, or pulmonary disease is significantly elevated beyond 30 years after the cancer diagnosis.[4,5] Almost half of long-term survivors will have moderate to extremely diminished health status, including limitations in activity and functional impairment.[6,7] Although some serious problems occur during the cancer therapy or soon thereafter (long-term effects), the majority do not become clinically apparent until many years after the cancer has been cured (late effects).[3] Contemporary therapy has evolved with a primary aim of not only improving cure but also decreasing the risk of long-term sequelae. It is

A version of this article was previously published in the *Pediatric Clinics of North America*, 55:1.
[a] Departments of Pediatrics and Medicine, Memorial Sloan-Kettering Cancer Center, 1275 York Avenue, New York, NY 10021, USA
[b] Division of Haematology/Oncology, The Hospital for Sick Children, 555 University Avenue, Toronto, ON M5G 1X8, Canada
[c] Department of Paediatric Oncology, Emma Children's Hospital/Academic Medical Center, Meibergdreef 9, 1105 AZ Amsterdam, the Netherlands
* Corresponding author.
E-mail address: oeffingk@mskcc.org (K.C. Oeffinger).

anticipated that children treated in the 21st century will not experience the frequency and severity of morbidity of those treated in the late 1900s. Furthermore, with proactive and anticipatory risk-based care and healthy lifestyles, the frequency and severity of many late effects of cancer therapy can be significantly reduced.[8,9]

Most childhood cancer survivors in North America and Europe are not followed at a cancer center.[10,11] Instead, over time, they generally drift back to the care of a primary care physician without a formal transition from the cancer center, generally unaware of their risks, without a summary of their cancer or cancer treatment, and with an inadequate understanding of their previous therapy.[11,12] In a routine year in a typical primary care practice, a clinician is likely to see fewer than five childhood cancer survivors, each with a different cancer treated with a different regimen. Recognizing the competing demands of a busy primary care practice and the relative infrequency of seeing a childhood cancer survivor, it can be difficult to stay up-to-date with the health risks associated with different types of cancer therapy, much less with the recommendations for surveillance. However, the primary care physician can play a pivotal role in the health and well being of a childhood cancer survivor by delivering risk-based health care.

This article is intended to assist the primary care physician in this role. With a focus on contemporary therapy, the authors begin by providing a brief discussion of four major types of late effects about which survivors and their families commonly have questions, including neurocognitive dysfunction, cardiovascular disease, infertility and gonadal dysfunction, and psychosocial problems. While these questions are often directed to the oncologist during therapy, families may seek further input from their primary care physician. In the authors' experience, these are also the most common questions that survivors or their families will ask years after the cancer therapy, often when they are no longer followed by the oncologist. Following these four topics, the authors discuss the concept of risk-based care, promote the use of recently developed evidence-based guidelines, describe current care in the United States, Canada, and the Netherlands, and articulate a model for shared survivor care that aims to optimize life-long health of survivors and improve two-way communication between the cancer center and the primary care physician. It is not the intent of this article to provide an exhaustive review of late effects, as recent publications have provided this information based upon treatment exposure[13] or affected organ system.[14,15] Two excellent books also provide much detail regarding late effects and the care of this population.[16,17] Rather, the goal of this article is to orient the reader regarding the key problems, highlight ways that a primary care physician can positively influence the health of childhood cancer survivors, and point toward reliable resources for further inquiry.

NEUROCOGNITIVE DYSFUNCTION

The potential for neurocognitive dysfunction is perhaps the most worrisome outcome to survivors and parents alike. When neurocognitive problems occur, children commonly present with school difficulties. Primary care physicians that deliver care for survivors should be aware of those at greatest risk, recognize the school difficulties associated with prior cancer therapy, and have an approach to screening, intervention and advocacy. Often this will involve helping the child and the family obtain the legally mandated supports required from the school system.[18] Survivors of central nervous system (CNS) tumors and acute lymphoblastic leukemia (ALL) are at particular risk of neurocognitive late effects, but difficulties have been observed in patients treated with a stem cell transplant[19] or with radiation for tumors of the head or neck. Cranial radiotherapy, particularly higher doses, is the major risk factor for adverse neurocognitive functioning,[20–22] and survivors of CNS tumors treated with radiation at a young age are at considerable risk of global neurocognitive difficulties. Fortunately, neurocognitive dysfunction is much less common and severe with contemporary ALL therapy, where cranial radiotherapy is no longer used in patients at low or standard risk of CNS relapse.[23] However, two-thirds of studies of children treated for ALL with chemotherapy alone demonstrate some degree of neurocognitive decline,[24] with methotrexate,[24–27] corticosteroids,[28] and high-dose cytarabine[29] most frequently associated with neurocognitive late effects. Female gender,[30–32] younger age at therapy (particularly children less than 3 years),[21,32–39] and increasing time from treatment increase the risk of these sequelae. Worsening academic performance is usually related to a reduced rate of skill acquisition rather than to loss of previously learned information,[40] and is independent of the number of days of school missed because of therapy.

Survivors may have impairment in any area of neurocognitive function, but problems with attention and concentration,[24,41,42] processing speed, visual perceptual skills,[43] executive function,[41] and memory[24] are most common. Deficits in attention often manifest without hyperactivity, and can be misinterpreted as disinterest or bad behavior. Careless errors, incomplete assignments, and inconsistent academic performance are common,[44] and these survivors often need extra time to complete their schoolwork. This can be compounded by difficulties with planning and organization.[41] Mathematics, reading, and spelling are the most frequently impacted academic areas,[24] and many survivors of ALL and CNS tumors require special education services.[45] School difficulties may not manifest during the primary grades when rote-learning (memorization by repetition) may be relatively intact, but become evident as children transition to middle or high school where organizational, reasoning, and time management skills become essential to successful school performance.[18]

When following a childhood cancer survivor, a primary care physician should assess school performance annually. Many pediatric cancer survivor programs obtain detailed neuropsychologic assessments in survivors at higher risk of difficulties, but in some circumstances these tests must be arranged by the survivor's primary care physician. Unfortunately, many insurance providers do not cover this service, and test results may be available only from evaluations performed through the school system. While school-based testing can be helpful in developing an individualized education program, some important, subtle late effects may be missed. The primary care physician can assist parents by educating school personnel about the academic challenges faced by survivors. Several United States federal laws protect the rights of children with mental and physical limitations to receive special education, accommodation, and related services within the school system, and in many cases, these statutes can be applied to cancer survivors with learning difficulties.[18]

Once completed, information from neuropsychologic assessments should be shared with the school. Simple educational accommodations include locating the child in the front of the classroom where there is less distraction, reducing the number of items on multiple choice tests, breaking assignments into discrete steps, and allowing more time for the completion of examinations.[46] Other interventions, such as cognitive remediation[42] and pharmacotherapy,[47] are currently undergoing investigation with multicenter trials. Even if no specific educational intervention is identified after an initial assessment, it is important to continually reassess a survivor's needs, because deficits may develop over time.

CARDIOVASCULAR DISEASE

The developing cardiovascular system of a child or adolescent is very vulnerable to cancer therapy. A cardiomyopathy may develop following exposure to anthracyclines.

Mantle radiotherapy promotes the development of coronary and carotid artery disease. In addition, perhaps most commonly, premature cardiovascular disease may result from alterations in multiple organ systems. The following sections describe each of these outcomes and emphasize the role of surveillance and prevention.

Anthracycline-Induced Cardiomyopathy

Anthracyclines, including doxorubicin and daunorubicin, are an important class of chemotherapeutic agents in the treatment of children with cancer. About half of those treated with contemporary therapy receive an anthracycline. Unfortunately, anthracycline cardiotoxicity is a major and generally unavoidable complication of childhood cancer therapy. The consequences of anthracycline cardiotoxicity for survivors are extensive. Late effects, resulting from myocardial damage, can manifest as left ventricular dysfunction, clinical heart failure, or as cardiac death. Anthracycline cardiotoxicity can be divided in asymptomatic (subclinical) and symptomatic (clinical) cardiotoxicity. Asymptomatic cardiotoxicity is defined as various cardiac abnormalities diagnosed with different diagnostic methods in asymptomatic patients; symptomatic cardiotoxicity is defined as clinical heart failure (CHF). Anthracycline-induced left ventricular dysfunction develops via two mechanisms: depressed contractility and an increased afterload.[48] Late-onset anthracycline cardiotoxicity, occurring after the first year of survivorship, is the direct result of damage done during therapy, and is progressive.[48]

Numerous studies have evaluated the cardiotoxic effects of anthracycline therapy in survivors of childhood cancer. As described in previous systematic reviews,[49,50] some studies have methodologic limitations: only a selected subgroup of survivors have been evaluated, follow-up is incomplete, or nonstandardized diagnostic measurements have been used. For asymptomatic cardiotoxicity in childhood cancer survivors, a wide variation in the prevalence, from 0% to 56%, has been described.[50–53] Differences in the selection of study groups, cumulative anthracycline dose, outcome definitions, and follow-up period could explain a part of this wide range. The risk of anthracycline-induced (A-) CHF in childhood cancer survivors has been evaluated in several cohort studies.[49] In a cohort study of 831 subjects treated with anthracyclines for childhood cancer, the estimated risk of A-CHF, 20 years after the first dose of anthracyclines, was 9.8% for subjects who received a cumulative dose of greater than or equal to 300 mg/m^2.[54] Risk factors for anthracycline cardiotoxicity include higher cumulative dose of anthracyclines, radiotherapy involving the heart region, and a few studies suggest younger age at treatment and the female sex.[49,50]

The risk of developing clinical heart failure for survivors treated with anthracyclines remains a life-long threat, and guidelines for long-term follow-up advise life-long cardiac monitoring for survivors treated with anthracycline.[55,56] However, management of childhood cancer survivors with asymptomatic cardiotoxicity is unclear.[57] Two studies have investigated the effect of angiotensin converting enzyme inhibitors in childhood cancer survivors.[58,59] Although the results were promising, the noncontrolled trial suggested that enalapril treatment could delay, but not completely prevent, progression of subclinical and clinical cardiotoxicity in survivors.[59] So primary prevention during treatment is essential, such as reducing the cumulative dose of anthracyclines, the use of possible less cardiotoxic anthracycline analogs, and reducing the peak dose or the use of cardioprotective agents.[60,61]

Coronary and Carotid Artery Disease Following Mantle Radiotherapy

Moderate dose mantle irradiation (3,500 centigray or cGy–4,500 cGy) was the mainstay for treatment of early stage supradiaphragmatic Hodgkin's disease from the

1960s to the 1980s. The mantle field encompasses the primary lymph node regions of the neck, supraclavicular, infraclavicular, axillary, and mediastinal areas. In a British cohort of 7,003 Hodgkin's survivors with an average of 11.2 years of follow-up, the standardized mortality risk secondary to myocardial infarction was 3.2 for those who were treated with mantle irradiation.[62] The absolute excess risk was 125.8 per 100,000 person-years. Aleman and colleagues[63] reported that by 30 years after mediastinal irradiation, the cumulative incidence of myocardial infarction was 12.9%. They reported a standardized incidence ratio of 3.6 for myocardial infarction, with 357 excess cases per 100,000 person-years. Traditional risk factors (smoking, hypercholesterolemia, diabetes) increased risk. In Dutch Hodgkin's survivors treated with moderate dose mediastinal irradiation (median, 3,720 cGy), Reinders and colleagues[64] reported an actuarial risk of symptomatic ischemic coronary artery disease of 21.2% by 20 years after irradiation. This increased risk of premature coronary artery disease and myocardial infarction following mediastinal irradiation has been consistently reported in several other well-designed studies.[65–70] Carotid artery disease has also been reported following mantle radiotherapy.[71,72]

In the past 15 years, modified mantle radiotherapy with a lower total dose (2,000 cGy–2,500 cGy) to involved fields has been used in combination with multiagent therapy. More recent methods, of shielding the heart and equally weighting the anterior and posterior fields, appear to decrease the risk of cardiac disease. However, even with current shielding techniques, the proximal coronary arteries are within the modified mantle fields. So, despite modifications in therapy aimed at reducing risk, children and adolescents treated on contemporary Hodgkin's disease protocols likely still face an increased risk of coronary and carotid artery disease. Longitudinal studies of survivors treated with contemporary therapy are needed to delineate the frequency, onset, and modifying factors of this risk. Aggressive risk reduction of traditional coronary artery disease risk factors (tobacco avoidance and cessation; optimum management of lipid disorders, diabetes mellitus, and hypertension; promotion of physical activity) should also reduce morbidity.

Cardiovascular Disease Following Childhood Acute Lymphoblastic Leukemia a Model for Multifactorial Cardiovascular Disease

Children who have survived ALL are more likely to be physically inactive[73,74] and obese,[75,76] have increased visceral adiposity,[77] develop insulin resistance[78,79] and dyslipidemia[75,80] at a young age, and have poor cardiorespiratory fitness.[81] These outcomes are in part related to cranial radiation, a therapy that is currently used in about 5% to 15% of children with ALL. However, children treated with chemotherapy alone also develop these outcomes, although the risk appears to be somewhat attenuated and possibly later in onset. This constellation of risk factors can be expected to lead to an increased incidence of cardiovascular disease, likely at a relatively young age. Similar outcomes have also been reported in brain tumor survivors[82] and in those treated with a stem cell transplant.[83,84] Research aimed at better understanding these relationships and the mechanisms leading to these outcomes is under way. In addition, the primary care physician should promote healthy behaviors (tobacco avoidance, healthy diet, and physical activity), screen for lipid disorders and insulin resistance, and closely monitor these survivors.

FERTILITY AND GONADAL DYSFUNCTION

When a child or adolescent is diagnosed with cancer, the discussion of cancer therapy is difficult and complicated, as the oncologist describes the response rates of various protocols, the associated acute toxicities of therapy, and the potential for future health problems related to the therapy. During this stress laden period when therapeutic decisions are made, as a parent faces the potential of losing a child, details regarding the potential for infertility and gonadal dysfunction are often not understood or remembered by families, and sometimes are not adequately provided by the cancer treating team.[85] Later, as the cancer is cured and the interval from completion of the cancer therapy lengthens, questions regarding fertility and gonadal function become more prevalent. The loss of fertility (or even the fear of impaired fertility) and alterations in gonadal function influence the survivor's developing body image, dating relationships, and marriage patterns.[86]

Fertility is the most difficult outcome to study in survivors, as the primary endpoint is pregnancy, an outcome that is influenced by many physical and societal factors beyond the direct effect of the cancer therapy on ovarian or testicular function. Fertility is particularly difficult to study in males, as many men are not willing to have a semen analysis and self-reporting a successful impregnation is subject to both over- and under-reporting biases. Further compounding the investigation of fertility in both genders are the often overlapping effects of different cancer therapies on the reproductive system, and the sometimes late recovery of function. Recognizing the complexity of this subject, a detailed description is beyond the scope of this article. Following is a brief overview; for the clinician interested in better understanding these outcomes, two excellent articles written by leading researchers in this area are helpful resources.[87,88]

Female Survivors, Acute Ovarian Failure, Premature Menopause, and Fertility Preservation

Though the ovaries during childhood and adolescence are relatively resistant to chemotherapy-induced damage, they are sensitive to radiation. Among 3,390 women in the Childhood Cancer Survivor Study (CCSS), loss of ovarian function during or shortly following completion of therapy (acute ovarian failure) was reported in 6.3%.[89] More than 70% of women who had been treated with 2,000 cGy or more of ovarian irradiation had acute ovarian failure. Doses of ovarian irradiation below 1,000 cGy were capable of inducing acute ovarian failure in women who received concomitant alkylating agents (eg, cyclophosphamide) or were older at exposure. Survivors at greatest risk for acute ovarian failure are those treated with total body irradiation (TBI) in preparation for a stem cell transplant. Virtually all women treated with TBI after age 10 years will develop acute ovarian failure.[90,91] In contrast, only 50% of those treated before 10 years of age will develop this outcome. In addition, women treated with high dose myeloablative therapy (eg, busulfan, melphalan, thiotepa), rather than TBI, before a stem cell transplant are at high risk of developing acute ovarian failure.[92,93]

Female survivors who do not develop acute ovarian failure are potentially at risk of developing premature menopause (ie, menopause before age 40 years) and having reduced ovarian reserve. Among 2,819 women in the CCSS cohort who did not have acute ovarian failure, Sklar and colleagues[94] reported a relative risk of nonsurgical premature menopause of 13.2, when compared with 1,065 siblings. Risk factors for premature menopause among survivors included older attained age, exposure to increasing dose of radiation to the ovaries, increasing dose of alkylating agents, and a diagnosis of Hodgkin's disease. For women treated with an alkylating agent plus abdominopelvic radiation, the cumulative incidence of nonsurgical menopause approached 30% by 40 years of age.

In an assessment of 100 Danish childhood cancer survivors with a median age of 26 years, Larsen and colleagues[95] reported that women with preserved menstrual cycles had sonographic and endocrine changes suggestive of diminished ovarian reserve. Decreased number of antral follicles per ovary was associated with treatment that included ovarian irradiation or use of alkylating agents, older age at diagnosis, and increasing years of therapy. With cranial radiation doses of 3,000 cGy or higher to the hypothalamic-pituitary axis, women may develop gonadotropin deficiency affecting fertility and sex hormone production.[96–98] The consequences of ovarian failure and premature menopause extend beyond the issue of fertility and may include alterations in bone metabolism, leading to osteoporosis, sexual dysfunction, and body image changes.

In recent years, much attention has been directed toward preserving fertility in females undergoing cancer therapy during their childhood years. When radiation fields include the pelvis, the ovaries can be surgically transposed to a more protected location.[99,100] However, even after transposition of the ovaries, some women will develop premature menopause secondary to their chemotherapy. Hormonal protection of the ovaries with a gonadotropin-releasing hormone analog has been attempted, with varying success, in small uncontrolled trials in patients undergoing therapy with moderate to high dose alkylating agents.[101] Because the success rate of cryopreservation of unfertilized oocytes is very low, and the necessary ovarian hormonal stimulation before removal of the oocytes may delay cancer therapy, this approach is used infrequently in adolescents with cancer.[102]

Lastly, ovarian tissue cryopreservation is an investigational method of fertility preservation that has the advantage of requiring neither a sperm donor nor ovarian stimulation.[85] The American Society of Clinical Oncology recommends that oncologists discuss fertility preservation options as appropriate, and to refer interested patients and their families to reproductive specialists.[85]

Encouragingly, women who become pregnant following childhood cancer generally have favorable outcomes. Among 1,953 women in the CCSS, 4,029 live births were reported and no association was found between chemotherapy and an adverse pregnancy outcome.[103] Previous pelvic irradiation was associated with lower birth weight.

Male Survivors, Infertility, Fertility Preservation, and Androgen Deficiency

The germinal epithelium of the testis is sensitive to radiation. Even low-dose testicular irradiation is associated with decreased spermatogenesis, with doses above 200 cGy invariably causing oligospermia or azoospermia.[87] Thus, males treated TBI, with a fractionated dose of 1,200 cGy to 1500 cGy, are often rendered infertile.[104] Similarly, males with ALL who are treated with irradiation of the testis for a testicular relapse will almost always be azoospermic. Though the testes are shielded with modern techniques, scatter radiation from high-dose radiation can result in oligospermia or azoospermia. Examples include pelvic, inguinal, or spinal radiation for a sarcoma, Hodgkin's disease, or CNS tumor, respectively.[105,106] Lastly, radiation to the hypothalamic-pituitary axis may result in a gonadotropin deficiency, thus indirectly affecting spermatogenesis and reproductive potential.

Spermatogenesis is also quite affected by several chemotherapeutic drugs, including alkylating agents (eg, cyclophosphamide and ifosfamide), procarbazine, and cisplatin. Outcomes are agent specific and dose-dependent. Treatment with moderate to high-dose cyclophosphamide or ifosfamide often results in azoospermia. The combination of these two agents, used in the treatment of patients with Ewing sarcoma, causes infertility in virtually all males.[107] Similarly, the combination of cisplatin with either ifosfamide or cyclophosphamide, used in the contemporary treatment of osteosarcoma, results in oligospermia or azoospermia in over 90% of males.[107] High-dose melphalan or busulfan, used in some preconditioning regimens before a stem cell transplant, also causes impaired spermatogenesis in the vast majority of males.[87] Early chemotherapeutic regimens used for Hodgkin's disease, including six courses of mechlorethamine, vincristine, procarbazine, and prednisone, generally resulted in a high incidence of azoospermia. To preserve fertility, contemporary multimodality therapy of Hodgkin's disease and non-Hodgkin lymphoma generally includes only three courses of an alkylating agent or procarbazine, alternating with another group of agents with a different set of toxicities.

Sperm cryopreservation is an effective method of fertility preservation in males.[85,108] Unfortunately, spermarche does not occur until about 13 to 14 years of age, thus limiting sperm banking to adolescent males. In general, methods to preserve fertility in younger males, including testicular tissue cryopreservation, have not been successful.[85] While it is recommended that the oncologist discuss sperm banking with all appropriate patients, it is also important for the primary care physician to be aware of this option if the patient or the family has any questions.

In comparison with the germinal epithelium, the Leydig cells are less affected by chemotherapy and radiotherapy. Testicular irradiation with doses of greater than 2,000 cGy and 3,000 cGy are associated with Leydig cell dysfunction in prepubertal and sexually mature males, respectively.[87] Even with high dose cyclophosphamide, frankly subnormal levels of testosterone are rare, though Leydig cell dysfunction may be evidenced by an elevated luteinizing hormone level.[109] Whether or not mild Leydig cell dysfunction will lead to premature androgen deficiency as this population ages is not known. Androgen deficiency can also result from hypogonadotropic hypogonadism following cranial radiotherapy.

PSYCHOSOCIAL ISSUES IN SURVIVORS AND THEIR FAMILIES

The experience of being diagnosed and treated for cancer during childhood exerts considerable psychologic strain on both the patient and the family. Despite this, many survivors report normal psychologic health, and some even demonstrate psychologic growth as a result of their cancer experience. Additionally, most studies suggest that survivors are less likely to exhibit risky behaviors, such as cigarette smoking or drug use.[110–112] However, on average, childhood cancer survivors are more likely to present with mental health disorders and to complain of chronic pain or fatigue than the general population. Hudson and colleagues[6] reported that 17% of 9,535 young adult survivors of childhood cancer in the CCSS had depressive, somatic, or anxiety symptoms, and 10% reported moderate to extreme pain as a result of their cancer. Approximately one out five young adult survivors of childhood cancer reports symptoms of posttraumatic stress disorder (PTSD),[113,114] characterized by re-experiencing elements of their prior cancer experience or its associated emotions, avoidance of people or places that remind them of their previous cancer, and increased anxiety or arousal. Avoidant behaviors may inhibit survivors from seeking appropriate follow-up care, particularly if care is delivered in the hospital where they received their cancer therapy. Additionally, both parents[115,116] and siblings[117] of survivors may develop symptoms of PTSD, and thus the primary care physician must extend their assessment of mental health to survivors' families. Rather than developing PTSD, some survivors demonstrate posttraumatic growth[118] and psychosocial thriving[119] as a result of their cancer experience. Many rate themselves highly on their ability to cope as a result of their prior cancer, suggesting that this life-altering event promotes resiliency.[120] When survivors do report psychologic distress, it is associated frequently with poorer health status, lower levels of income, and poorer social functioning.[121,122]

Physicians need to be sensitive to the concerns expressed by survivors who often worry about fertility and parenthood, obtaining health and life insurance, educational difficulties, job availability after completing school, and their risk for future health problems, including second cancers.[123,124] Although most survivors become socially independent and leave home at a similar age to the general population, rates of marriage are slightly lower.[125–127] Survivors of CNS tumors are at particular risk of not marrying, and many are unable to live independently.[128] Additionally, survivors of CNS tumors (but not other cancers) may be at increased risk of hospitalization for a psychiatric disorder.[129] Primary care physicians can support these patients by providing interventions that improve health, support educational or occupational advancement to improve income potential, and promote social interaction.[121] In particular, the development of a social network has been shown to enhance quality of life in survivors.[130]

Several organizations provide services that can assist survivors, their parents, and their health care providers in dealing with the various challenges that may arise as these children and adolescents move beyond their primary cancer (**Table 1**). Two books written for survivors or their families provide quality information and address the specific challenges of the cancer experience and survivorship.[131,132]

RISK-BASED HEALTH CARE AND SHARED CARE OF CANCER SURVIVORS

Because the risk and severity of many late effects is modifiable, and some are preventable, life long health care is recommended for all childhood cancer survivors.[9] A systematic plan for longitudinal screening, surveillance, and prevention that incorporates risks based on the previous cancer, cancer therapy, genetic predispositions, lifestyle behaviors, and comorbid health conditions should be developed for all childhood cancer survivors.

To facilitate and standardize risk-based care of childhood cancer survivors, several evidence-based guidelines have been developed.[55,56,133,134] In the development of these guidelines, the evidence of the association between a therapeutic exposure and a late effect is generally of high quality. However, with a relatively small population of childhood cancer survivors limiting prospective study design, there are no studies that have estimated the reduction in morbidity or mortality with surveillance. Thus, principles of screening in the general population and other high-risk groups have been applied, in addition to the collective clinical experience of expert panels, in the development of surveillance recommendations.[55]

In North America, the 240-institution Children's Oncology Group (COG) "Long-Term Follow-Up Guidelines for Survivors of Childhood, Adolescent, and Young Adult Cancers" (available at www.survivorshipguidelines.org) are widely used.[55] Recommendations for periodic evaluations are based upon different treatment exposures or therapeutic modalities and include modifying risk factors. For each late effect, a score of the quality of the evidence is provided, along with supporting references. In addition, over 40 different patient education handouts (Health Links) that discuss frequent problems or questions are accessible through the Web site. The guidelines are periodically reviewed by the COG Late Effects Committee and updated as new evidence becomes available.

In the Netherlands, 16 multidisciplinary teams summarized the evidence in existing guidelines, systematic reviews, books, and papers based on clinical questions regarding the magnitude of the risk of selected late effects, the efficacy of screening, and possible treatments. Ten nationwide meetings were held to define the final Dutch

Table 1
Resources for childhood cancer survivors, their parent and caregivers

Service and Disability Organizations	Service Provided
National Childhood Cancer Foundation 440 E. Huntington Dr, Arcadia, CA 91066-6012, (800) 458-6223. http://www.curesearch.org	Provides information and resources for pediatric cancer survivors.
American Cancer Society 1599 Clifton Rd NE, Atlanta, GA 30329-4215, (800) ACS-2345. http://www.cancer.org	Programs include equipment and supplies, support groups, educational literature, and summer camps for childhood cancer survivors.
Canadian Cancer Society 565 West 10th Avenue, Vancouver, BC V5Z 4J4 Canada. http://www.bc.cancer.ca	Programs include those that the American Cancer Society provides.
Association of Cancer Online Resources http://www.acor.org	Online information and electronic support groups for pediatric cancer survivors and their caregivers.
Candlelighters Childhood Cancer Foundation 3910 Warner Street, Kensington, MD 20895, (800) 366-CCCF. http://www.candlelighters.org	Provides resource guides, quarterly newsletters, referrals, information, and publishes books for pediatric cancer survivors, including *Educating the Child with Cancer.*
Candlelighters Childhood Cancer Foundation Canada 55 Eglington Avenue East, Suite 401, Toronto, Ontario M4P 1G8 Canada, (800) 363-1062. http://www.candlelighters.org.ca	Provides resource guides, newsletters, and information.

Childhood Cancer Ombudsman Program 27 Witch Duck Lane, Heathsville, VA 22473. gpmonaco@rivnet.net	Provides help for pediatric cancer survivors experiencing problems getting access to appropriate education, medical care, health care cost coverage, and employment.
Federation for Children with Special Needs 1135 Tremont Street, Suite 420, Boston, MA 02120, (617) 236-7210. http://www.fcsn.org	Federally funded organization providing information on special education rights and laws, conferences, referrals for services, parent training workshops, publications, and advocacy information.
Lance Armstrong Foundation PO Box 161150, Austin, TX 78716, (866) 235-7205. www.livestrong.org	A nonprofit organization that offers extensive education, advocacy and public health resources.
National Center for Learning Disabilities 381 Park Avenue South, Suite 1401, New York, NY 10016, (888) 575-7373. http://www.ncld.org	Offers extensive resources, referral services, and educational programs related to learning disabilities.
US Department of Justice ADA Information Line, Civil Rights Division, PO Box 66738, Washington, DC 20035, (800) 514-0301. http://www.usdoj.gov/crt/ada/adahom1.htm	Answers questions about the Americans with Disabilities Act, explains how to file a complaint, and provides dispute resolution information.

Data from Nathan PC, Patel SK, Dilley K, et al. Guidelines for identification of, advocacy for, and intervention in neurocognitive problems in survivors of childhood cancer: a report from the Children's Oncology Group. Arch Pediatr Adolesc Med 2007;161(8):798–806.

recommendations based on available evidence.[134] These recommendations led to standardization and improvement of patient care for survivors in the Netherlands.[2]

Long-term follow up practices vary across the United States, Canada, and the Netherlands. In the United States, most COG institutions have a specialized long-term follow up (LTFU) program that delivers risk-based health care for survivors during their childhood years.[135,136] However, because of insurance limitations, travel distances, and other barriers, survivors are gradually lost to follow-up over time. More-over, very few LTFU programs in the United States provide care for childhood cancer survivors who are in their adult years. In Canada, Ontario is the only province with a coordinated system of care for both pediatric and adult survivors of childhood cancer. The province funds a group of coordinated Aftercare Clinics, located in cancer centers in five major cities across the province (see http://www.pogo.ca/care/after-careclinics/, accessed August 29, 2007). Although the majority of survivors receive their medical care in such a program during their childhood years, many adult survi-vors are not seen regularly in these Aftercare programs, despite such care being provided free of charge. The majority of adult survivors of childhood cancer in Canada report receiving care from a family physician.[137] In the Netherlands, all pediatric oncology centers have an LTFU program and most children are followed through these programs. As in the United States, financial support limits the care of adult survivors.

The majority of late effects become clinically apparent many years after the cancer therapy, generally when survivors are in their adult years.[3] This is the time period when most survivors in North America and Europe are no longer followed in a specialized LTFU program. Formal transition of survivors to their primary care physician, with proper communication, is rare. Instead, follow-up care tends to be haphazard for most survivors. If our common goal is to optimize the life-long health of survivors, it is imperative that LTFU programs implement strategies that efficiently allocate limited resources where they are most needed.

As illustrated in **Fig. 1**, one potential strategy is to integrate primary care physicians into a risk-stratified shared care model.[11,138,139] This strategy stratifies survivors into three groups based upon their risk of late effects (see **Fig. 1** for potential groupings). Given their expertise in this area, the stratification would be determined by the LTFU staff. All survivors would continue to have their noncancer-related care delivered by the primary care physician. At the time of diagnosis, the primary oncologist would mail (or fax) the primary care physician a summary of the cancer treatment plan. At 2 years following the completion of therapy, the survivor would be transitioned from the oncology team to the LTFU program for a single visit. At this visit, a cancer summary would be developed and include information about the cancer, cancer therapy, and recommended surveillance. A copy of the summary would be sent to the primary care physician, with a lay version provided to the survivor (and his or her family). After this single LTFU visit, the survivor at low risk would be transitioned to the primary care physician for periodic risk-based care. The LTFU staff would communicate with the primary care physician every 3 to 5 years and inquire about changes in the survivor's health and any new findings that might change surveillance recommendations. Survivors at moderate risk would be followed annually through the LTFU program for their risk-based care until 5 to 10 years after the completion of cancer therapy. During this time period, in addition to monitoring for late effects and surveillance for recurrence, age- and developmental stage-appropriate education and counseling highlighting the benefits of healthy lifestyles would be provided. At 5 to 10 years after cancer therapy, depending upon the program, the survivor would be transitioned to their primary care physician for the delivery of risk-based care. At

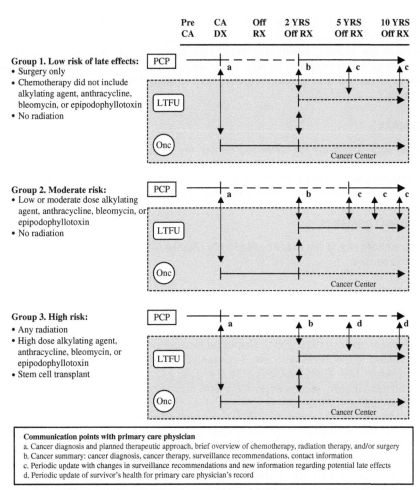

Fig. 1. Proposed risk-stratified shared care model for childhood cancer survivors. Solid line denotes primary responsibility for risk-based care; risk stratification based upon determination of the LTFU staff. CA, cancer; DX, diagnosis; Onc, oncologist; PCP, primary care provider; RX, therapy. (*Adapted from* Oeffinger KC, McCabe MS. Models for delivering survivorship care. J Clin Oncol 2006;24(32):5119; with permission from the American Society of Clinical Oncology.)

the time of transition, the LTFU staff would provide the primary care physician with an updated treatment summary and surveillance plan, and then annually communicate with the primary care physician (and survivor if needed) to document any new late effects, changes in lifestyle behaviors and family history, and update the surveillance recommendations. The LTFU program would also serve in a consultative mode, as needed, for survivors at low or moderate risk who develop a late effect or need further evaluation. A survivor at high risk of developing late effects would continue to be monitored through the LTFU program, with continued communication with the primary care physician regarding any new health problems and planned surveillance (to avoid duplication of testing).

This strategy would allow LTFU programs to concentrate their resources on the survivors at highest risk and provide foundational education and counseling to those at moderate risk. Furthermore, the standardized and systematic communication between the LTFU staff and the primary care physician would serve to inform both groups of the evolving health and health care needs of the survivor. To implement this strategy, LTFU programs located at a children's hospital that restricts care of adult patients would need to develop an alternative strategy for the care of their high risk survivors.

SUMMARY

Late effects of therapy for childhood cancer are frequent and serious. Fortunately, many late effects are also modifiable. Proactive and anticipatory risk-based care can reduce the frequency and severity of treatment-related morbidity. The primary care physician should be an integral component in risk-based care of survivors.

ACKNOWLEDGMENTS

The authors would like to acknowledge Dr Charles Sklar for his insightful comments with this review.

REFERENCES

1. Ries LAG, Melbert D, Krapcho M, et al. SEER cancer statistics review, 1975–2004. Bethesda (MD): National Cancer Institute; 2007. Available at: http://seer.cancer.gov/csr/1975_2004/. Based on November 2006 SEER data submission, posted to the SEER Web site. Accessed September 1, 2007.
2. Geenen MM, Cardous-Ubbink MC, Kremer LC, et al. Medical assessment of adverse health outcomes in long-term survivors of childhood cancer. JAMA 2007;297(24):2705–15.
3. Oeffinger KC, Mertens AC, Sklar CA, et al. Chronic health conditions in adult survivors of childhood cancer. N Engl J Med 2006;355(15):1572–82.
4. Mertens AC, Yasui Y, Neglia JP, et al. Late mortality experience in five-year survivors of childhood and adolescent cancer: the Childhood Cancer Survivor Study. J Clin Oncol 2001;19(13):3163–72.
5. Moller TR, Garwicz S, Barlow L, et al. Decreasing late mortality among five-year survivors of cancer in childhood and adolescence: a population-based study in the Nordic countries. J Clin Oncol 2001;19(13):3173–81.
6. Hudson MM, Mertens AC, Yasui Y, et al. Health status of adult long-term survivors of childhood cancer: a report from the Childhood Cancer Survivor Study. JAMA 2003;290(12):1583–92.
7. Ness KK, Mertens AC, Hudson MM, et al. Limitations on physical performance and daily activities among long-term survivors of childhood cancer. Ann Intern Med 2005;143(9):639–47.
8. Oeffinger KC. Longitudinal risk-based health care for adult survivors of childhood cancer. Curr Probl Cancer 2003;27(3):143–67.
9. Hewitt M, Weiner SL, Simone JV, editors. Childhood cancer survivorship: improving care and quality of life. Washington, DC: National Academies Press; 2003.
10. Oeffinger KC, Mertens AC, Hudson MM, et al. Health care of young adult survivors of childhood cancer: a report from the Childhood Cancer Survivor Study. Ann Fam Med 2004;2(1):61–70.
11. Oeffinger KC, Wallace WH. Barriers to follow-up care of survivors in the United States and the United Kingdom. Pediatr Blood Cancer 2006;46(2):135–42.

12. Kadan-Lottick NS, Robison LL, Gurney JG, et al. Childhood cancer survivors' knowledge about their past diagnosis and treatment: Childhood Cancer Survivor Study. JAMA 2002;287(14):1832–9.
13. Oeffinger KC, Hudson MM. Long-term complications following childhood and adolescent cancer: foundations for providing risk-based health care for survivors. CA Cancer J Clin 2004;54(4):208–36.
14. Bhatia S, Landier W. Evaluating survivors of pediatric cancer. Cancer J 2005; 11(4):340–54.
15. Friedman DL, Meadows AT. Late effects of childhood cancer therapy. Pediatr Clin North Am 2002;49(5):1083–106.
16. Wallace WH, Green DM, editors. Late effects of childhood cancer. London: Arnold Publishers; 2004.
17. Schwartz CL, Hobbie WL, Constine LS, et al, editors. Survivors of childhood and adolescent cancer: a multidisciplinary approach. Berlin: Springer-Verlag; 2005.
18. Nathan PC, Patel SK, Dilley K, et al. Guidelines for identification of, advocacy for, and intervention in neurocognitive problems in survivors of childhood cancer: a report from the Children's Oncology Group. Arch Pediatr Adolesc Med 2007;161(8):798–806.
19. Kramer JH, Crittenden MR, DeSantes K, et al. Cognitive and adaptive behavior 1 and 3 years following bone marrow transplantation. Bone Marrow Transplant 1997;19(6):607–13.
20. Grill J, Renaux VK, Bulteau C, et al. Long-term intellectual outcome in children with posterior fossa tumors according to radiation doses and volumes. Int J Radiat Oncol Biol Phys 1999;45(1):137–45.
21. Mulhern RK, Kepner JL, Thomas PR, et al. Neuropsychologic functioning of survivors of childhood medulloblastoma randomized to receive conventional or reduced-dose craniospinal irradiation: a Pediatric Oncology Group study. J Clin Oncol 1998;16(5):1723–8.
22. Ris MD, Packer R, Goldwein J, et al. Intellectual outcome after reduced-dose radiation therapy plus adjuvant chemotherapy for medulloblastoma: a Children's Cancer Group study. J Clin Oncol 2001;19(15):3470–6.
23. Pui CH, Evans WE. Treatment of acute lymphoblastic leukemia. N Engl J Med 2006;354(2):166–78.
24. Moleski M. Neuropsychological, neuroanatomical, and neurophysiological consequences of CNS chemotherapy for acute lymphoblastic leukemia. Arch Clin Neuropsychol 2000;15(7):603–30.
25. Espy KA, Moore IM, Kaufmann PM, et al. Chemotherapeutic CNS prophylaxis and neuropsychologic change in children with acute lymphoblastic leukemia: a prospective study. J Pediatr Psychol 2001;26(1):1–9.
26. Riva D, Giorgi C, Nichelli F, et al. Intrathecal methotrexate affects cognitive function in children with medulloblastoma. Neurology 2002;59(1):48–53.
27. Brown RT, Madan-Swain A, Walco GA, et al. Cognitive and academic late effects among children previously treated for acute lymphocytic leukemia receiving chemotherapy as CNS prophylaxis. J Pediatr Psychol 1998;23(5): 333–40.
28. Waber DP, Carpentieri SC, Klar N, et al. Cognitive sequelae in children treated for acute lymphoblastic leukemia with dexamethasone or prednisone. J Pediatr Hematol Oncol 2000;22(3):206–13.
29. Nand S, Messmore HL Jr, Patel R, et al. Neurotoxicity associated with systemic high-dose cytosine arabinoside. J Clin Oncol 1986;4(4):571–5.

30. von der Weid N, Mosimann I, Hirt A, et al. Intellectual outcome in children and adolescents with acute lymphoblastic leukaemia treated with chemotherapy alone: age- and sex-related differences. Eur J Cancer 2003;39(3): 359–65.

31. Waber DP, Tarbell NJ, Kahn CM, et al. The relationship of sex and treatment modality to neuropsychologic outcome in childhood acute lymphoblastic leukemia. J Clin Oncol 1992;10(5):810–7.

32. Christie D, Leiper AD, Chessells JM, et al. Intellectual performance after presymptomatic cranial radiotherapy for leukaemia: effects of age and sex. Arch Dis Child 1995;73(2):136–40.

33. Ronning C, Sundet K, Due-Tonnessen B, et al. Persistent cognitive dysfunction secondary to cerebellar injury in patients treated for posterior fossa tumors in childhood. Pediatr Neurosurg 2005;41(1):15–21.

34. Palmer SL, Goloubeva O, Reddick WE, et al. Patterns of intellectual development among survivors of pediatric medulloblastoma: a longitudinal analysis. J Clin Oncol 2001;19(8):2302–8.

35. Copeland DR, deMoor C, Moore BD 3rd, et al. Neurocognitive development of children after a cerebellar tumor in infancy: a longitudinal study. J Clin Oncol 1999;17(11):3476–86.

36. Packer RJ, Sutton LN, Atkins TE, et al. A prospective study of cognitive function in children receiving whole-brain radiotherapy and chemotherapy: 2-year results. J Neurosurg 1989;70(5):707–13.

37. Radcliffe J, Bunin GR, Sutton LN, et al. Cognitive deficits in long-term survivors of childhood medulloblastoma and other noncortical tumors: age-dependent effects of whole brain radiation. Int J Dev Neurosci 1994;12(4):327–34.

38. Radcliffe J, Packer RJ, Atkins TE, et al. Three- and four-year cognitive outcome in children with noncortical brain tumors treated with whole-brain radiotherapy. Ann Neurol 1992;32(4):551–4.

39. Kaleita TA, Reaman GH, MacLean WE, et al. Neurodevelopmental outcome of infants with acute lymphoblastic leukemia: a Children's Cancer Group report. Cancer 1999;85(8):1859–65.

40. Mabbott DJ, Spiegler BJ, Greenberg ML, et al. Serial evaluation of academic and behavioral outcome after treatment with cranial radiation in childhood. J Clin Oncol 2005;23(10):2256–63.

41. Mulhern RK, Palmer SL. Neurocognitive late effects in pediatric cancer. Curr Probl Cancer 2003;27(4):177–97.

42. Butler RW, Copeland DR. Attentional processes and their remediation in children treated for cancer: a literature review and the development of a therapeutic approach. J Int Neuropsychol Soc 2002;8(1):115–24.

43. Said JA, Waters BG, Cousens P, et al. Neuropsychological sequelae of central nervous system prophylaxis in survivors of childhood acute lymphoblastic leukemia. J Consult Clin Psychol 1989;57(2):251–6.

44. Armstrong FD, Briery BG. Childhood cancer and the school. In: Brown RT, editor. Handbook of pediatric psychology in school settings. Mahwah (NJ): Lawrence Erlbaum Associates, Inc; 2004. p. 263–81.

45. Kingma A, van Dommelen RI, Mooyaart EL, et al. Slight cognitive impairment and magnetic resonance imaging abnormalities but normal school levels in children treated for acute lymphoblastic leukemia with chemotherapy only. J Pediatr 2001;139(3):413–20.

46. Butler RW, Mulhern RK. Neurocognitive interventions for children and adolescents surviving cancer. J Pediatr Psychol 2005;30(1):65–78.

47. Mulhern RK, Khan RB, Kaplan S, et al. Short-term efficacy of methylphenidate: a randomized, double-blind, placebo-controlled trial among survivors of childhood cancer. J Clin Oncol 2004;22(23):4743–51.
48. Lipshultz SE, Lipsitz SR, Sallan SE, et al. Chronic progressive cardiac dysfunction years after doxorubicin therapy for childhood acute lymphoblastic leukemia. J Clin Oncol 2005;23(12):2629–36.
49. Kremer LC, van Dalen EC, Offringa M, et al. Frequency and risk factors of anthracycline-induced clinical heart failure in children: a systematic review. Ann Oncol 2002;13(4):503–12.
50. Kremer LC, van der Pal HJ, Offringa M, et al. Frequency and risk factors of subclinical cardiotoxicity after anthracycline therapy in children: a systematic review. Ann Oncol 2002;13(6):819–29.
51. Lipshultz SE, Colan SD, Gelber RD, et al. Late cardiac effects of doxorubicin therapy for acute lymphoblastic leukemia in childhood. N Engl J Med 1991; 324(12):808–15.
52. Rammeloo LA, Postma A, Sobotka-Plojhar MA, et al. Low-dose daunorubicin in induction treatment of childhood acute lymphoblastic leukemia: no long-term cardiac damage in a randomized study of the Dutch Childhood Leukemia Study Group. Med Pediatr Oncol 2000;35(1):13–9.
53. Hudson MM, Rai SN, Nunez C, et al. Noninvasive evaluation of late anthracycline cardiac toxicity in childhood cancer survivors. J Clin Oncol 2007;25(24):3635–43.
54. van Dalen EC, van der Pal HJ, Kok WE, et al. Clinical heart failure in a cohort of children treated with anthracyclines: a long-term follow-up study. Eur J Cancer 2006;42(18):3191–8.
55. Landier W, Bhatia S, Eshelman DA, et al. Development of risk-based guidelines for pediatric cancer survivors: the Children's Oncology Group long-term follow-up guidelines from the Children's Oncology Group Late Effects Committee and nursing discipline. J Clin Oncol 2004;22(24):4979–90.
56. Scottish Intercollegiate Guidelines Network (SIGN). Long term follow up of survivors of childhood cancer. Guideline no. 76. Available at: www.sign.ac.uk/pdf/sign76.pdf. Accessed September 1, 2007.
57. van Dalen EC, Caron HN, Kremer LC. Prevention of anthracycline-induced cardiotoxicity in children: the evidence. Eur J Cancer 2007;43(7):1134–40.
58. Silber JH, Cnaan A, Clark BJ, et al. Enalapril to prevent cardiac function decline in long-term survivors of pediatric cancer exposed to anthracyclines. J Clin Oncol 2004;22(5):820–8.
59. Lipshultz SE, Lipsitz SR, Sallan SE, et al. Long-term enalapril therapy for left ventricular dysfunction in doxorubicin-treated survivors of childhood cancer. J Clin Oncol 2002;20(23):4517–22.
60. van Dalen EC, van der Pal HJ, Reitsma JB, et al. Management of asymptomatic anthracycline-induced cardiac damage after treatment for childhood cancer: a postal survey among Dutch adult and pediatric cardiologists. J Pediatr Hematol Oncol 2005;27(6):319–22.
61. Wouters KA, Kremer LC, Miller TL, et al. Protecting against anthracycline-induced myocardial damage: a review of the most promising strategies. Br J Haematol 2005;131(5):561–78.
62. Swerdlow AJ, Higgins CD, Smith P, et al. Myocardial infarction mortality risk after treatment for Hodgkin disease: a collaborative British cohort study. J Natl Cancer Inst 2007;99(3):206–14.
63. Aleman BM, van den Belt-Dusebout AW, De Bruin ML, et al. Late cardiotoxicity after treatment for Hodgkin lymphoma. Blood 2007;109(5):1878–86.

64. Reinders JG, Heijmen BJ, Olofsen-van Acht MJ, et al. Ischemic heart disease after mantlefield irradiation for Hodgkin's disease in long-term follow-up. Radiother Oncol 1999;51(1):35–42.

65. Boivin JF, Hutchison GB, Lubin JH, et al. Coronary artery disease mortality in patients treated for Hodgkin's disease. Cancer 1992;69(5):1241–7.

66. Constine LS, Schwartz RG, Savage DE, et al. Cardiac function, perfusion, and morbidity in irradiated long-term survivors of Hodgkin's disease. Int J Radiat Oncol Biol Phys 1997;39(4):897–906.

67. Hancock SL, Tucker MA, Hoppe RT. Factors affecting late mortality from heart disease after treatment of Hodgkin's disease. JAMA 1993;270(16):1949–55.

68. Heidenreich PA, Schnittger I, Strauss HW, et al. Screening for coronary artery disease after mediastinal irradiation for Hodgkin's disease. J Clin Oncol 2007; 25(1):43–9.

69. Hull MC, Morris CG, Pepine CJ, et al. Valvular dysfunction and carotid, subclavian, and coronary artery disease in survivors of Hodgkin lymphoma treated with radiation therapy. JAMA 2003;290(21):2831–7.

70. King V, Constine LS, Clark D, et al. Symptomatic coronary artery disease after mantle irradiation for Hodgkin's disease. Int J Radiat Oncol Biol Phys 1996; 36(4):881–9.

71. Bowers DC, McNeil DE, Liu Y, et al. Stroke as a late treatment effect of Hodgkin's disease: a report from the Childhood Cancer Survivor Study. J Clin Oncol 2005; 23(27):6508–15.

72. Meeske KA, Nelson MD, Lavey RS, et al. Premature carotid artery disease in long-term survivors of childhood cancer treated with neck irradiation: a series of 5 cases. J Pediatr Hematol Oncol 2007;29(7):480–4.

73. Florin TA, Fryer GE, Miyoshi T, et al. Physical inactivity in adult survivors of childhood acute lymphoblastic leukemia: a report from the Childhood Cancer Survivor Study. Cancer Epidemiol Biomarkers Prev 2007;16(7):1356–63.

74. Reilly JJ, Ventham JC, Ralston JM, et al. Reduced energy expenditure in preobese children treated for acute lymphoblastic leukemia. Pediatr Res 1998;44(4): 557–62.

75. Jarfelt M, Lannering B, Bosaeus I, et al. Body composition in young adult survivors of childhood acute lymphoblastic leukaemia. Eur J Endocrinol 2005;153(1): 81–9.

76. Oeffinger KC, Mertens AC, Sklar CA, et al. Obesity in adult survivors of childhood acute lymphoblastic leukemia: a report from the Childhood Cancer Survivor Study. J Clin Oncol 2003;21(7):1359–65.

77. Janiszewski PM, Oeffinger KC, Church TS, et al. Abdominal obesity, liver fat and muscle composition in survivors of childhood acute lymphoblastic leukemia. J Clin Endocrinol Metab 2007;92:3816–21.

78. Gurney JG, Ness KK, Sibley SD, et al. Metabolic syndrome and growth hormone deficiency in adult survivors of childhood acute lymphoblastic leukemia. Cancer 2006;107(6):1303–12.

79. Trimis G, Moschovi M, Papassotiriou I, et al. Early indicators of dysmetabolic syndrome in young survivors of acute lymphoblastic leukemia in childhood as a target for preventing disease. J Pediatr Hematol Oncol 2007;29(5):309–14.

80. Moschovi M, Trimis G, Apostolakou F, et al. Serum lipid alterations in acute lymphoblastic leukemia of childhood. J Pediatr Hematol Oncol 2004;26(5): 289–93.

81. van Brussel M, Takken T, Lucia A, et al. Is physical fitness decreased in survivors of childhood leukemia? A systematic review. Leukemia 2005;19(1):13–7.

82. Heikens J, Ubbink MC, van der Pal HP, et al. Long term survivors of childhood brain cancer have an increased risk for cardiovascular disease. Cancer 2000; 88(9):2116–21.

83. Baker KS, Ness KK, Steinberger J, et al. Diabetes, hypertension, and cardiovascular events in survivors of hematopoietic cell transplantation: a report from the Bone Marrow Transplantation Survivor Study. Blood 2007;109(4):1765–72.

84. Neville KA, Cohn RJ, Steinbeck KS, et al. Hyperinsulinemia, impaired glucose tolerance, and diabetes mellitus in survivors of childhood cancer: prevalence and risk factors. J Clin Endocrinol Metab 2006;91(11):4401–7.

85. Lee SJ, Schover LR, Partridge AH, et al. American Society of Clinical Oncology recommendations on fertility preservation in cancer patients. J Clin Oncol 2006; 24(18):2917–31.

86. Schover LR. Sexuality and fertility after cancer. Hematology Am Soc Hematol Educ Program 2005;1:523–7.

87. Critchley H, Thomson AB, Wallace WH. Ovarian and uterine function and reproductive potential. In: Wallace WH, Green DM, editors. Late effects of childhood cancer. London: Arnold Publishers; 2004. p. 225–38.

88. Thomson AB, Wallace WH, Sklar CA. Testicular function. In: Wallace WH, Green DM, editors. Late effects of childhood cancer. London: Arnold Publishers; 2004. p. 239–53.

89. Chemaitilly W, Mertens AC, Mitby P, et al. Acute ovarian failure in the Childhood Cancer Survivor Study. J Clin Endocrinol Metab 2006;91(5):1723–8.

90. Sklar C. Maintenance of ovarian function and risk of premature menopause related to cancer treatment. J Natl Cancer Inst Monogr 2005;34:25–7.

91. Sklar C. Growth and endocrine disturbances after bone marrow transplantation in childhood. Acta Paediatr Suppl 1995;411:57–61 [discussion: 62].

92. Michel G, Socie G, Gebhard F, et al. Late effects of allogeneic bone marrow transplantation for children with acute myeloblastic leukemia in first complete remission: the impact of conditioning regimen without total-body irradiation— a report from the Societe Francaise de Greffe de Moelle. J Clin Oncol 1997; 15(6):2238–46.

93. Thibaud E, Rodriguez-Macias K, Trivin C, et al. Ovarian function after bone marrow transplantation during childhood. Bone Marrow Transplant 1998;21(3): 287–90.

94. Sklar CA, Mertens AC, Mitby P, et al. Premature menopause in survivors of childhood cancer: a report from the Childhood Cancer Survivor Study. J Natl Cancer Inst 2006;98(13):890–6.

95. Larsen EC, Muller J, Schmiegelow K, et al. Reduced ovarian function in long-term survivors of radiation- and chemotherapy-treated childhood cancer. J Clin Endocrinol Metab 2003;88(11):5307–14.

96. Constine LS, Woolf PD, Cann D, et al. Hypothalamic-pituitary dysfunction after radiation for brain tumors. N Engl J Med 1993;328(2):87–94.

97. Rappaport R, Brauner R, Czernichow P, et al. Effect of hypothalamic and pituitary irradiation on pubertal development in children with cranial tumors. J Clin Endocrinol Metab 1982;54(6):1164–8.

98. Sklar CA, Constine LS. Chronic neuroendocrinological sequelae of radiation therapy. Int J Radiat Oncol Biol Phys 1995;31(5):1113–21.

99. Bisharah M, Tulandi T. Laparoscopic preservation of ovarian function: an underused procedure. Am J Obstet Gynecol 2003;188(2):367–70.

100. Williams RS, Littell RD, Mendenhall NP. Laparoscopic oophoropexy and ovarian function in the treatment of Hodgkin disease. Cancer 1999;86(10):2138–42.

101. Blumenfeld Z, Dann E, Avivi I, et al. Fertility after treatment for Hodgkin's disease. Ann Oncol 2002;13(Suppl 1):138–47.
102. Oktay K, Cil AP, Bang H. Efficiency of oocyte cryopreservation: a meta-analysis. Fertil Steril 2006;86(1):70–80.
103. Green DM, Whitton JA, Stovall M, et al. Pregnancy outcome of female survivors of childhood cancer: a report from the Childhood Cancer Survivor Study. Am J Obstet Gynecol 2002;187(4):1070–80.
104. Rovo A, Tichelli A, Passweg JR, et al. Spermatogenesis in long-term survivors after allogeneic hematopoietic stem cell transplantation is associated with age, time interval since transplantation, and apparently absence of chronic GvHD. Blood 2006;108(3):1100–5.
105. Howell SJ, Shalet SM. Spermatogenesis after cancer treatment: damage and recovery. J Natl Cancer Inst Monogr 2005;34:12–7.
106. Sklar CA, Robison LL, Nesbit ME, et al. Effects of radiation on testicular function in long-term survivors of childhood acute lymphoblastic leukemia: a report from the Children Cancer Study Group. J Clin Oncol 1990;8(12):1981–7.
107. Mansky P, Arai A, Stratton P, et al. Treatment late effects in long-term survivors of pediatric sarcoma. Pediatr Blood Cancer 2007;48(2):192–9.
108. Ginsberg JP, Ogle SK, Tuchman LK, et al. Sperm banking for adolescent and young adult cancer patients: sperm quality, patient, and parent perspectives. Pediatr Blood Cancer; 2007, in press.
109. Kenney LB, Laufer MR, Grant FD, et al. High risk of infertility and long term gonadal damage in males treated with high dose cyclophosphamide for sarcoma during childhood. Cancer 2001;91(3):613–21.
110. Clarke SA, Eiser C. Health behaviours in childhood cancer survivors: a systematic review. Eur J Cancer 2007;43(9):1373–84.
111. Larcombe I, Mott M, Hunt L. Lifestyle behaviours of young adult survivors of childhood cancer. Br J Cancer 2002;87(11):1204–9.
112. Bauld C, Toumbourou JW, Anderson V, et al. Health-risk behaviours among adolescent survivors of childhood cancer. Pediatr Blood Cancer 2005;45(5):706–15.
113. Rourke MT, Hobbie WL, Schwartz L, et al. Posttrauamatic stress disorder (PTSD) in young adult survivors of childhood cancer. Pediatr Blood Cancer 2007;49(2):177–82.
114. Schwartz L, Drotar D. Posttraumatic stress and related impairment in survivors of childhood cancer in early adulthood compared to healthy peers. J Pediatr Psychol 2006;31(4):356–66.
115. Alderfer MA, Cnaan A, Annunziato RA, et al. Patterns of posttraumatic stress symptoms in parents of childhood cancer survivors. J Fam Psychol 2005;19(3):430–40.
116. Kazak AE, Alderfer M, Rourke MT, et al. Posttraumatic stress disorder (PTSD) and posttraumatic stress symptoms (PTSS) in families of adolescent childhood cancer survivors. J Pediatr Psychol 2004;29(3):211–9.
117. Alderfer MA, Labay LE, Kazak AE. Brief report: does posttraumatic stress apply to siblings of childhood cancer survivors? J Pediatr Psychol 2003;28(4):281–6.
118. Barakat LP, Alderfer MA, Kazak AE. Posttraumatic growth in adolescent survivors of cancer and their mothers and fathers. J Pediatr Psychol 2006;31(4):413–9.
119. Parry C, Chesler MA. Thematic evidence of psychosocial thriving in childhood cancer survivors. Qual Health Res 2005;15(8):1055–73.
120. Zebrack BJ, Chesler MA. Quality of life in childhood cancer survivors. Psychooncology 2002;11(2):132–41.

121. Zebrack BJ, Zevon MA, Turk N, et al. Psychological distress in long-term survivors of solid tumors diagnosed in childhood: a report from the Childhood Cancer Survivor Study. Pediatr Blood Cancer 2007;49(1):47–51.

122. Zebrack BJ, Gurney JG, Oeffinger K, et al. Psychological outcomes in long-term survivors of childhood brain cancer: a report from the Childhood Cancer Survivor Study. J Clin Oncol 2004;22(6):999–1006.

123. Langeveld NE, Stam H, Grootenhuis MA, et al. Quality of life in young adult survivors of childhood cancer. Support Care Cancer 2002;10(8):579–600.

124. Langeveld NE, Grootenhuis MA, Voute PA, et al. Quality of life, self-esteem and worries in young adult survivors of childhood cancer. Psychooncology 2004; 13(12):867–81.

125. Rauck AM, Green DM, Yasui Y, et al. Marriage in the survivors of childhood cancer: a preliminary description from the Childhood Cancer Survivor Study. Med Pediatr Oncol 1999;33(1):60–3.

126. Langeveld NE, Ubbink MC, Last BF, et al. Educational achievement, employment and living situation in long-term young adult survivors of childhood cancer in the Netherlands. Psychooncology 2003;12(3):213–25.

127. Frobisher C, Lancashire ER, Winter DL, et al. Long-term population-based marriage rates among adult survivors of childhood cancer in Britain. Int J Cancer 2007;121(4):846–55.

128. Koch SV, Kejs AM, Engholm G, et al. Leaving home after cancer in childhood: a measure of social independence in early adulthood. Pediatr Blood Cancer 2006;47(1):61–70.

129. Ross L, Johansen C, Dalton SO, et al. Psychiatric hospitalizations among survivors of cancer in childhood or adolescence. N Engl J Med 2003;349(7):650–7.

130. Lim JW, Zebrack B. Social networks and quality of life for long-term survivors of leukemia and lymphoma. Support Care Cancer 2006;14(2):185–92.

131. Keene N, Hobbie W, Ruccione K. Childhood cancer survivors: a practical guide to your future. Sebastopol (CA): O'Reilly & Associates; 2007.

132. Keene N. Educating the child with cancer: a guide for parents and teachers. Bethesda (MD): Candlelighters Childhood Cancer Foundation; 2003.

133. Skinner R, Wallace WHB, Levitt GA, editors. Therapy based long term follow up. 2nd edition. Leicester (UK): United Kingdom Children's Cancer Study Group: Late effects group; 2005.

134. Kremer LCM, Jaspers MWM, van Leeuwen FE, et al. [Landelijke richtlijnen voor follow-up van overlevenden van kinderkanker]. Tijdschrift voor Kindergeneeskunde 2006;74:214–8 [in Dutch].

135. Aziz NM, Oeffinger KC, Brooks S, et al. Comprehensive long-term follow-up programs for pediatric cancer survivors. Cancer 2006;107(4):841–8.

136. Friedman DL, Freyer DR, Levitt GA. Models of care for survivors of childhood cancer. Pediatr Blood Cancer 2006;46(2):159–68.

137. Shaw AK, Pogany L, Speechley KN, et al. Use of health care services by survivors of childhood and adolescent cancer in Canada. Cancer 2006;106(8): 1829–37.

138. Oeffinger KC, McCabe MS. Models for delivering survivorship care. J Clin Oncol 2006;24(32):5117–24.

139. Skinner R, Wallace WH, Levitt GA. Long-term follow-up of people who have survived cancer during childhood. Lancet Oncol 2006;7(6):489–98.

Venous Thromboembolism in Children

Neil A. Goldenberg, MD[a,b,*], Timothy J. Bernard, MD[a,b,c]

KEYWORDS

- Children • Venous • Thromboembolism • Anticoagulation
- Post-thrombotic syndrome

With improved pediatric survival from serious underlying illnesses, greater use of invasive vascular procedures and devices, and a growing (albeit still suboptimal) awareness that vascular events do occur among the young, venous thromboembolism (VTE) increasingly is recognized as a critical pediatric concern. The focus of this review is on providing background on etiology and epidemiology in this disorder, followed by an in-depth discussion of approaches to the clinical characterization, diagnostic evaluation, and management of pediatric VTE. Prognostic indicators and long-term outcomes are considered, with emphasis placed on available evidence underlying present knowledge and key questions for further investigation.

CHARACTERIZATION

VTE is classified clinically by various relevant descriptors, including first episode versus recurrent, symptomatic versus asymptomatic, acute versus chronic (a distinction that can be difficult at times), veno-occlusive versus nonocclusive, and idiopathic versus risk associated. This last category includes clinical prothrombotic risk factors (eg, exogenous estrogen administration, indwelling central venous catheter, and reduced mobility) and blood-based thrombophilic conditions (eg, transient or persistent antiphospholipid antibodies [APAs], acquired or congenital anticoagulant deficiencies, and factor V Leiden or prothrombin G20210A mutations); the latter are discussed in greater detail later. Because of the frequency of indwelling central venous

A version of this article was previously published in the *Pediatric Clinics of North America*, 55:2.
[a] Mountain States Regional Hemophilia and Thrombosis Center, PO Box 6507, Mail-Stop F-416, Aurora, CO 80045-0507, USA
[b] Pediatric Stroke Program, University of Colorado and The Children's Hospital, 13123 East 16th Avenue, Aurora, CO 80045, USA
[c] Department of Child Neurology, University of Colorado and The Children's Hospital, 13123 East 16th Avenue, Aurora, CO 80045, USA
* Corresponding author. Mountain States Regional Hemophilia and Thrombosis Center, PO Box 6507, Mail-Stop F-416, Aurora, CO 80045-0507.
E-mail address: neil.goldenberg@uchsc.edu (N.A. Goldenberg).

Hematol Oncol Clin N Am 24 (2010) 151–166
doi:10.1016/j.hoc.2009.11.005
0889-8588/10/$ – see front matter © 2010 Elsevier Inc. All rights reserved.

hemonc.theclinics.com

catheters as a major clinical risk factor for VTE in children, VTE also may be classified as catheter-related thromboembolism (CRT) versus non-CRT. VTEs also are distinguished anatomically by vascular type (ie, venous versus arterial); vascular distribution (eg, distal lower extremity versus proximal lower extremity versus central or superficial versus deep vasculature); and organ system affected, if applicable (eg, cerebral sinovenous thrombosis [CSVT] or pulmonary embolism). The use of systematic nomenclature and precise descriptors for VTE assists in optimizing clinical care and in evaluating clinical research evidence in the field.

EPIDEMIOLOGY

Several years ago, registry data revealed an estimated cumulative incidence of 0.07 per 10,000 (5.3 per 10,000 hospitalizations) for extremity deep venous thrombosis (DVT) or pulmonary embolism (PE) among non-neonatal Canadian children[1] and an incidence rate of 0.14 per 10,000 Dutch children per year for VTE in general.[2] More recently, an evaluation of the National Hospital Discharge Survey and census data for VTE in the United States disclosed an overall incidence rate of 0.49 per 10,000 per year.[3]

Epidemiologic data have revealed that the age distribution of the incidence rate for VTE in children is bimodal, with peak rates in the neontal period and adolescence. The Dutch registry, for example, indicated a VTE incidence rate of 14.5 per 10,000 per year in the neonatal period, approximately 100 times greater than the overall rate in childhood,[2] whereas the VTE-specific incidence rate in the United States among adolescents 15 to 17 years of age was determined as 1.1 per 10,000 per year, a rate nearly threefold that observed overall in children.[3]

ETIOLOGY

The pathogenesis of VTE readily can be appreciated by considering the Virchow triad, consisting of venous stasis, endothelial damage, and the hypercoagulable state. In children, greater than 90% of VTEs are risk associated[2,4,5] (compared with approximately 60% in adults), with risk factors often disclosed from more than one component of this triad. Specific examples of VTE risk factors in children are shown in (**Fig. 1**). One of the most common clinical prothrombotic risk factors in childhood is an indwelling central venous catheter. More than 50% of cases of DVT in children and more than 80% of cases in newborns occur in association with central venous

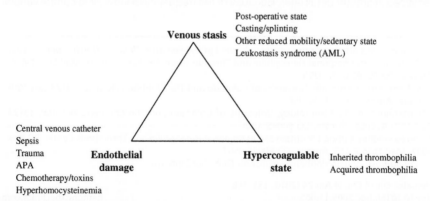

Venous stasis
Post-operative state
Casting/splinting
Other reduced mobility/sedentary state
Leukostasis syndrome (AML)

Central venous catheter
Sepsis
Trauma
APA
Chemotherapy/toxins
Hyperhomocysteinemia

Endothelial damage

Hypercoagulable state
Inherited thrombophilia
Acquired thrombophilia

Fig. 1. Clinical prothrombotic risk factors: the Virchow triad applied to VTE in children.

catheters.[1,6] The presence of an indwelling central venous catheter, underlying malignancy or disorder for which bone marrow transplantation was undertaken, and congenital cardiac disease and its corrective surgery all were highly prevalent in the Canadian pediatric thrombosis registry,[4] whereas underlying infectious illness and the presence of an indwelling central venous cathether were identified as pervasive clinical risk factors in a recent cohort study analysis from the United States.[5] It is likely that differences in the composition of referral populations contribute strongly to differences in the composition of VTE etiologies across major pediatric thrombosis centers.

With regard to the third component of the Virchow triad, the hypercoagulable state, blood-based risk factors for VTE in children include inherited and acquired thrombophilic conditions and markers of coagulation activation (discussed later). Potent thrombophilic conditions (eg, APAs) in children frequently are acquired and, more rarely, may be congenital (eg, severe anticoagulant deficiencies). By contrast, mild congenital thrombophilia traits (eg, the factor V Leiden and prothrombin G20210A mutations) are common in white populations, with prevalences of approximately 5% and 2%, respectively. Thrombophilia potentially can be caused by any alteration in the hemostatic balance that increases thrombin production, enhances platelet activation or aggregation, mediates endothelial activation or damage, or inhibits fibrinolysis. Common examples of acquired thrombophilia in children include increased factor VIII activity with significant infection and inflammatory states, anticoagulant deficiencies resulting from consumption in bacterial sepsis and disseminated intravascular coagulation (DIC) or production of inhibitory antibodies in acute viral infection, and parainfectious development of APAs. To provide an appreciation of the magnitude of VTE risk increase associated with several congenital or genetically influenced thrombophilia traits, population-based VTE risk estimates derived from the adult literature are shown in **Table 1**. As seen in **Table 1**, the addition of standard-dose estrogen oral contraceptive pill to an underlying heterozygous factor V Leiden (in large part by virtue of a "double-hit" to the protein C pathway) substantially increases the risk for VTE from a baseline risk of 15 per 10,000 women in the United States, ages 15 to 17, per year[3] to a risk of more than 500 per 10,000 (or 5%) per year.

CLINICAL PRESENTATION

The degree of clinical suspicion for acute VTE in children should be influenced principally by (1) clinical prothrombotic risk factors and family history of early VTE or other vascular disease elicited on thorough interview; (2) known thrombophilia traits and risk factors; and (3) clinical signs and symptoms. The signs and symptoms of VTE depend

Table 1
Venous thromboembolism risk estimates for selected thrombophilia traits and conditions

Trait/Condition	Venous Thromboembolism Risk Estimate (× Baseline)
Hyperhomocysteinemia	2.5
Prothrombin 20,210 mutation, heterozygous	3
Oral contraceptive pill (tandard dose estrogen)	4
Factor V Leiden mutation, heterozygous	2–7
OCP + factor V Leiden mutation, heterozygous	35
Factor V Leiden mutation, homozygous	80

on anatomic location and organ system affected and are influenced by characteristics of veno-occlusiveness and chronicity. The classic manifestation of acute extremity DVT is painful unilateral limb swelling. The lack of other physical examination findings (eg, Homans' sign or presence of a palpable cord in the popliteal fossa) should not reduce the clinical index of suspicion of DVT. In upper extremity DVT with extension into, and occlusion of, the superior vena cava (SVC), signs and symptoms may include swelling of neck and face, bilateral periorbital edema, and headache. PE classically is manifest by sudden-onset, unexplained shortness of breath with pleuritic chest pain. When PE is proximal or extensive bilaterally in the distal pulmonary arterial tree, hypoxemia often is demonstrated. Associated right heart failure may manifest with hepatomegaly or peripheral edema. Proximal PE and especially saddle embolus can present with cyanosis or sudden collapse. In many cases, however, PE may be asymptomatic or produce only subtle symptoms in children,[7–10] especially when involving limited segmental branches of the pulmonary arteries. In one retrospective series, only 50% of affected children had clinical symptoms attributable to PE.[8] Acute CSVT may present with unusually severe and persistent headache, blurred vision, neurologic signs (eg, cranial nerve palsy and papilledema), or seizures. The classic findings in renal vein thrombosis (RVT) are hematuria and thrombocytopenia, sometimes associated with uremia (especially when bilateral). Presenting signs include oliguria (especially when bilateral) and, in the neonatal period (the time at which RVT is most common during childhood), a flank mass that often is palpable on examination. RVT in older children often is associated with nephrotic syndrome (a risk factor for VTE in general) and, hence, may present with associated stigmata of peripheral and periorbital edema when diagnosed at presentation of nephrosis.[11] Thrombocytopenia may be a presenting manifestation not only of RVT but also of an intracardiac (eg, right atrial) thrombus, especially as in cases of CRT associated with sepsis and DIC. Portal vein thrombosis characteristically presents with splenomegaly and is associated with thrombocytopenia and, often, anemia; gastrointestinal bleeding at presentation typically signals the presence of gastroesophageal varices as a result of portal hypertension. Internal jugular vein thrombosis may manifest with neck pain or swelling and, in the Lemierre syndrome, also is associated classically with fever, trismus, and a palpable mass in the lateral triangle of the neck. Isolated intracardiac thrombosis in association with cardiac surgery or central venous catheter placement most often is asymptomatic.

Chronic VTE may be diagnosed incidentally without signs or symptoms (as sometimes occurs for CSVT during unrelated brain imaging) or, alternatively, may present with signs and symptoms of chronic venous obstruction or post-thrombotic syndrome (PTS) secondary to central venous or extremity thrombosis, including limb pain and edema, dilated superficial collateral veins, venous stasis dermatitis, or frank ulceration of the skin.

DIAGNOSTIC EVALUATION
Radiologic Imaging

Historically, venography has been the gold standard for diagnosis of venous thrombosis but limited by its invasiveness. In recent years, this modality has experienced a diminishing role with the development of effective noninvasive or minimally invasive radiologic imaging techniques. Radiologic imaging is used not only to confirm the clinical diagnosis of VTE but also to define the extent and occlusiveness of thrombosis. For suspected DVT of the distal or proximal lower extremity, compression ultrasonography with Doppler imaging typically is used for objective confirmation. When the thrombus may affect or extend into deep pelvic or abdominal veins, CT or MRI often is required. In suspected DVT of the upper extremity, compression ultrasound with Doppler effectively evaluates the limb, but other modalities (eg, echocardiography, CT, and MRI) are needed to disclose involvement of more central vasculature (eg, right atrial thrombosis and SVC thrombosis). In the case of asymptomatic nonocclusive extremity DVT, conventional venography may be used as an alternative to CT or MRI. To establish a diagnosis of DVT of the jugular venous system (such as in suspected cases of the Lemierre syndrome),[12] compression ultrasound with Doppler imaging typically is used.

PE in children commonly is disclosed by spiral CT or, alternatively, ventilation-perfusion scan, the latter generally is suboptimal in cases wherein other lung pathology exists and at centers wherein availability of (and expertise with) this modality is limited. CSVT typically is diagnosed by standard CT or CT venography or, alternatively, MRI or MR venography. The diagnosis of RVT most often is made clinically in neonates and supported by Doppler ultrasound findings of intrarenal vascular resistive indices; however, in some cases a discrete thrombus may be suggested by Doppler ultrasound (especially when extending into the inferior vena cava [IVC]) or disclosed further via MR venography. When RVT occurs in older children, Doppler ultrasound or CT often is diagnostic. Similarly, portal vein thrombosis typically is visualized by Doppler ultrasound or CT.

When new-onset venous thrombosis is evaluated in patients in areas of anatomic abnormality of the venous system (eg, extensive collateral venous circulation due to a prior VTE episode, May-Thurner anomaly, or atretic IVC with azygous continuation), more sensitive methods, such as CT venography or magnetic resonance (MR) venography, often are required to delineate the vascular anatomy adequately and the presence, extent, and occlusiveness of thrombosis. In some cases, conventional venography may be required.

MR venography is more expensive than CT venography, typically requires sedation in children less than 8 years of age or those who are developmentally delayed or very anxious, and its feasibility during acute VTE evaluation may be limited by availability of MR-trained technologists. MR venography offers a significant advantage over CT venography, however, in that it provides diagnostic sensitivity at least as great as CT venography, without engendering the significant radiation exposure of the latter modality.

Laboratory Evaluation

Diagnostic laboratory evaluation for pediatric acute VTE includes a complete blood count, comprehensive thrombophilia evaluation (discussed previously), and beta-hCG testing in postmenarchal women. Additional laboratory studies may be warranted depending on associated medical conditions and VTE involvement of specific organ systems. **Table 2** summarizes a panel of thrombophilia traits and markers identified as risk factors for VTE in pediatric studies and recommended by the Scientific and Standardization Committee Subcommitee on Perinatal and Pediatric Haemostasis of the International Society on Thrombosis and Haemostasis for the diagnostic laboratory evaluation of acute VTE in children.[13] The panel is comprised of testing for states of anticoagulant (eg, protein C, protein S, and antithrombin) deficiency and procoagulant (eg, factor VIII) excess, mediators of hypercoagulablity or endothelial damage (eg, APAs, lipoprotein(a), and homocysteine), and markers of coagulation activation (eg, D-dimer).

Table 2
Thrombophilic conditions and markers tested during comprehensive diagnostic laboratory evaluation of acute venous thromboembolism in children

Condition/Marker	Testing Methods
Genetic	
Factor V Leiden polymorphism	PCR
Prothrombin G20210A polymorphism	PCR
Elevated plasma lipoprotein(a) concentration[a]	ELISA
Acquired or genetic	
Antithrombin deficiency	Chromogenic (functional) assay
Protein C deficiency	Chromogenic (functional) assay
Protein S deficiency	ELISA for free (ie, functionally active) protein S antigen
Elevated plasma factor VIII activity[b]	One-stage clotting assay (aPTT-based)
Hyperhomocysteinemia	Mass spectroscopy
APAs	ELISA for anticardiolipin and anti-β2-glycoprotein I IgG and IgM; clotting assay (dilute Russell viper venom time or aPTT-based phospholipid neutralization method) for LA
DIC	Includes platelet count, fibrinogen by clotting method (Clauss), and D-dimer by semiquantitative or quantitative immunoassay (eg, latex agglutination)
Activated protein C resistance	Clotting assay (aPTT based)

[a] Although desginated here as genetic, lipoprotein(a) also may be elevated as part of the acute phase response.
[b] Noted as worthy of consideration in original International Society on Thrombosis and Haemostasis recommendations;[13] this since has been shown a prognostic marker in pediatric thrombosis.[6] Additional testing involving the fibrinolytic system and systemic inflammatory response also is noted as worthy of consideration.

TREATMENT

A summary of conventional antithrombotic agents and corresponding target anticoagulant levels, based on recent pediatric recommendations,[14] is provided in **Table 3** for initial (ie, acute phase) and extended (ie, subacute phase) treatment. Conventional anticoagulants attenuate hypercoagulability, decreasing the risk for thrombus progression and embolism, and rely on intrinsic fibrinolytic mechanisms to dissolve the thrombus over time. The conventional anticoagulants used most commonly in children include heparins and warfarin. Heparins, including unfractionated heparin (UFH) and low molecular weight heparin (LMWH), enhance the activity of antithrombin, an intrinsic anticoagulant protein that serves as a key inhibitor of thrombin. Warfarin acts through antagonism of vitamin K, thereby interfering with γ-carboxylation of the vitamin K–dependent procoagulant factors II, VII, IX, and X and intrinsic anticoagulant proteins C and S.

Initial anticoagulant therapy (ie, acute phase) for VTE in children uses UFH or LMWH. LMWH increasingly is used as a first-line agent for initial anticoagulant therapy in children given the relative ease of subcutaneous over intravenous administration, the decreased need for blood monitoring of anticoagulant efficacy, and a decreased

Table 3
Recommended intensities and durations of conventional antithrombotic therapies in children, by etiology and treatment agent

| Episode | Agents and Target Anticoagulant Activities | | Duration of Therapy, by Etiology |
	Initial Treatment	Extended Treatment	
First	UFH 0.3–0.7 anti-Xa U/mL	Warfarin INR 2.0–3.0	Resolved risk factor: 3–6 months
	LMWH 0.5–1.0 anti-Xa U/mL	LMWH 0.5–1.0 anti-Xa U/mL	No known clinical risk factor: 6–12 months Chronic clinical risk factor: 12 months Potent congenital thrombophilia: indefinite
Recurrent	UFH 0.3–0.7 anti-Xa U/mL	Warfarin INR 2.0–3.0	Resolved risk factor: 6–12 months
	LMWH 0.5–1.0 anti-Xa U/mL	LMWH 0.5–1.0 anti-Xa U/mL	No known clinical risk factor: 12 months Chronic clinical risk factor: indefinite Potent congenital thrombophilia: indefinite

risk for the development of heparin-induced thrombocytopenia (HIT). UFH (which has a shorter half-life than LMWH) typically is preferred in circumstances of heightened bleeding risk or labile acute clinical status, given the rapid extinction of anticoagulant effect after cessation of the drug. In addition, UFH often is used for acute VTE therapy in the setting of significant impairment or lability in renal function because of the relatively greater renal elimination of LMWH. Common initial maintenance dosing for UFH in non-neonatal children begins with an intravenous loading dose (50 to 75 U/kg) followed by a continuous intravenous infusion (15 to 25 U/kg per hour). In full-term neonates, a maintenance dose (up to 50 U/kg per hour) may be required, especially if the clinical condition is complicated by antithrombin consumption. The starting dose for the LMWH enoxaparin in non-neonatal children commonly ranges between 1.0 and 1.25 mg/kg subcutaneously on an every-12-hour schedule; no bolus dose is given. In full-term neonates, a higher dose of enoxaparin (1.5 mg/kg) typically is necessary.[15] Some recent research has investigated whether once-daily enoxaparin dosing may be suitable for acute VTE therapy in children. For the LMWH dalteparin, initial maintenance dosing of100–150 antifactor Xa (anti-Xa) U/kg seems appropriate based on available pediatric data;[16] however, further studies are warranted (with more robust representation of all age groups within the pediatric age range) to determine the optimal intensity and frequency of dosing of dalteparin. Heparin therapy, UFH or LMWH, is monitored most accurately by anti-Xa activity. Anti-Xa level is obtained 6 to 8 hours after initiation of UFH infusion and 4 hours after one of the first few doses of LMWH. Clinical laboratories must be made aware of the type of heparin administered so that the appropriate assay standard (eg, UFH or enoxaparin) is used. For UFH, the therapeutic range is 0.3 to 0.7 anti-Xa activity U/mL, whereas for LMWH the therapeutic range is 0.5 to 1.0 U/mL. When the anti-Xa assay is not available, the activated partial thromboplastin time (aPTT) may be used (with a goal aPTT of 60–85 seconds or approximately 1.5–2 times the upper limit of age-appropriate normal values); however, this approach is suboptimal especially in the pediatric age group, in which transient APAs are common and may alter the clotting endpoint. One study of pediatric heparin monitoring demonstrated inaccuracy of aPTT approximately 30% of the time.[17] When dosed by weight in childhood, LMWH does not require frequent monitoring, but anti-Xa activity should be evaluated with changes in renal function. In addition, in cases of acute VTE in which acquired antithrombin deficiency is related to consumption in acute infection or inflammation, anti-Xa activity may rise as antithrombin levels normalize with resolution of the acute illness; in this circumstance, follow-up evaluation of anti-Xa activity is warranted in the subacute period.

The recommended duration of heparinization of 5 to 10 days during the initial therapy for acute VTE has been extrapolated from adult data.[18] UFH treatment rarely is maintained beyond the acute period, given the risk for osteoporosis with extended administration[14] and the inconvenience of continuous intravenous administration. Although adult data suggest efficacy of subcutaneous administration of UFH for acute VTE,[19] this has been evaluated only for the acute therapy period before extended therapy with warfarin, and the appropriateness of such an approach in children is not established.

Extended anticoagulant therapy (ie, subacute phase) for VTE in children may use LMWH or warfarin. For warfarin anticoagulation, warfarin may be started during the acute phase; however, because severe congenital deficiencies involving the protein C pathway can present as VTE in early childhood and are associated with warfarin skin necrosis, warfarinization ideally should be initiated only after therapeutic anticoagulation is achieved with a heparin agent. Warfarin is available in tablet form in a variety of doses (eg, 5 mg, 2 mg, or 1 mg) and as an oral liquid formulation at many pediatric tertiary care hospitals. Commonly, the starting dose for warfarin in children is 0.1 mg/kg orally once daily. Warfarin is monitored by international normalized ratio (INR), derived from the measured prothrombin time. The therapeutic INR range for warfarin anticoagulation in VTE is 2.0 to 3.0. Recent adult data do not agree with the historical evidence for maintaining a higher INR (2.5–3.5) in the presence of an APA; however, pediatric data are lacking with regard to optimal dose intensity and duration in children who have APA syndrome. The INR typically is checked after the first 5 days of initiation of (or dosing change in) warfarin therapy and weekly thereafter until stable; gradually, less frequent monitoring often is feasible, with continued stability. The INR also should be evaluated at the time of any bleeding manifestations or increased bruising. Warfarin must be discontinued at least 5 days before invasive procedures, with an INR obtained preprocedurally. Often, an anticoagulant transition (bridge) to LMWH can be performed. The development of pediatric anticoagulation monitoring and transition algorithms can assist in optimizing patient care.

Pediatric recommendations for the duration of antithrombotic therapy in acute VTE[14] largely are derived from evidence in adult trials. For first-episode VTE in children in the absence of potent chronic thrombophilia (eg, APA syndrome, homozygous anticoagulant deficiency, and homozygous factor V Leiden or prothrombin G20210A), the recommended duration of anticoagulant therapy is 3 to 6 months in the presence of an underlying reversible risk factor (eg, postoperative VTE), 6 to 12 months when idiopathic, and 12 months to lifelong when a chronic risk factor persists (eg, systemic lupus erythematosus [SLE]). Recurrent VTE is treated for 6 to 12 months in the presence of an underlying reversible risk factor, 12 months to lifelong when idiopathic, and lifelong when a chronic risk factor persists. In the setting of APA syndrome or potent congenital thrombophilia, the treatment duration for first-episode VTE often is indefinite. Some evidence suggests that children who have SLE and persistence of the lupus anticoagulant (LA) have a 16- to 25-fold greater risk for VTEs than children who have SLE and no LA.[20] In children who have primary (ie, idiopathic) or secondary (ie, associated with SLE or other underlying chronic inflammatory condition) APA syndrome, however, it is possible that the autoimmune disease will become quiescent in later years, such that the benefit of continued therapeutic anticoagulation as secondary VTE prophylaxis may be re-evaluated. Some experts recommend consideration of low-dose anticoagulation as secondary VTE prophylaxis after a conventional 3- to 6-month course of therapeutic anticoagulation for VTE in children who have SLE and who have APA syndrome.[21] Such low-dose anticoagulation might, for example, consist of enoxaparin 1.0–1.5 mg/kg subcutaneously once daily, enoxaparin 0.5 mg/kg subcutaneously twice daily, or daily warfarin with a goal INR of approximately 1.5. Further study to optimize the intensity and duration of therapy or secondary prophylaxis for VTE in children who have APA syndrome urgently is needed, however, especially given the recent evidence in adult VTE that secondary prophylaxis with low-dose warfarin not only may offer little risk reduction beyond no anticoagulation but also is associated with bleeding complications despite a reduced warfarin dose.[22,23]

Thrombolytic approaches are gaining increasing attention and use during acute VTE therapy in children, particularly in patients who have hemodynamically significant PE or extensive limb-threatening VTE. Unlike conventional anticoagulants, which attenuate hypercoagulability, thrombolytics promote fibrinolysis directly. Tissue-type plasminogen activator is an intrinsic activator of the fibrinolytic system and is administered as a recombinant agent by various routes (eg, systemic bolus, systemic short-duration infusion, systemic low-dose continuous infusion, or local catheter-directed infusion with or without interventional mechanical thrombectomy/thrombolysis). A recent cohort study analysis of children who had acute lower extremity DVT and who had an a priori high risk for poor post-thrombotic outcomes by virtue of completely veno-occlusive thrombus and plasma FVIII activity greater than 150 U/dL or D-dimer concentration greater than 500 ng/mL revealed that a thrombolysis regimen followed by standard anticoagulation may reduce the risk for PTS substantially compared with standard anticoagulation alone.[24] Further investigation in clinical trials is necessary to confirm these findings.

Other antithrombotic agents include factor Xa inhibitors and direct thrombin inhibitors. Factor Xa inhibitors, including fondaparinux, inhibit the activation of factor X, thereby inhibiting thrombin indirectly. Direct thrombin inhibitors, by contrast, inhibit thrombin directly via its active site or by binding to its target on fibrin and include such drugs as hirudin, recombinant hirudins (eg, lepirudin), and argatroban, all of which are administered intravenously. Intravenous direct thrombin inhibitors are indicated for the treatment of HIT, in particular HIT with associated acute thrombosis, and are used in patients who have a history of HIT. The aforementioned factor Xa inhibitors and direct thrombin inhibitors routinely are monitored by aPTT, with the therapeutic goal ranging from a 1.5- to 3.0-fold aPTT prolongation. A variety of factor Xa inhibitors and oral direct thrombin inhibitors are undergoing preclinical development or evaluation in adult clinical trials.

Other products may have antithrombotic roles in selected circumstances but await demonstration of efficacy in clinical trials. For example, plasma replacement with protein C concentrate is a useful adjunctive therapy to conventional anticoagulant for VTE or purpura fulminans because of microvascular thrombosis in severe congenital protein C deficiency[25–28] and may play a beneficial role in the treatment of purpura fulminans resulting from microvascular thrombosis in children who have sepsis, in particular meningococcemia.[29–31] In addition, case series suggest a role for antithrombin replacement in prevention of VTE in children and young adults who have congenital severe antihrombin deficiency[32] for the prevention of L-asparaginase–associated VTE in pediatric acute lymphoblastic leukemia[33,34] and as combination therapy with defibrotide in the prevention and treatment of hepatic sinusoidal obstruction syndrome (formerly termed veno-occlusive disease) in children undergoing hematopoietic stem cell transplantation.[35] The potential benefit for VTE risk reduction using a regimen of antithrombin replacement combined with daily prophylactic LMWH during induction and consolidation phases of therapy in acute lymphoblastic leukemia also is suggested by a historically controlled cohort study of the BFM 2000 protocol experience in Europe.[36] As discussed previously, antithrombin replacement also may be worthy of consideration in patients who have acute VTE and are undergoing heparinization in whom significant antithrombin deficiency prevents the achievement of therapeutic anti-Xa levels (ie, heparin "resistance"). This may be the case in nephrotic syndrome–associated VTE. Additionally, neonates who have clinical conditions complicated by antithrombin consumption in particular are predisposed to such heparin "resistance" because of a physiologic relative deficiency of this key intrinsic thrombin inhibitor.

The use of vena caval filters should be considered in children of appropriate size in whom recurrent VTE (especially PE) occurrs on therapeutic anticoagulation in the presence of a persistent prothrombotic risk factor. In addition, temporary vena caval filters may be considered during times of especially heightened risk for PE. With regard to long-standing vena caval filters, although a case series has suggested that these devices are effective when used with concomitant therapeutic anticoagluation for primary and secondary prevention of PE in teens,[37] the impact of such nonretrievable devices on the vena cava of developing children is not well studied, and experience with surgical removal of permanent vena caval filters is limited. Consequently, the use of nonretrievable vena caval filters in pediatrics should be undertaken with great caution.

OUTCOMES

Complications of VTEs can occur acutely and over the long term. Short-term adverse outcomes include major hemorrhagic complications of antithrombotic interventions and of the thrombotic event itself (eg, post-thrombotic hemorrhage in the brain, testis, or adrenal gland); early recurrent VTE (including DVT and PE); SVC syndrome in DVT of the upper venous system; acute renal insufficiency in RVT; catheter-related sepsis, PE, and catheter malfunction (sometimes necessitating surgical replacement) in CRT; severe acute venous insufficiency leading to venous infarction with limb gangrene in rare cases of occlusive DVT involving the extremities; and death from hemodynamic instability in extensive intracardiac thrombosis or proximal PE. Given the long-term risks for recurrence, disease sequelae, and functional impairment, however, VTE arguably is best considered a chronic disorder in children. Long-term adverse outcomes in pediatric VTE recently have been reviewed[38] and include recurrent VTE; chronic hypertension and renal insufficiency in RVT; variceal hemorrhage in portal vein thrombosis; chronic SVC syndrome in CRT involving SVC occlusion; loss of availability for venous access in recurrent or extensive CRT of the upper venous system; and development of the PTS, a condition of chronic venous insufficiency after DVT. The manifestations of PTS may include edema, visibly dilated superficial collateral veins (**Fig. 2**A), venous stasis dermatitis (see **Fig. 2**B), and (in the most severe cases) venous stasis ulcers.

Registry[1,4,39] and cohort study[5] data in pediatric VTE of all types indicate that children seem to have a lower risk for recurrent thrombembolism than adults (cumulative

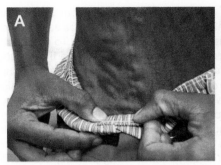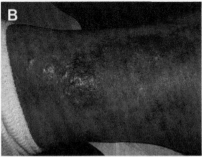

Fig. 2. PTS: dilated collateral superficial venous circulation and venous stasis dermatitis. (*A*) Dilated collaterals in a 14-year-old boy who had ileofemoral to IVC DVT. (*B*) Stasis dermatitis in a 13-year-old boy who had iliofemoral to IVC DVT.

incidences at 1 to 2 years of 6% to 11% versus 12% to 22%, respectively).[40,41] The risk for PTS in children who have DVT of the limbs, however, seems at least as great as that in adults (cumulative incidences at 1 to 2 years of 33% to 70%[2,5] versus 29%, respectively[41]). In addition, a German cohort study of children who had spontaneous VTE (ie, VTE in the absence of identified clinical risk factors), the cumulative incidence of recurrent VTE at a median follow-up time of 7 years was 21%,[42] suggesting that, in this subgroup of pediatric VTE, the risk for recurrent events is long-lived. Although VTE-specific mortality in children is low, ranging from 0% to 2%,[43,44] considerably higher all-cause mortality reflects the severity of underlying conditions (eg, sepsis, cancer, and congenital cardiac disease) in pediatric VTE. Neonate-specific outcomes data in pediatric non-RVT VTE reflect an all-cause mortality of 12% to 18%,[6,45,46] including one series of premature infants who had CRT treated with enoxaparin.[46] With regard to major bleeding complications occurring during the anticoagulation period, frequencies in children range from 0% to 9% [5,43] in recent studies.

As indicated previously, outcomes of VTE in children may differ among specific anatomic sites. In a Canadian study of CRT in children from 1990 to 1996,[47] VTE-specific mortality was 4% among all children and 20% among those children in whom CRT was complicated by PE. No major bleeding episodes were observed. At a median follow-up of 2 years, the cumulative incidence of symptomatic recurrent VTE was 6.5%, and PTS developed in 9% of children. In other series of RVT[48-52] (primarily among neonates), VTE-related death has been uncommon, and the cumulative incidence of recurrent VTE ranged from 0% to 4%. The cumulative incidence of chronic hypertension in RVT in these studies was reported at 22% to 33%. For CSVT, the pediatric literature reflects a VTE-specific mortality ranging from 4% to 20%, with a cumulative incidence of recurrent VTE of 8% for neonatal CSVT cases and 17% for CSVT occurring in older children.[53-56] Long-term neurologic sequelae were noted in 17% to 26% of neonatal CSVT cases and the cumulative incidence of such sequelae in childhood (ie, non-neonatal) CSVT ranged widely between 8% and 47%. In the aforementioned pediatric series of RVT and CSVT, the proportion of children who received anticoagulation and the duration of the anticoagulation course varied considerably across studies. With regard to portal vein thrombosis, few pediatric series reporting outcomes have been published; however, it seems that the risk for developing recurrent gastrovariceal bleeding in this population is substantial, occurring in many cases even after surgical interventions have been undertaken to reduce portal hypertension.[57] For PE in childhood, long-term outcomes, such as chronic pulmonary hypertension and pulmonary function, have yet to be established.

An additional VTE outcome of interest is residual thrombus burden. To date, data (principally in adults) suggest that the persistence of thrombosis after a therapeutic course of anticoagulation of appropriate duration does not increase the risk for recurrent VTE, including PE, appreciably. Some evidence[58] indicates, however, that persistent thrombosis is associated with the development of venous valvular insufficiency, an important risk factor for (albeit an imperfect correlate of)[59] the development of PTS. The prevalence of residual thrombosis despite adequate anticolagulation in neonatal VTE has ranged from 12% in a small series of premature newborns who had CRT[46] to 62% in full-term neonatal VTE survivors.[4] Among primarily older children, the prevalence of persistent thrombosis has ranged broadly from 37% to 68% in the few longitudinal studies that have used systematic radiologic evaluation of thrombus evolution.[5,16]

The ability to predict clinically relevant long-term outcomes of VTE at diagnosis and during the acute and subacute phases of treatment is essential to establishing a future risk-stratified approach to antithrombotic management in children. Early work defined strong associations of homozygous anticoagulant deficiencies and APA syndrome with recurrent VTE. Over the past several years, the presence of multiple thromophilia traits has been identified as prognostic for recurrent VTE,[42] and the radiologic finding of complete veno-occlusion at diagnosis of DVT is associated with an increased risk for persistent thrombosis[60] (which, in turn, is associated with the development of venous valvular insufficiency,[58] as discussed previously). Most recently, plasma FVIII activity greater than 150 U/dL and D-dimer concentration greater than 500 ng/mL at the time of diagnosis of VTE in children and after 3 to 6 months of standard anticoagulation are shown to predict a composite adverse thrombotic outcome, characterized by persistent thrombosis, recurrent VTE, or the development of PTS,[5] adding to evidence for the prognostic usefulness of these markers in adult VTE.[61–63]

FUTURE DIRECTIONS

VTE has emerged in recent years as a critical pediatric concern with acute and chronic sequelae. Important and highly clinically relevant questions on its etiology, pathogenesis, and natural history remain to be addressed via collaborative cohort studies. For example, what are the mechanisms by which distinct APA mediate the prothrombotic state and, in turn, confer distinct risks for relevant outcomes of thrombus progression, recurrence, and embolism? Do criteria for APA syndrome established in adults—and the implications for indefinite anticoagulation—readily apply to children? Pediatric recommendations for antithrombotic management in acute VTE in general are derived largely from evidence from adult trials. The ability to predict clinically relevant long-term outcomes of pediatric VTE at diagnosis and during the acute and subacute phases of treatment, however, is essential to establishing a risk-stratified approach to antithrombotic management specific to children. Key evidence in this area is beginning to emerge. Using such evidence, multicenter randomized controlled trials are proposed (or already are underway) to evaluate the duration of standard anticoagulant therapy for first-episode VTE in children who do not have an increased a priori risk for recurrent VTE and PTS and to investigate thrombolytic therapeutic approaches in children who have acute DVT of the proximal lower extremities and who are at high risk for adverse outcomes. Finally, increased regulatory emphasis for devoted pediatric study of agents newly approved in adult populations promises to add diversity to the available antithrombotic strategies for pediatric VTE in the future. New agents will be important particularly in rare but life-threatening circumstances, such as catastrophic APA syndrome and HIT, for which alternative approaches to conventional anticoagulants are needed.

REFERENCES

1. Andrew M, David M, Adams M, et al. Venous thromboembolic complications (VTE) in children: first analyses of the Canadian Registry of VTE. Blood 1994; 83:1251–7.
2. van Ommen CH, Heijboer H, Buller HR, et al. Venous thromboembolism in childhood: a prospective two-year registry in the Netherlands. J Pediatr 2001;139: 676–81.
3. Stein PD, Kayali R, Olson RE, et al. Incidence of venous thromboembolism in infants and children: data from the National Hospital Discharge Survey. J Pediatr 2004;145:563–5.
4. Monagle P, Adams M, Mahoney M, et al. Outcome of pediatric thromboembolic disease: a report from the Canadian Childhood Thrombophilia Registry. Pediatr Res 2000;47:763–6.
5. Goldenberg NA, Knapp-Clevenger R, Manco-Johnson MJ, et al. Elevated plasma factor VIII and D-dimer levels as predictors of poor outcomes of thrombosis in children. N Engl J Med 2004;351:1081–8.
6. Schmidt B, Andrew M. Neonatal thrombosis: report of a prospective Canadian and international registry. Pediatrics 1995;96:939–43.
7. David M, Andrew M. Venous thromboembolic complications in children. J Pediatr 1993;123:337–46.
8. Buck JR, Connor RH, Cook WW, et al. Pulmonary embolism in children. J Pediatr Surg 1981;16:385–91.
9. Van Ommen CH, Peters M. Acute pulmonary embolism in childhood. Thromb Res 2006;118(1):13–25.
10. Hoyer PF, Gonda S, Barthels M, et al. Thromboembolic complications in children with nephritic syndrome. Risk and incidence. Acta Paediatr Scand 1986;75: 804–10.
11. Lewy PR, Jao W. Nephrotic syndrome in association with renal vein thrombosis in infancy. J Pediatr 1974;85:359–65.
12. Goldenberg NA, Knapp-Clevenger R, Hays T, et al. Lemierre's and Lemierre's-like syndromes in children: survival and thromboembolic outcomes. Pediatrics 2005; 116:e543–8.
13. Manco-Johnson MJ, Grabowski EF, Hellgreen M, et al. Laboratory testing for thrombophilia in pediatric patients. On behalf of the Subcommittee for Perinatal and Pediatric Thrombosis of the Scientific and Standardization Committee of the International Society on Threombosis and Haemostasis (ISTH). Thromb Haemost 2002;88:155–6.
14. Monagle P, Chan A, Massicotte P, et al. Antithrombotic therapy in children: the Seventh ACCP Conference on Antithrombotic and Thrombotic Therapy. Chest 2004;126(Suppl 3):645S–87S.
15. Manco-Johnson M. How I treat venous thrombosis in children. Blood 2006;107: 21–9.
16. Nohe N, Flemmer A, Rumler R, et al. The low molecular weight heparin dalteparin for prophylaxis and therapy of thrombosis in childhood: a report on 48 cases. Eur J Pediatr 1999;158:S134–9.

17. Andrew M, Marzinotto V, Massicotte P, et al. Heparin therapy in pediatric patients: a prospective cohort study. Pediatr Res 1994;35:78–83.

18. Hull RD, Raskob GE, Rosenbloom D, et al. Heparin for 5 days as compared with 10 days in the initial treatment of proximal venous thrombosis. N Engl J Med 1990;322:1260–4.

19. Kearon C, Ginsberg JS, Julina JA, et al. Comparison of fixed-dose weight-adjusted unfractionated heparin and low-molecular-weight heparin for acute treatment of venous thromboembolism. JAMA 2006;296:935–42.

20. Berube C, Mitchell L, Silverman E, et al. The relationship of antiphospholipid antibodies to thromboembolic events in pediatric patients with systemic lupus erythematosus: a cross-sectional study. Pediatr Res 1998;44:351–6.

21. Monagle P, Andew M. Acquired disorders of hemostasis. In: Nathan DG, Stuart H, Orkin A, editors. Nathan and Oski's hematology of infancy and childhood. 6th edition. Philadelpia: Saunders; 2003.

22. Kearon C, Ginsberg JS, Kovacs MJ, et al. Comparison of low-intensity warfarin therapy with conventional-intensity warfarin therapy for long-term prevention of recurrent venous thromboembolism. N Engl J Med 2003;349:631–9.

23. Kovacs MJ. Long-term low-dose warfarin use is effective in the prevention of recurrent venous thromboembolism: no. J Thromb Haemost 2004;2:1041–3.

24. Goldenberg NA, Knapp-Clevenger R, Durham JD, et al. A thrombolytic regimen for high-risk deep venous thrombosis may substantially reduce the risk of post-thrombotic syndrome in children. Blood 2007;110:45–53.

25. Vukovich T, Auberger K, Weil J, et al. Replacement therapy for a homozygous protein C deficiency state using a concentrate of human protein C and S. Br J Haematol 1988;70:435–40.

26. Dreyfus M, Masterson M, David M, et al. Replacement therapy with a monoclonal antibody purified protein C concentrate in newborns with severe congenital protein C deficiency. Semin Thromb Hemost 1995;21:371–81.

27. Dreyfus M, Magny JF, Bridey F, et al. Treatment of homozygous protein C deficiency and neonatal purpura fulminans with a purified protein C concentrate. N Engl J Med 1991;325:1565–8.

28. Muller FM, Ehrenthal W, Hafner G, et al. Purpura fulminans in severe congenital protein C deficiency: monitoring of treatment with protein C concentrate. Eur J Pediatr 1996;155:20–5.

29. de Kleijn ED, de Groot R, Hack CE, et al. Activation of protein C following infusion of protein C concentrate in children with severe meningococcal sepsis and purpura fulminans: a randomized, double-blinded, placebo-controlled, dose-finding study. Crit Care Med 2003;31:1839–47.

30. Ettingshausen CE, Veldmann A, Beeg T, et al. Replacement therapy with protein C concentrate in infants and adolescents with meningococcal sepsis and purpura fulminans. Semin Thromb Hemost 1999;25:537–41.

31. Rivard GE, David M, Farrell C, et al. Treatment of purpura fulminans in meningococcemia with protein C concentrate. J Pediatr 1995;126(4):646–52.

32. Konkle BA, Bauer KA, Weinstein R, et al. Use of recombinant human antithrombin in patients with congenital antithrombin deficiency undergoing surgical procedures. Transfusion 2003;43:390–4.

33. Zaunschirm A, Muntean W. Correction of hemostatic imbalances induced by L-asparaginase therapy in children with acute lymphoblastic leukemia. Pediatr Hematol Oncol 1986;3:19–25.

34. Mitchell L, Andrew M, Hanna K, et al. Trend to efficacy and safety using antithrombin concentrate in prevention of thrombosis in children receiving

L-asparaginase for acute lymphoblastic leukemia. Results of the PARKAA study. Thromb Haemost 2003;90:235–44.

35. Haussmann U, Fischer J, Eber S, et al. Hepatic veno-occlusive disease in pediatric stem cell transplantation: impact of pre-emptive antithrombin III replacement and combin antithrombin III/defibrotide therapy. Haematologica 2006;91: 795–800.

36. Meister B, Kropshofer G, Klein-Franke A, et al. Comparison of low-molecular-weight heparin and antithrombin versus antithrombin alone for the prevention of thrombosis in children with acute lymphoblastic leukemia. Pediatr Blood Cancer 2008;50(2):298–303.

37. Cahn MD, Rohrer MJ, Martella MB, et al. Long-term follow-up of Greenfield inferior vena cava filter placement in children. J Vasc Surg 2001;34:820–5.

38. Goldenberg NA. Long-term outcomes of venous thrombosis in children. Curr Opin Hematol 2005;12:370–6.

39. van Ommen CH, Heijboer H, van den Dool EJ, et al. Pediatric venous thromboembolic disease in one single center: congenital prothrombotic disorders and the clinical outcome. J Thromb Haemost 2003;1:2516–22.

40. Bick RL. Prothrombin G20210A mutation, antithombin, heparin cofactor II, protein C, and protein S defects. Hematol Oncol Clin North Am 2003;17:9–36.

41. Prandoni P, Lensing AW, Cogo A, et al. The long-term clinical course of acute deep venous thrombosis. Ann Intern Med 1996;125:1–7.

42. Nowak-Göttl U, Junker R, Kruez W, et al. Risk of recurrent venous thrombosis in children with combined prothrombotic risk factors. Blood 2001;97:858–62.

43. Massicotte P, Julian JA, Gent M, et al. An open label randomized controlled trial of low molecular weight heparin compared to heparin and Coumadin for the treatment of venous thromboembolic events in children: the REVIVE trial. Thromb Res 2003;109:85–92.

44. Oren H, Devecioglu O, Ertem M, et al. Analysis of pediatric thrombotic patients in Turkey. Pediatr Hematol Oncol 2004;21:573–83.

45. Nowak-Göttl U, Von Kries R, Gobel U. Neonatal symptomatic thromboembolism in Germany: two year survey. Arch Dis Child Fetal Neonatal Ed 1997;76:F163–7.

46. Michaels LA, Gurian M, Hagyi T, et al. Low molecular weight heparin in the treatment of venous and arterial thromboses in the premature infant. Pediatrics 2004; 114:703–7.

47. Massicotte MP, Dix D, Monagle P, et al. Central venous catheter related thrombosis in children: analysis of the Canadian Registry of Venous Thromboembolic Complications. J Pediatr 1998;133:770–6.

48. Mocan H, Beattie TJ, Murphy AV, et al. Renal venous thrombosis in infancy: long-term follow-up. Pediatr Nephrol 1991;5:45–9.

49. Nuss R, Hays T, Manco-Johnson M. Efficacy and safety of heparin anticoagulation for neonatal renal vein thrombosis. Am J Pediatr Hematol Oncol 1994;16:127–31.

50. Keidan I, Lotan D, Gazit G, et al. Early neonatal renal venous thrombosis: long-term outcome. Acta Paediatr 1994;83:1225–7.

51. Kuhle S, Massicotte P, Chan A, et al. A case series of 72 neonates with renal vein thrombosis: data from the 1-800-NO-CLOTS Registry. Thromb Haemost 2004;92: 929–33.

52. Kosch A, Kuwertz-Broking E, Heller C, et al. Renal venous thrombosis in neonates: prothrombotic risk factors and long-term follow-up. Blood 2004;104: 1356–60.

53. deVeber G, Andrew M, Adams C, et al. Cerebral sinovenous thrombosis in children. N Engl J Med 2001;345:417–23.

54. deVeber GA, MacGregor D, Curtis R, et al. Neurologic outcome in survivors of childhood arterial ischemic stroke and sinovenous thrombosis. J Child Neurol 2000;15:316–24.
55. Kenet G, Waldman D, Lubetsky A, et al. Paediatric cerebral sinus vein thrombosis. Thromb Haemost 2004;92:713–8.
56. De Schryver EL, Blom I, Braun KP, et al. Long-term prognosis of cerebral venous sinus thrombosis in childhood. Dev Med Child Neurol 2004;46:514–9.
57. Gurakan F, Eren M, Kocak N, et al. Extrahepatic portal vein thrombosis in children: etiology and long-term follow-up. J Clin Gastroenterol 2004;38:368–72.
58. Meissner MH, Manzo RA, Bergelin RO, et al. Deep venous insufficiency: the relationship between lysis and subsequent reflux. J Vasc Surg 1993;18:596–605.
59. Kahn SR, Dsmarais S, Ducruet T, et al. Comparison of the Villalta and Ginsberg clinical scales to diagnose the post-thrombotic syndrome: correlation with patient-reported disease burden and venous valvular reflux. J Thromb Haemost 2006;4:907–8.
60. Revel-Vilk S, Sharathkumar A, Massicotte P, et al. Natural history of arterial and venous thrombosis in children treated with low molecular weight heparin: a longitudinal study by ultrasound. J Thromb Haemost 2004;2:42–6.
61. Kyrle PA, Minar E, Hirschl M, et al. High plasma levels of factor VIII and the risk of recurrent venous thromboembolism. N Engl J Med 2000;343:457–62.
62. Palareti G, Legnani C, Cosmi B, et al. Risk of venous thromboembolism recurrence: high negative predictive value of D-dimer performed after oral anticoagulation is stopped. Thromb Haemost 2002;87:7–12.
63. Eichinger S, Minar E, Bialonczyk C, et al. D-dimer levels and risk of recurrent venous thromboembolism. JAMA 2003;290:1071–4.

Pediatric Arterial Ischemic Stroke

Timothy J. Bernard, MD[a,b,c,]*, Neil A. Goldenberg, MD[a,b]

KEYWORDS

- Pediatric stroke • Pediatric arterial ischemic stroke
- Neonatal stroke

Arterial ischemic stroke (AIS) is a rare, but increasingly recognized, disorder in children. Research in this area suggests that risk factors, outcomes, and even presentation are different from those of adult stroke. In particular, prothrombotic abnormalities and large vessel arteriopathies that are nonatherosclerotic seem to play a large role in the pathogenesis of childhood AIS. The purpose of this review is first to examine the epidemiology and etiologies of neonatal and childhood AIS and then provide a detailed discussion of approaches to the clinical characterization, diagnostic evaluation, and management of this disorder in pediatric patients. Long-term outcomes of recurrent AIS and neuromotor, speech, cognitive, and behavioral deficits are considered. Emphasis is on available evidence underlying current knowledge and key questions for further investigation.

CHARACTERIZATION

AIS is characterized by a clinical presentation consistent with stroke combined with radiographic evidence of ischemia or infarction in a known arterial distribution. Unless otherwise specified, throughout this article the term, "stroke," is used synonymously with AIS. AIS in pediatrics is divided into two main categories: neonatal AIS and childhood (non-neonatal) AIS. Neonatal AIS is defined as any ischemic stroke occurring within the first 28 days of life and is subdivided further into prenatal, perinatal, and postnatal. Acute perinatal stroke usually presents with neonatal seizures during the first week of life. This differs from a presumed prenatal stroke, which typically presents at 4 to 8 months of life with an evolving hemiparesis.[1] Because of the difficulty in

A version of this article was previously published in the *Pediatric Clinics of North America*, 55:2.
[a] Mountain States Regional Hemophilia and Thrombosis Center, PO Box 6507, Mail-Stop F-416, Aurora, CO 80045-0507, USA
[b] Pediatric Stroke Program, University of Colorado and The Children's Hospital, 13123 East 16th Avenue, Aurora, CO 80045, USA
[c] Department of Child Neurology, University of Colorado and The Children's Hospital, 13123 East 16th Avenue, Aurora, CO 80045-0507, USA
* Corresponding author. Department of Child Neurology, University of Colorado and The Children's Hospital, PO Box 6507, Mail Stop F-416, Aurora, CO 80045-0507.
E-mail address: timothy.bernard@uchsc.edu (T.J. Bernard).

Hematol Oncol Clin N Am 24 (2010) 167–180
doi:10.1016/j.hoc.2009.11.007
0889-8588/10/$ – see front matter © 2010 Elsevier Inc. All rights reserved.

determining the exact timing of presumed prenatal AIS, some investigators combine the two classifications as presumed prenatal/perinatal AIS. In contrast to neonatal stroke, childhood AIS typically presents with sudden onset of focal neurologic symptoms and signs and (given the broad differential diagnosis) requires an MRI of the brain with diffusion-weighted images to confirm the diagnosis of AIS (AIS presentation discussed later).

EPIDEMIOLOGY

The incidence of neonatal AIS recently is estimated at approximately 1 in 4000 live births annually.[2] Similar estimates are provided by the United States National Hospital Discharge Survey, which recently published an incidence of 18 neonatal strokes per 100,000 births per year.[3] Childhood AIS is less common than neonatal stroke, occurring one third to one tenth as often. The incidence of childhood stroke is approximately 2 to 8 in 100,000 per year in North America.[4,5] Before the advent of MRI techniques, a Mayo Clinic retrospective analysis of cases in Rochester, Minnesota, in the late 1970s yielded an incidence of 2.5 strokes per 100,000 children per year.[6] Although pre-MRI data likely underestimate the incidence of AIS because of the low sensitivity of CT for ischemia, more recent retrospective analyses using medical record review are subject to well-documented inaccuracies engendered by the *International Statistical Classification of Diseases, 9th Revision* coding.[7] In addition, given the low index of suspicion for cerebrovascular events in children, the true incidence of pediatric AIS likely remains underdiagnosed.

ETIOLOGY

The etiology of neonatal and childhood AIS is in many instances poorly understood, largely owing to the low incidence of the disease in the pediatric population and the lack of sufficient multicenter data on causal factors. The traditional ischemic stroke risk factors in adults, such as hypertension, atherosclerosis, diabetes, smoking, obesity, and hypercholesterolemia, are infrequent among neonates and older children who have AIS. In some instances of childhood AIS, such as congenital heart disease, sickle cell disease, and arterial dissection, the etiology readily is understood. For instance, with regard to cardiac risk factors, the Canadian Pediatric Stroke Registry found heart disease in 25% of patients who had pediatric AIS,[8] whereas the prevalence of patent foramen ovale (PFO) in patients who had cryptogenic stroke was 40% to 50% compared with 10% to 27% in the general population.[9,10] Some additional important risk factors for childhood AIS are identified, including vasculopathy, infection, head and neck trauma, previous transient ischemic attack (TIA) (defined as a focal neurologic deficit lasting less than 24 hours), and prothrombotic disorders.[11–21] Often more than one risk factor is identified. Nevertheless, in the majority of childhood AIS cases, the etiology remains unclear, resulting in a broad subgroup of idiopathic childhood AIS.

Increasingly, arteriopathy (characterized by a disturbance of arterial blood flow within the vessel) is identified as a prevalent risk factor for childhood AIS, occurring in as many as 50% to 80% of cases.[13,22] Often this arteriopathy is secondary to dissection of carotid or vertebral arteries, which accounts for 7% to 20% of all cases of childhood AIS,[12,22] and may be caused by neck manipulation or head and neck trauma[23–26] (although this association may be influenced by recall bias) and in rare cases may be related to underlying connective tissues disorders (eg, collagen defects).[27] Nondissective arteriopathy also is related to certain infections. For example, there is a threefold increased risk for AIS within 1 year of acute varicella zoster virus (VZV) infection in childhood.[28] Postvaricella arteriopathy typically exhibits a characteristic pattern of intracranial narrowing of the internal carotid artery (ICA), middle cerebral artery (MCA), and anterior cerebral artery (ACA), classically causing basal ganglia infarctions.[29]

Increasingly, however, angiographic studies in childhood AIS identify MCA, ICA, and ACA arteriopathy without a known infectious or alternative cause; such cases consequently are characterized as idiopathic arteriopathies (**Fig. 1**).[13] A minority of these cases represent early moyamoya syndrome (defined as stenosis in the terminal portion of the ICAs bilaterally with the formation of tenuous collateral arteries, producing the classic angiographic "puff of smoke") or possible moyamoya syndrome (recently characterized as unilateral stenosis in the terminal segment of an ICA with collaterals or the presence of bilateral stenosis of the terminal portion of the ICAs without collaterals) (**Fig. 2**).[12] Moyamoya, in turn, may be associated with sickle cell

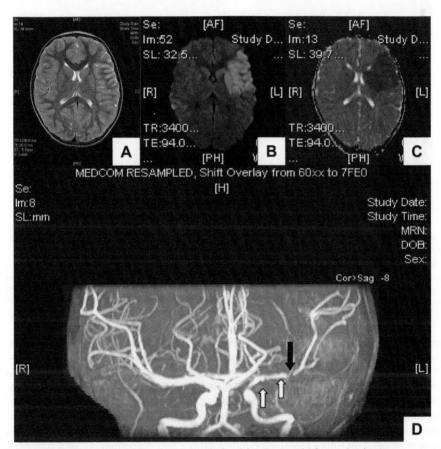

Fig. 1. Idiopathic arteriopathy. A previously healthy 6-year-old boy who had acute-onset right hemiparesis and aphasia. MRI T2 sequences (*A*) are unrevealing 5 hours after onset, but diffusion-weighted imaging (*B*) and ADC mapping (*C*) demonstrate cytotoxic edema, consistent with AIS in the left MCA territory. From the same examination, an anterior-posterior MRA (slightly oblique) image (*D*) demonstrates irregularity of the distal left ICA, extending to the proximal MCA (*white arrows*). There also seems to be an occlusion in the proximal MCA (*black arrow*).

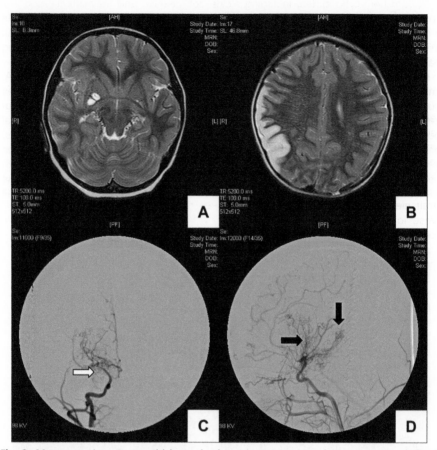

Fig. 2. Moyamoya in a 4-year-old boy who has trisomy 21. MRI demonstrates multifocal infarctions on T2 sequencing; one image reveals an old right-sided basal ganglia infarction (*A*), whereas another illustrates a subacute right parietal infarction (*B*). Follow-up angiogram of the right anterior circulation demonstrates ICA narrowing (*white arrow*) and the classic puff-of-smoke appearance of collateral circulation (*black arrows*) on anterior (*C*) and lateral (*D*) images.

anemia, trisomy 21, a history of cranial irradiation for malignancy,[30] or fibromuscular dysplasia; in many cases, however, moyamoya is of unclear etiology. In the majority of idiopathic arteriopathies, in which there is no progression to moyamoya, the phenomenon is termed, "transient cerebral arteriopathy," in cases of a monophasic transient lesion that resolves or stabilizes within 6 months, and "chronic cerebral arteriopathy" in progressive cases.[12] An elucidation of the etiology of these currently idiopathic arteriopathies will enhance the understanding of childhood stroke and may have an impact on future therapeutic management and outcomes in these patients.

Thrombophilia may contribute to AIS risk via arterial thrombosis or cerebral embolism of a venous thrombus through a cardiac lesion with right-to-left shunt. Thrombophilia risk factors in pediatric AIS include antiphospholipid antibodies,[19,20] anticoagulant deficiencies,[21] and hyperhomocysteinemia.[31,32] Protein C is the most commonly associated anticoagulant deficiency, although in cases of AIS (and venous thromboembolism [VTE]) after acute varicella infection, antibody-mediated acquired protein S deficiency seems prevalent.[33] It is likely that anticoagulant deficiencies are acquired most commonly secondary to viral-mediated inflammation, as is the case in varicella. As in VTE, however, severe congenital anticoagulant deficiencies also may be contributory. Although homozygosity for factor V Leiden or prothrombin G20210A polymorphism is a strong risk factor for thrombotic events, it remains unclear whether or not the factor V Leiden or prothrombin G20210A variant in heterozygous form confers a meaningful increase in the risk for pediatric AIS.[18–21] Greatly elevated homocysteine levels classically are associated with metabolic disorders, such as homocysteinuria (resulting from cystathionine β-synthase deficiency), and mild to moderately elevated levels also occur in homozygous carriers of the methylenetetraydrofolate reductase mutation (MTHFR C677T). Among heterozgyotes, the latter cause of hyperhomocysteinemia is evident particularly in countries where routine folate supplementation of the diet is not undertaken. Another prothrombotic trait, elevated lipoprotein(a) concentration, is associated with increased odds of otherwise idiopathic (ie, apart from thrombophilia) childhood AIS.[18] Other suspected blood-based risk factors for pediatric AIS, supported thus far by evidence from case series or case-control studies, include iron deficiency anemia,[34] polycythemia, and thrombocytosis.[35]

Given that focal arteriopathy is an uncommon finding in neonatal AIS, stroke etiology is less clear for this group than for childhood AIS. Nevertheless, congenital cardiac anomalies are established risk factors, and thrombophilia investigation has provided additional meaningful contributions. Similar thrombophilic risk factors are identified for neonatal AIS as for childhood stroke, including factor V Leiden, protein C deficiency, and elevated lipoprotein(a).[36] The possibility of vertical transmission of prothrombotic molecular entities or vasoconstrictive agents (eg, antiphospholipid antibodies or cocaine, respectively) also is important to consider in the etiology of neonatal AIS but has not been studied systematically. In addition, maternal pregestational and gestational factors, such as infertility, placental infection, premature rupture of membranes, and preeclampsia, in the past few years have been found independently associated with neonatal AIS.[37] Recent birth registry data are further suggestive of maternal vascular disease risk factors contributing to neonatal AIS, given the finding of an association with the development of seizures in term neonates (a common manifestation of neonatal AIS);[38] however, further work is necessary to establish this potential risk factor. In addition, emerging data suggest a combination of maternal- and fetal-specific molecular risk factors in the development of placental pathology may be worthy of additional study regarding perinatal stroke risk.[39]

CLINICAL PRESENTATION

The clinical presentation of AIS differs greatly among presumed prenatal, perinatal, postnatal, and childhood stroke. Within each classification, further variance of presentation exists and depends largely on the territory, extent, and timing of ischemia. The most common presentation for presumed prenatal stroke is evolving hemiparesis at 4 to 8 months of life.[1] Typically, the hand is more involved than the arm, because of the high incidence of MCA distribution infarction, and the left hemisphere is affected more commonly than the right.[36] Perinatal AIS has a similar predilection for the left MCA but often presents with focal neonatal seizures during the first week of life. Postnatal stroke may present similarly to perinatal AIS; in other instances, it presentation is like that of childhood stroke (discussed later).

The clinical presentation of childhood AIS is less stereotypical than that of pre- and perinatal AIS and is more dependent on the territory of ischemia. As a general rule, patients who have small- to medium-sized events present with sudden-onset focal neurologic deficits (such as hemiparesis, visual field deficits, aphasia, cranial nerve palsies, dyspahagia, and unilateral ataxia) without major alterations of consciousness. Focal neurologic deficit in the presence of preserved consciousness can aid in the diagnosis, as many more common pediatric illnesses, such as complex partial and generalized seizures or encephalitis, often have alteration of awareness. Larger strokes tend to have multiple deficits and alteration of consciousness. As discussed previously, a history of head or neck trauma, recent varicella infection, and the presence of sickle cell disease or cardiac disease may aid in understanding the underlying etiology. A recent single-center retrospective series of AIS in non-neonatal children found that a nonabrupt pattern of neurologic symptoms or signs (including those in whom the maximum severity of symptoms or signs developed more than 30 minutes from the time of symptom onset, the presentation of symptoms or signs was waxing and waning, or the presentation was preceded by recurrent transient symptoms or signs with intercurrent resolution) often was associated with findings of arteriopathy on diagnostic neuroimaging.[40]

Strokes of metabolic etiology frequently manifest a progressive course of stroke-like episodes. Often, there is a family history of early-onset strokes, early-onset dementia, or severe migraines. A classic example of a metabolic stroke occurs in mitochondrial myopathy, encephalopathy, lactic acidosis, and stroke-like episodes (MELAS). MELAS is caused by mitochondrial DNA defects encoding tRNA involved in the generation of ATP and the majority of cases (80%) have the mt3243 mutation.[41] In addition to a maternal history of migraine and stroke, there often is a history of short stature, diabetes, hearing loss, occipital lobe seizures, and optic atrophy.[41] The presentation often is characterized by stroke-like episodes with complete resolution of neurologic function. Over time, however, neurologic deficits persist, often in the form of hemianopia.[42] Acute lesions observed by MRI can be distinguished from typical AIS by virtue of their paradoxic bright appearance on apparent diffusion coefficient (ADC) maps. In cases of a family history of cryptogenic stroke or atypical presentation of stroke, other inherited disorders (eg, non-MELAS mitochondrial DNA defects, organic acidemias, lysosomal diseases, severe congenital thrombophilias, and cerebral autosomal dominant arteriopathy with subcortical infarctions and leukoencephalopathy [CADASIL]), should be considered.[41]

DIAGNOSTIC EVALUATION

Diagnostic evaluation of pediatric AIS is more extensive than in adult stroke because of the broad differential diagnosis at presentation and the higher incidence of ateriopathies in childhood AIS. In a child presenting with an acute focal neurologic deficit, multiple alternative etiologies must be considered, including hypoglycemia, prolonged focal seizures, prolonged postictal paresis (Todd's paralysis), acute disseminated encephalomyelitis, meningitis, encephalitis, and brain abscess.[43] For this reason, MRI brain with diffusion-weighted images is becoming the radiographic modality of choice in most cases of childhood AIS. Acutely, CT can rule out hemorrhage, tumor, and abscess and may be an appropriate first-line evaluation in some cases. Typically, this needs to be followed by an MRI with diffusion-weighted images to assess for cytotoxic edema, the hallmark of acute ischemia (see **Fig. 1**). The use of perfusion-weighted imaging largely is experimental in children[44] but as acute interventions become more available in childhood AIS, this modality likely will be used increasingly as a means by which to identify potentially preservable territories of at-risk functioning brain. Furthermore, the pattern of infarction also may be suggestive of etiology. For example, a case of multiple infarctions in separate arterial distributions likely is thromboembolic, findings of occipital and parietal strokes that cross vascular territories may suggest MELAS, a distribution between vascular territories is consistent with watershed infarction suggestive of a hypotensive etiology, and a pattern of small multifocal lesions at the gray-white junction is suspicious for vasculitis.

Although routine CT and MRI evaluate for ischemia, hemorrhage, mass/mass effect, and other non-AIS pathologies, vascular imaging (magnetic resonance angiography [MRA], CT angiography [CTA], or conventional angiography) can demonstrate arteriopathy, including dissection, stenosis, irregular contour, or intra-arterial thrombosis of the head and neck. Typically, MRA or CTA is the modality used as first-line arterial imaging, unless MRI reveals a pattern consistent with small vessel vasculitis, in which case conventional angiography is indicated. If MRA or CTA suggests moyamoya or atypical vasculature, conventional angiography is warranted, as MRA or CTA may underestimate or overestimate the degree of disease.[45]

An additional important component of diagnostic imaging in pediatric AIS is echocardiography with peripheral venous saline injection. In addition to disclosing a septal defect and other congenital cardiac anomalies, echocardiography with saline injection may disclose a small lesion, including a PFO that otherwise may not be detected by conventional transthoracic echocardiography. The prevalence of PFO in patients who have cryptogenic stroke is 40% to 50% compared with 10% to 27% in the general population.[9,10] The use of Doppler imaging during echocardiography assists in determining the direction of shunt through a lesion, although the prognostic significance of the direction of shunt is not well established in pediatric stroke.

At a minimum, diagnostic laboratory evaluation in pediatric acute AIS involves a complete blood count, toxicology screen, complete metabolic panel, erythrocyte sedimentation rate/C-reactive protein (ESR/CRP) to assess for biochemical evidence of systemic inflammation that may suggest vasculitis or infection in the etiology of AIS, β-hCG testing in postmenarchal women, fasting lipid profile, and a comprehensive thrombophilia panel (**Box 1**). Further investigation into metabolic, genetic, infectious, or rheumatologic diseases should be considered in cases of atypical presentation. In the setting of arteritis, arthritis, or elevated ESR/CRP, rheumatologic evaluation should be considered and include testing of antinuclear antibodies and rheumatoid factor. In childhood AIS with encephalopathy of unclear etiology, nonarterial distribution, or other multisystem disorders of unclear etiology (eg, hearing loss, myopathy, or endocrinopathy), testing should include lactate and pyruvate to screen for metabolic disorders and mitochondrial DNA testing for MELAS and related disorders. A lumbar puncture is indicated if infectious signs and symptoms are present and in other inflammatory states of unclear etiology. If cerebrospinal fluid (CSF) abnormalities are present, further infectious work-up and routine chemistries and blood counts are warranted. It may be prudent to test routinely for VZV, herpes simplex virus (HSV), enterovirus, and other known viral etiologies in the CSF when a lumbar puncture is performed in addition to performing routine bacterial cultures.

Because the etiology and pathogenesis of childhood AIS often are unclear at the time of diagnosis, thrombophilia testing during the diagnostic evaluation of AIS should be comprehensive (see **Box 1**). Given the association between recurrence of neonatal AIS and thrombophilia,[46] a similar investigation is warranted in neonatal AIS. A particularly important issue of thrombophilia testing specific to neonatal AIS involves antiphospholipid antibody (APA) testing (see **Box 1**). When APAs are positive in neonates who have AIS, it is informative to evaluate for APA in the mothers, as many case reports have identified vertical (ie, transplacental) transmission of IgG APA in association with neonatal AIS.[47]

Box 1
Suggested diagnostic laboratory evaluation in children who have acute arterial ischemic stroke

Complete blood count

Comprehensive metabolic panel (including hepatic indices)

ESR

CRP

Antinuclear antibody screen

Disseminated intravascular coagulation screen[a]

Thrombophilia panel[b]

Urine toxicology screen

Urine β-hCG (in postmenarchal woman)

Viral evaluation (if suspected by clinical presentation or if cerebral arteriopathy is demonstrated)[c]

Metabolic disease screening (if suspected by clinical presentation)[d]

Mitochondrial DNA mutational analyses (if suspected by clinical presentation)

[a] Includes prothrombin time, activated partial thromboplastin time, fibrinogen, and D-dimer.
[b] Includes protein C activity, free protein S antigen or protein S activity, antithrombin activity, factor VIII activity, factor V Leiden mutation, prothrombin 20,210 mutation, homocysteine concentration (± methylenetetrahydrofolate reductase mutations), antiphospholipid antibody evaluation (lupus anticoagulant testing [eg, dilute Russell's viper venom time or StaClot-LA], anticardiolipin IgG and IgM levels, anti–β2-glycoprotein I IgG and IgM levels), and lipoprotein(a) concentration.
[c] Consider blood titers of VZV, HSV, Epstein-Barr virus (EBV), enterovirus, and parvovirus; blood viral culture; CSF viral culture; CSF VZV, HSV, EBV, enterovirus, and parvovirus testing by polymerase chain reaction (PCR); *Helicobacter pylori* testing; and enteroviral PCR from oral and rectal swabs.
[d] Includes blood lactate concentration, blood pyruvate concentration, serum carnitine concentration, urine organic acids profile, and serum amino acids profile.

TREATMENT

Initial management of childhood stroke should emphasize supportive measures, such as airway stabilization, administration of oxygen, maintenance of euglycemia, and treatment of seizures if they are present. Currently there are no randomized controlled trials on which to base management of medical therapies in childhood or neonatal AIS, with the exception of AIS in the setting of sickle cell disease. Guidelines exist from the American College of Chest Physicians (ACCP)[48] and the Royal College of Physicians,[49] with recommendations based on consensus, cohort studies, and extrapolation from adult studies.

Most commonly, childhood AIS is treated with antithrombotic agents, such as aspirin or heparins (unfractionated heparin [UFH] or low-molecular-weight heparin [LMWH]), unless a stroke is a complication of sickle cell anemia. The ACCP recommendations suggest treatment of all nonsickle cell childhood AIS with UFH or LMWH for 5 to 7 days and until cardioembolic stroke and dissection are excluded. For cases of cardioembolic stroke or dissection, the ACCP recommends anticoagulation for 3 to 6 months. After discontinuation of anticoagulation in all patients who have childhood AIS, long-term aspirin therapy is recommended. These ACCP recommendations are based on grade 2C data.[48] In contrast, the Royal College of Physicians recommends initial treatment with aspirin rather than anticoagulation in all childhood AIS. A nonrandomized prospective cohort study of low-dose LMWH versus aspirin in the treatment of AIS (ie, as secondary AIS prophylaxis) in children detected no significant difference in the cumulative incidence of recurrent AIS or significant side effects between these two therapies.[50]

Treatment of stroke in sickle cell disease is based largely on clinical experience and retrospective analysis. Recommendations (from ACCP)[48] include exchange transfusion to reduce hemoglobin S to levels less than 30% for acute stroke and maintaining a long-term transfusion program after initial stroke. Based on results from the Stroke Prevention Trial in Sickle Cell Anemia (STOP), which showed that regular transfusions can prevent primary stroke in high-risk children who have sickle cell anemia and whose transcranial Doppler time–averaged maximum velocities exceed 200 cm per second,[51] ACCP also recommends primary prevention of AIS through annual transcranial Doppler sceening for arteriopathy in children who have sickle cell disease and are older than 2 years.

Pediatric AIS with moyamoya syndrome usually is treated with surgical intervention. Anticoagulation and antiplatelet agents are considered possible therapies but typically are temporizing measures before surgery. Given heightened risks for recurrent AIS and bleeding, neurosurgical approaches at revascularization (including indirect means, such as encephaloduroarteriomyosyangiosis [EDAMS], and direct means, such as superficial temporal artery branch to MCA branch bypass) generally are preferred as first-line therapy.[52,53] Given the bleeding risk inherent in moyamoya, long-term antithrombotic therapy perhaps best is reserved for children who have appropriately defined "possible moyamoya" in the absence of recurrent symptoms or recurrent AIS/TIA despite appropriate surgical intervention.

Case reports and case series describe the use of systemic intravenous and selective interventional arterial thrombolytic therapy in acute childhood stroke, in many instances used beyond the 3- to 6-hour window from symptom onset for which safety and efficacy is established in adult trials.[54–57] Bleeding risks, efficacy, and outcomes are defined poorly in these studies, making it difficult to assess risk-benefit considerations of this therapy. A multicenter collaborative clinical trial approach with stringent uniform exclusion criteria ultimately will be required to address whether or not adult evidence for a beneficial role of systemic tissue plasminogen activator administration in the immediate period after onset of AIS and the optimal time window for this intervention also apply to children.

In contrast to childhood stroke, neonatal stroke usually is treated acutely with supportive measures only. Antiplatelet therapy and anticoagulation rarely are used, given the low risk for recurrence (cumulative incidence of approximately 3% at a median follow-up duration of 3.5 years).[46] In the largest follow-up series to date evaluating recurrence in neonatal AIS, all of the recurrent events were associated with an identifiable prothrombotic or cardiac risk factor.[46] Therefore, most neonates who have AIS unlikely benefit from anticoagulation or antiplatelet therapy when these risk factors are evaluated and excluded appropriately. In the event that a potent thrombophilic risk factor is identified, antithrombotic therapy should be considered on a case-by-case basis.

Long-term management of childhood and neonatal AIS ideally should be coordinated by a multidisciplinary team that has pediatric stroke expertise and includes a neurologist, hematologist, rehabilitation physician (along with physical, occupational, and speech therapy services), and neuropsychologist. Children who have hemiparesis should be considered for constraint therapy, a method in which the unaffected arm is restrained, thereby training use of the paretic arm. Recent studies have demonstrated a potential benefit of this therapy.[58] Furthermore, the impact of rehabilitative and neuropsychologic interventions on the neuromotor and academic progress and future needs of patients who have pediatric AIS should be reassessed regularly during extended follow-up. Finally, attention should be given to assessing and monitoring the psychologic impact of AIS on patients and their families.

OUTCOMES

Recurrent AIS is one of the principal outcomes for which current medical therapies are undertaken (ie, secondary stroke prophylaxis), and the risk for recurrence after non-neonatal AIS varies between approximately 20% and 40% at a fixed follow-up duration of 5 years.[17,59] Certain risk factors in the childhood population are associated with a higher recurrence risk. A recent United States population-based cohort study demonstrated a 66% recurrence risk in children who have abnormal vascular imaging as compared with a neglible recurrence risk in AIS victims who have normal vascular imaging at presentation.[60] Previously, a large multicenter German prospective cohort study of childhood AIS demonstrated a similar increased risk for recurrence in AIS patients who had vasculopathy.[61] It has become clear, therefore, over the past several years that arterial abnormalities impart an increased risk for recurrence. Patients who have moyamoya, in particular, are at greatly increased risk for recurrent AIS and persistent neurologic deficits.[17,22,62]

The risk of recurrent AIS also seems to increase with the number of AIS risk factors.[59] In particular, elevated serum levels of lipoprotein(a), congenital protein C deficiency, and vasculopathy are independent risk factors for recurrent AIS.[61] Some studies also suggest a possible relationship between anticardiolipin IgG antibodies and recurrence, although this association has not reached statistical significance.[63]

Neuromotor, language, and cognitive outcomes of childhood and neonatal AIS are highly variable and dependent on stroke size, comorbid conditions, and age at diagnosis. Long-term sequelae include residual neurologic deficits (especially hemiparesis), learning disabilities, seizures, and cognitive impairments. The magnitude of these outcomes and their prediction are less clear in childhood AIS than neonatal stroke, perhaps because of the greater heterogeneity in stroke subtypes and distributions (primarily MCA territory) in the former group. A few cohort study analyses indicate that 30% of survivors of childhood AIS have normal motor function at an average follow-up of 6 months to 2.5 years.[22,64] The cumulative incidence of seizure after childhood AIS seems to be 25% to 33% and of behavioral concerns from 29% to 44% at 5 to 7 years of follow-up.[65,66]

In neonatal AIS, the risk for recurrence is approximately 0% to 3% at an average follow-up of 3.5 to 6 years.[46,59] As discussed previously, recurrence in neonatal AIS seems confined primarily to patients who have prothrombotic abnormalities and congenital heart disease.[46] Much evidence has emerged recently with regard to prediction of outcomes in neonatal AIS. An abnormal background on early neonatal encephalography and an ischemia distribution that includes the internal capsule, basal ganglia, and the surrounding cortex are associated with the development of hemiplegia or asymmetry of tone without hemiplegia.[67,68] Acute findings on MRI are predictive of hemiparesis in several series. The presence of signal abnormalities in the posterior limb of the internal capsule or the cerebral peduncles on magnetic resonance with diffusion-weighted imaging and ADC mapping in neonatal acute AIS is associated with the development of unilateral motor deficit.[69,70] Most recently, abnormal signal in the descending corticospinal tract on magnetic resonance with diffusion-weighted imaging in neonates who have AIS has been evaluated; the percentage of cerebral peduncle affected and the total length of descending cortico-spinal tract involved correlates with the development of hemiparesis.[71]

Expressive speech impairments were noted in 12% of perinatal/neonatal and 18% of non-neonatal AIS cases in a single study.[53] As for neuropsychologic outcomes, cognitive or behavioral deficits were discerned in 3% to 14% of children who had neonatal AIS at an average follow-up of 2 to 6 years.[68,72]

Despite important work to date in the field, prediction of outcomes and risk stratification in neonatal and childhood stroke remain largely in their infancy. Given the current limited knowledge of prognostic factors in pediatric AIS, it is hoped that within the next few years, large multicenter cohort analyses will permit further risk stratification, laying the foundation for interventional clinical trials.

ACKNOWLEDGMENTS

The authors thank Dr Marilyn Manco-Johnson for helpful comments on the manuscript and Dr Laura Fenton for expert review of the radiologic imaging studies presented in **Figs. 1** and **2**.

REFERENCES

1. Golomb MR, MacGregor DL, Domi T, et al. Presumed pre- or perinatal arterial ischemic stroke: risk factors and outcomes. Ann Neurol 2001;50(2):163–8.
2. Nelson K, Lynch JK. Stroke in newborn infants. Lancet Neurol 2004;3:150.
3. Lynch JK, Hirtz DG, DeVeber G, et al. Report of the National Institute of Neurological Disorders and Stroke workshop on perinatal and childhood stroke. Pediatrics 2002;109:116–23.
4. Kittner SJ, Adams RJ. Stroke in children and young adults. Curr Opin Neurol 1996;9:53–6.
5. Giroud M, Lemesle M, Gouyon JB, et al. Cerebrovascular disease in children under 16 years of age in the city of Dijon, France: a study of incidence and clinical features from 1985 to 1993. J Clin Epidemiol 1995;48:1343–8.
6. Schoenberg BS, Mellinger JF, Schoenberg DG, et al. Cerebrovascular disease in infants and children: a study of incidence, clinical features, and survival. Neurology 1978;8:763–8.
7. Golomb MR, Garg BP, Saha C, et al. Accuracy and yield of ICD-9 codes for identifying children with ischemic stroke. Neurology 2006;67:2053–5.
8. DeVeber G. Risk factors for childhood stroke: little folks have different strokes! Ann Neurol 2003;52(3):167–73.
9. Wu LA, Malouf JF, Dearani JA, et al. Patent foramen ovale in cryptogenic stroke. Arch Intern Med 2004;164:950–6.
10. Lechat P, Mas MJ, Lascault P, et al. Prevalence of patent foramen ovule in patients with stroke. N Engl J Med 1988;318:1148–52.
11. Chabrier S, Lasjaunias P, Husson B, et al. Ischaemic stroke from dissection of the craniofacial arteries in childhood: report of 12 patients. Eur J Paediatr Neurol 2003;7:39–42.
12. Sebire G, Fullerton H, Riou E, et al. Toward the definition of cerebral arteriopathies in childhood. Curr Opin Pediatr 2004;16:617–22.
13. Danchaivijitr N, Cox TC, Saunders DE, et al. Evolution of cerebral arteriopathies in childhood arterial ischemic stroke. Ann Neurol 2006;59:620–6.
14. Shaffer L, Rich PM, Pohl KRE, et al. Can mild head injury cause ischaemic stroke? Arch Dis Child 2003;88:267–9.

15. Kieslich M, Fiedler A, Heller C, et al. Minor head injury as cause and co-factor in the aetiology of stroke in childhood: a report of eight cases. J Neurol Neurosurg Psychiatry 2002;73:13–6.
16. Ganesan V, Prengler M, McShane MA, et al. Investigation of risk factors in children with arterial ischemic stroke. Ann Neurol 2003;53:167–73.
17. Ganesan V, Prengler M, Wade A, et al. Clinical and radiological recurrence after childhood arterial ischemic stroke. Circulation 2006;114:2170–7.
18. Nowak-Göttl U, Sträter R, Heinecke A, et al. Lipoprotein (a) and genetic polymorphisms of clotting factor V, prothrombin, and methylenetetrahydrofolate reductase are risk factors of spontaneous ischemic stroke in childhood. Blood 1999; 94:3678–82.
19. Kenet G, Sadetzki S, Murad H, et al. Factor V Leiden and antiphospholipid antibodies are significant risk factors for ischemic stroke in children. Stroke 2000;31:1283–8.
20. Sträter R, Vielhaber H, Kassenböhmer R, et al. Genetic risk factors of thrombophilia in ischaemic childhood stroke of cardiac origin. A prospective ESPED survey. Eur J Pediatr 1999;158(Suppl 3):S122–5.
21. Haywood S, Liesner R, Pindora S, et al. Thrombophilia and first arterial ischaemic stroke: a systematic review. Arch Dis Child 2005;90:402–5.
22. Chabrier S, Husson B, Lasjaunias P, et al. Stroke in childhood: outcome and recurrence risk by mechanism in 59 patients. J Child Neurol 2000;15:290–4.
23. Rubinstein SM, Peerdeman SM, van Tulder MW, et al. A systematic review of the risk factors for cervical artery dissection. Stroke 2005;36:1575–80.
24. Patel H, Smith RR, Garg BP. Spontaneous extracranial carotid artery dissection in children. Pediatr Neurol 1995;13:55–60.
25. Reess J, Pfandl S, Pfeifer T, et al. Traumatic occlusion of the internal carotid artery as an injury sequela of soccer. Sportverletz Sportschaden 1993;2:88–9.
26. Tekin S, Aykut-Bingol C, Aktan S. Case of intracranial vertebral artery dissection in young age. Pediatr Neurol 1997;16:67–70.
27. Brandt T, Orberk E, Weber R, et al. Pathogenesis of cervical artery dissections. Association with connective tissue abnormalities. Neurology 2001;57:24–30.
28. Askalan R, Laughlin S, Mayank S, et al. Chickenpox and stroke in children. Stroke 2002;32:1257–62.
29. Lanthier S, Armstron D, Doni T, et al. Post-varicella arteriopathy of childhood. Neurology 2005;64:660–3.
30. Bowers DC, Liu Y, Leisenring W, et al. Late-occuring stroke among long-term survivors of childhood leukemia and brain tumors: a report form the childhood cancer survivor study. J Clin Oncol 2006;24:5277–82.
31. van Beynum IM, Smeitink JAM, den Heijer M, et al. Hyperhomocysteinemia. A risk factor for ischemic stroke in children. Circulation 1999;99:2070–2.
32. Cardo E, Vilaseca MA, Campistol J, et al. Evaluation of hyperhomocysteinemia in children with stroke. Eur J Paediatr Neurol 1999;3:113–7.
33. Josephson C, Nuss R, Jacobson L, et al. The varicella autoantibody syndrome. Pediatr Res 2001;50:345–52.
34. Maguire JL, deVeber G, Parkin PC. Association between iron-deficiency anemia and stroke in young children. Pediatrics 2007;120:1053–7.
35. Alvarez-Larran A, Cervantes F, Bellosillo B, et al. Essential thrombocythemia in young individuals: frequency and risk factors for vascular events and evolution to myelofibrosis in 126 patients. Leukemia 2007;21:1218–23.
36. Kirton A, deVeber G. Cerebral palsy secondary to perinatal ischemic stroke. Clin Perinatol 2006;33(2):367–86.

37. Lee J, Croen LA, Backstrand KH, et al. Maternal and infant characteristics associated with perinatal arterial stroke in the infant. JAMA 2005;293:723.
38. Hall DA, Wadwa RP, Goldenberg NA, et al. Maternal cardiovascular risk factors for term neonatal seizures: a population-based study in Colorado 1989–2003. J Child Neurol 2006;21:795–8.
39. Sood R, Zogg M, Westrick RJ, et al. Fetal and maternal thrombophilia genes cooperate to influence pregnancy outcomes. J Exp Med 2007;204:1049–56.
40. Braun KPJ, Rafay MF, Uiterwaal CSPM, et al. Mode of onset predicts etiological diagnosis of arterial ischemic stroke in children. Stroke 2007;38:298–302.
41. Pavlakis SG, Kingsley PB, Bialer MG. Stroke in children: genetic and metabolic issues. J Child Neurol 2000;15:308–15.
42. Hirano M, Pavlakis SG. Mitochondrial myopathy, encephalopathy, lactic acidosis, and stroke-like episodes (MELAS): current concepts. J Child Neurol 1994;9:4–13.
43. Shellhaas R, Smith SE, O'Tool E, et al. Mimics of childhood stroke: characteristics of a prospective cohort. Pediatrics 2006;118:704.
44. Gadian DG, Calamante F, Kirkham FJ, et al. Diffusion and perfusion magnetic resonance imaging in childhood stroke. J Child Neurol 2000;15:279–83.
45. Bernard TJ, Mull BR, Handler MH, et al. An 18-year-old man with fenestrated vertebral arteries, recurrent stroke and successful angiographic coiling. J Neurol Sci 2007;260:279–82.
46. Kurnik K, Kosch A, Sträter R, et al. Recurrent thromboembolism in infants and children suffering from symptomatic neonatal arterial stroke. A prospective follow-up study. Stroke 2003;34:2887–93.
47. Boffa MC, Lachassinne E. Review: infant perinatal thrombosis and antiphospholipid antibodies: a review. Lupus 2007;16:634–41.
48. Monagle P, Chan A, Massicotte P, et al. Antithrombotic therapy in children: the Seventh ACCP Conference on Antithrombotic and Thrombotic Therapy. Chest 2004;126(Suppl 3):645S–87S.
49. Paediatric Stroke Working Group. Stroke in childhood: Clinical guidelines for diagnosis, management and rehabilitation. Royal College of Physicians; 2004. Available at: http://www.rcplondon.ac.uk/pubs/books/childstroke/childstroke_guidelines.pdf. Accessed February 25, 2008.
50. Sträter R, Kurnik K, Heller C, et al. Aspirin versus low-dose molecular-weight heparin: antithrombotic therapy in pediatric ischemic stroke patients. A propsective follow-up study. Stroke 2001;32:2554–8.
51. Adams R, McKie V, Hsu L, et al. Prevention of a first stroke by transfusion in children with abnormal results of transcranial Doppler ultrasonography. N Engl J Med 1998;339:5–11.
52. Ozgur BM, Aryan HE, Levy ML. Indirect revascularization for paediatric moyamoya disease: the EDAMS technique. J Clin Neurosci 2006;13:105–8.
53. Khan N, Schuknecht B, Boltshauser E, et al. Moyamoya disease and Moyamoya syndrome: experience in Europe; choice of revascularization procedures. Acta Neurochir (Wien) 2003;145:1061–71.
54. Amlie-Lefond C, Benedict SL, Benard T, et al. Thrombolysis in children with arterial ischemic stroke: initial results from the International Paediatric Stroke Study [abstract]. Stroke 2007;38:485.
55. Golomb MR, Rafay M, Armstrong D, et al. Intra-arterial tissue plasminogen activator for thrombosis complicating cerebral angiography in a 17-year-old girl. J Child Neurol 2003;18:420–3.
56. Benedict SL, Ni OK, Schloesser P, et al. Intra-arterial thrombolysis in a 2-year-old with cardioembolic stroke. J Child Neurol 2007;22:225–7.

57. Thirumalai SS, Shubin RA. Successful treatment for stroke in a child using recombinant tissue plasminogen activator. J Child Neurol 2000;15:558.
58. Taub E, Griffin A, Nick J, et al. Pediatric CI therapy for stroke-induced hemiparesis in young children. Dev Neurorehabil 2007;10:3.
59. Lanthier S, Carmant L, David M, et al. Stroke in children. The coexistence of multiple risk factors predicts poor outcome. Neurology 2000;54:371–8.
60. Fullerton HJ, Wu YW, Sidney S, et al. Risk of recurrent childhood arterial ischemic stroke in a population-based cohort: the importance of cerebrovascular imaging. Pediatrics 2007;119:495–501.
61. Sträter R, Becker S, von Eckardstein A, et al. Prospective assessment of risk factors for recurrent stroke during childhood—a 5-year follow-up study. Lancet 2002;360:1540–5.
62. Nagata S, Matsushima T, Morioka T, et al. Unilaterally symptomatic moyamoya disease in children: long-term follow-up of 20 patients. Neurosurgery 2006;59: 830–6.
63. Lanthier S, Kirkham FJ, Mitchell LG, et al. Increased anticardiolipin antibody IgG titers do not predict recurrent stroke or TIA in children. Neurology 2004;62: 194–200.
64. Steinlin M, Pfister I, Pavlovic J, et al. The first three years of the Swiss Neuropaediatric Stroke Registry (SNPSR): a population-based study of incidence, symptoms and risk factors. Neuropediatrics 2005;36:90–7.
65. DeSchryver EL, Kappelle LJ, Jennekens-Schinkel A, et al. Prognosis of ischemic stroke in childhood: a long term follow up study. Dev Med Child Neurol 2000;42: 313–8.
66. Steinlin M, Roellin K, Schroth G. Long-term follow-up after stroke in childhood. Eur J Pediatr 2004;163:245–50.
67. Mercuri E, Rutherford M, Cowan F, et al. Early prognostic indicators of outcome in infants with neonatal cerebral infarction: a clinical electroencephalogram, and magnetic resonance imaging study. Pediatrics 1999;103:1–15.
68. Mercuri E, Barnett A, Rutherford M, et al. Neonatal cerebral infarction and neuromotor outcome at school age. Pediatrics 2004;113:95–100.
69. De Vries LS, Van der Grond J, Van Haastert IC, et al. Prediction of outcome in new-born infants with arterial ischaemic stroke using diffusion-weighted magnetic resonance imaging. Neuropediatrics 2005;36:12–20.
70. Boardman JP, Ganesan V, Rutherford MA, et al. Magnetic resonance image correlates of hemiparesis after neonatal and childhood middle cerebral artery stroke. Pediatrics 2005;115:321–6.
71. Kirton A, Shroff M, Visvanathan T, et al. Quantified corticospinal tract diffusion restriction predicts neonatal stroke outcome. Stroke 2007;38:974–80.
72. deVeber GA, MacGregor D, Curtis R, et al. Neurologic outcome in survivors of childhood arterial ischemic stroke and sinovenous thrombosis. J Child Neurol 2000;15:316–24.

Advances in Hemophilia: Experimental Aspects and Therapy

Nidra I. Rodriguez, MD[a,b,*], W. Keith Hoots, MD[a,b]

KEYWORDS

• Hemophilia • Inhibitors • Prophylaxis

Hemophilia A or B is an X-linked recessive disorder that results from the deficiency of blood coagulation factor VIII or IX, respectively (**Fig. 1**). Hemophilia is classified based on the level of factor VIII or IX activity as severe (<1%), moderate (1%–5%), or mild (>5%–40%). The type and frequency of bleeding in hemophilia vary according to its severity. For example, patients who have severe hemophilia present with spontaneous bleeding into the joints or muscles, soft tissue bleeding, and life-threatening hemorrhage in addition to episodes of minor bleeding. Patients who have moderate hemophilia present less commonly with spontaneous bleeding but frequently experience bleeding after minor trauma. Finally, patients who have mild hemophilia typically present bleeding only after surgery or major trauma.

Musculoskeletal bleeding is the most common type of bleeding in hemophilia. Such bleeding can result in arthropathy, a common complication seen in the patient population that has this disease. In general, hemophilia treatment consists of replacing the missing coagulation protein with clotting factor concentrates when bleeding episodes occur (treatment on demand) or by scheduled infusions of clotting factor several times per week (prophylaxis). The development of neutralizing antibodies or inhibitors against factor VIII or IX is another complication encountered as a result of hemophilia treatment.

Multiple factor VIII and IX concentrates are available and categorized based on their source (plasma derived versus recombinant), purity, and viral inactivation methods.[1] Recombinant products are categorized further based on the presence or absence of animal/human protein in the cell culture media or in the final stabilized product

A version of this article was previously published in the *Pediatric Clinics of North America*, 55:2.
[a] Division of Pediatrics, Hematology Section, The University of Texas Health Science Center, 6411 Fannin, Houston, TX 77030, USA
[b] Gulf States Hemophilia and Thrombophilia Center, 6655 Travis, Suite 400 HMC, Houston, TX 77030, USA
* Corresponding author. Gulf States Hemophilia and Thrombophilia Center, 6655 Travis, Suite 400 HMC, Houston, TX 77030.
E-mail address: nidra.i.rodriguez@uth.tmc.edu (N.I. Rodriguez).

Hematol Oncol Clin N Am 24 (2010) 181–198
doi:10.1016/j.hoc.2009.11.003
0889-8588/10/$ – see front matter

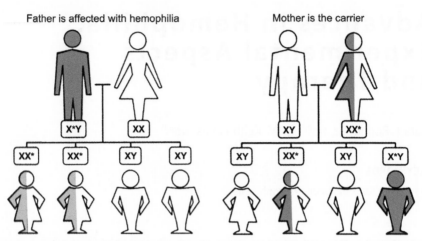

Fig. 1. X-linked recessive inheritance of hemophilia. Asterisk (*) designates affected chromosome. (*From* Pruthi RK. Hemophilia: a practical approach to genetic testing. Mayo Clin Proc 2005;80(11):1485–99; with permission.)

(Table 1).[1] Treatment of patients who develop inhibitors against factor VIII or IX is significantly more challenging than treatment of patients who do not have such antibodies. For patients who have high-titer inhibitors, the use of bypassing agents, such as recombinant factor VIIa or activated prothrombin complex concentrates, may be necessary to achieve hemostasis. In these particular patients, however, the ultimate therapeutic goal is to eradicate the inhibitor by means of immune tolerance induction (ITI). With this approach, patients receive repetitive doses of factor VIII or IX, usually once a day, with or without associated immunosuppresion. Typically, there is an initial rise in the antibody titers as a result of anamnestic response. Subsequently, however, a gradual reduction in titer is seen until in the end the inhibitor becomes undetectable. After successful immune tolerance, patients continue on regular factor infusions several times per week.

This article focuses on recent advances. From a clinical standpoint, different prophylactic regimens, including primary, secondary, and tailored prophylaxis, for severe hemophilia are discussed. Some of these regimens may serve as alternatives to primary prophylaxis in developing countries where the high cost of factor concentrates precludes its regular use. Adjuvant treatment options for bleeding management in hemophilia also are discussed along with the role of radionuclide synovectomy with isotopes, such as phosphorus 32 sulfur colloid (P^{32}) to treat joint arthropathy. Current challenges in hemophilia care, including inhibitor development and approaches to achieve ITI, are addressed.

From a research standpoint, some of the mechanisms believed to lead to blood-induced joint disease are discussed. Data suggest that iron deposition in the synovium plays an important role in this process. This article discusses the experimental aspects of synovitis, including the role of iron and cytokines, in inducing an inflammatory response that stimulates angiogenesis and contributes to bone destruction.

APPROACHES TO THE MEDICAL MANAGEMENT OF HEMOPHILIA

Despite improvements in hemophilia therapy, arthropathy remains a significant clinical problem. The Medical and Scientific Advisory Council of the National Hemophilia

Foundation, the World Federation of Hemophilia, and the World Health Organization all recommend that prophylaxis (intravenous factor replacement at least 46 weeks per year through adulthood infused in anticipation of and to prevent bleeding)[2] be considered standard of care to prevent complications, such as arthropathy. Based on this recommendation, a major goal of hemophilia therapy is to prevent any joint disease.

Observational studies support that prophylaxis is superior to on-demand therapy in delaying or preventing the development of hemophilic arthropathy.[2] There are different types of prophylaxis. Primary prophylaxis refers to therapy initiated in young patients who have hemophilia before joint damage (preventive therapy), whereas secondary prophylaxis refers to therapy initiated after joint abnormalities develop.

Since the 1990s, the standard of care for children who have severe hemophilia A or B in developed countries has been long-term prophylaxis, mainly primary, even though there is insufficient data to provide level A evidence of efficacy.[3] Although experience over the past years shows the benefits of such approach, the high cost associated with primary prophylaxis has prevented it from being adopted in developing countries.

Manco-Johnson and colleagues[4] recently published the results of the first prospective, randomized, controlled clinical trial in the United States evaluating the progression of arthropathy in children who have hemophilia treated with prophylaxis versus on-demand therapy. In this multicenter Joint Outcome Study, 65 children who had severe hemophilia (ages 30 months or less) were randomized to receive prophylaxis (25 IU/kg every other day) or an intense, episodic factor replacement (40 IU/kg initially, followed by 20 IU/kg at 24 and 72 hours after a joint bleed). Patients were followed until 6 years of age. Joint damage, the primary outcome of this study, was evaluated by MRI or plain radiographs. An 83% reduction in the risk for joint damage was shown by MRI in the prophylaxis group, supporting that such approach is effective in preventing joint damage. In 14% of cases of MRI changes, there was no evidence of any previous clinical hemarthrosis, suggesting that subclinical bleeding into the joints or the subchondral bone may cause joint damage. Further longitudinal imaging data likely are required to determine whether or not the use of continuous prophylaxis can prevent this subclinical bleeding from producing even minimal arthropathy years later.

Timing of Prophylaxis

The question of when to start primary prophylaxis has been a subject of controversy among hemophilia caregivers worldwide. To date, there is no consensus. Several studies show that children who have hemophilia and few or no joint bleeds[5–8] who are started on prophylaxis early (mean age of 3 years) exhibit a better musculoskeletal outcome. Progression of joint arthropathy, even after starting prophylaxis, is described in patients who have at least five joint bleeds occurring at the same or different joints.[5–8]

In a study published by Astermark and colleagues,[5] the only significant predictor for development of hemophilic arthropathy was the age of patients when prophylaxis was started. Using the Pettersson score, a scoring system that allows radiologic evaluation of the joints in patients who have hemophilia, Fischer and colleagues[9] described the Pettersson scores increasing by 8% each year that prophylaxis was postponed after the first occurrence of hemarthrosis. These studies show that irreversible joint damage may follow after a few joint bleeds and that even early prophylaxis may not abrogate that process completely. Therefore, worldwide recommendations to start prophylaxis

Table 1
Clotting factor concentrates available in the United States in 2008

Product Name (Manufacturer)	Viral Inactivation Procedures	Purity/Specific Activity (IU Factor VIII Activity/mg Total Protein) Before Addition of Stabilizer
Human plasma–derived factor VIII concentrates		
Humate-P (ZLB Behring, Inc) (contains functional VWF protein)	Pasteurization (heating in solution, 60°C, 10 h)	Intermediate (1–10 IU/mg)
Alphanate SD (Grifols, Inc) (contains some functional VWF protein)	Solvent detergent (TNBP/polysorbate 80) Affinity chromatography Dry heat (80°C, 72 h)	High (50–100 IU/mg) (>400 IU/mg after correcting for VWF content)
Koate-DVI (Bayer, Inc) (contains VWF protein)	Solvent detergent (TNBP/polysorbate 80) Dry heat (80°C, 72 h)	High (50–100 IU/mg)
Monoclonal antibody–purified factor VIII concentrates (immunoaffinity purified from human plasma, no intact VWF protein)		
Monarc-M (Baxter/Immuno, Inc using recovered plasma from the American Red Cross)	Solvent detergent (TNBP/octoxynol 9) Immunoaffinity chromatography	Ultra high (>3000 IU/mg)
Hemofil-M (Baxter/Immuno, Inc)	Solvent detergent (TNBP/octoxynol 9) Immunoaffinity chromatography	Ultra high (>3000 IU/mg)
Monoclate-P (ZLB Behring, Inc)	Pasteurization (heated in solution, 60°C, 10 h) Immunoaffinity chromatography	Ultra high (>3000 IU/mg)
Recombinant (genetic-engineered)/first-generation factor VIII concentrates		
Recombinate (Baxter/Immuno, Inc) (human albumin as a stabilizer)	Immunoaffinity, ion exchange chromatography Bovine serum albumin used in culture medium for Chinese hamster ovary cells	Ultra high (>4000 IU/mg)
Recombinant/second-generation factor VIII concentrates (human albumin-free final formulations)		
Kogenate FS (Bayer, Inc) Helixate FS (Bayer for ZLB Behring, Inc) (sucrose as a stabilizer)	Immunoaffinity chromatography Ion exchange Solvent detergent (TNBP/polysorbate 80) Ultrafiltration	Ultra high (>4000 IU/mg)

Product	Purification/viral inactivation	Specific activity
Refacto (Wyeth, Inc) B-domain deleted (sucrose as a stabilizer)	Ion exchange Solvent detergent (TNBP/Triton X-100) Nanofiltration	Ultra high (>11,200–15,500 IU/mg), measured via chromogenic assay technique
Recombinant/third-generation factor VIII concentrates (no human or animal protein used in the culture medium or manufacturing process; does contain trace amounts of murine monoclonal antibody)		
Advate (Baxter/Immuno, Inc) (trehalose as a stabilizer)	Immunoaffinity chromatography Ion exchange Solvent detergent (TNBP/polysorbate 80)	Ultra high (>4000–10,000 IU/mg)
Plasma-derived prothrombin complex concentrates/factor IX complex concentrates (nonactivated, also contain factor X and prothrombin but only traces of factor VII)		
Bebulin VH (Baxter/Immuno, Inc)	Vapor heat (60°C, 10 h at 190 mbar pressure plus 1 h at 80°C, 375 mbar)	Intermediate (<50 IU/mg)
Profilnine SD (Grifols, Inc)	Solvent detergent (TNBP/polysorbate 80)	Intermediate (<50 IU/mg)
Proplex-T (Baxter/Immuno, Inc)	Dry heat (60°C, 144 h)	Intermediate (<50 IU/mg)
Plasma-derived prothrombin complex concentrates/factor IX complex concentrates (activated)		
FEIBA (Baxter/Immuno, Inc)	Vapor heating (60°C, 10 h, 1160 mbar)	Intermediate (<50 U/mg)
Plasma-derived coagulation factor IX (human) concentrates		
AlphaNine SD (Grifols, Inc)	Dual affinity chromatography Solvent detergent (TNBP/polysorbate 80) Nanofiltration (viral filter)	High (>200 IU/mg)
Mononine (ZLB Behring, Inc)	Monoclonal antibody immunoaffinity chromatography Sodium thiocyanate Ultrafiltration	High (>160 IU/mg)
Recombinant factor IX concentrates		
BeneFIX (Wyeth, Inc) (no animal or human-derived protein in cell line; no albumin added to final product)	Affinity chromatography Ultrafiltration	Ultra high (>200 IU/mg)

(continued on next page)

Table 1
(continued)

Product Name (Manufacturer)	Viral Inactivation Procedures	Purity/Specific Activity (IU Factor VIII Activity/mg Total Protein) Before Addition of Stabilizer
Factor VIII (or factor IX) concentrates useful in treatment of alloantibody and autoantibody inhibitor-related bleeding		
Product name (manufacturer)	Viral inactivation method	Dosage
Recombinant factor VIIa (genetic engineered)		
NovoSeven (Novo Nordisk, Inc) (stabilized in mannitol; bovine calf serum used in culture medium)	Affinity chromatography Solvent/detergent (TNPB/polysorbate 80)	90-µg/kg intravenous bolus every 2–3 h until bleeding ceases (larger dosing regimens are experimental but may be useful in refractory bleeding). This product is the treatment of choice for individuals who have allofactor IX antibody inhibitors and anaphylaxis or renal disease associated with the use of factor IX containing concentrates.
FEIBA-VH (Baxter Immuno, Inc) (human plasma derived)	Vapor heated (10 h, 60°C, 190 mbar plus 1 h, 80°C, 375 mbar)	50–100 IU/kg not to exceed 200 IU/kg/24 h (for factor VIII and IX inhibitors)
Porcine plasma-derived factor VIII concentrate		
Hyate C (Ibsen Biomeasure, Inc)	No longer available	>50 IU/mg (for factor VIII inhibitors only)

Adapted from Kessler CM. New perspectives in hemophilia treatment. Hematology Am Soc Hematol Educ Program 2005;429–35; with permission.

before joint damage are favored to promote joint integrity, ideally before 3 years of age.

Secondary Prophylaxis

Patients who have preexisting joint disease and who experience frequent acute hemarthroses may be treated with periodic use of factor concentrates for a short or long period of time to curtail bleeding recurrence. This approach is known as secondary prophylaxis and is used commonly to minimize bleeding frequency and lessen the progression of joint disease. Even though secondary prophylaxis cannot reverse the changes of chronic arthropathy, it may be beneficial by reducing frequency of bleeding, hospital admissions, and lost days from school or work and by decreasing damage progression.

The use of secondary prophylaxis versus on-demand therapy has been the subject of various studies done in children and adults who have severe hemophilia.[10–12] In summary, the results indicate that patients treated with secondary prophylaxis have decreased number of joint bleeds at the expense of higher clotting factor consumption. A recent study, however, does not confirm the higher cost of this approach.

A long-term outcome study (follow-up of 22 years) published by Fischer and colleagues[13] compared the costs of prophylaxis (primary and secondary) versus secondary prophylaxis alone versus on-demand therapy in patients who had severe hemophilia. In this study, short-term prophylaxis was administered for 7.5 months (range 3 to 12 months) and long-term prophylaxis was administered over 12 months. Almost half of patients in the on-demand group occasionally had received short-term prophylaxis for several months to a year. This study showed that clotting factor consumption per year was similar for both treatment regimens (on-demand group: median of 1260 IU/kg per /year; prophylaxis group: median 1550 IU/kg per year). A significant difference, however, was that patients treated on demand presented a 3.2-fold increase in the frequency of joint bleeds, a 2.7-fold increase in clinical severity, and a 1.9-fold increase in Pettersson scores. Not surprisingly, the quality of life for this group of patients was decreased. Hence, these data support that the concept that prophylaxis may improve clinical outcomes without significantly increasing treatment costs.

Tailored Prophylaxis: Individualizing Therapy to Patients' Needs

Because the natural history of arthropathy varies in patients who have hemophilia, even considering those who are classified as having severe hemophilia, tailoring prophylaxis to a patient's bleeding pattern, joint involvement, and individual needs seems a reasonable approach.

As discussed previously, data support initiating prophylaxis at an early age to prevent joint damage. Particularly in young children, however, establishing venous access commonly is a challenge and not surprisingly central venous catheters (CVCs) often are required in this population for the administration of multiple dosages of factor. The benefit of easy access provided by such catheters must be balanced by their risks, in particular catheter-related infection.

Several studies have described different regimens to initiate prophylaxis early on with a dual goal of preventing joint damage and minimizing the need for CVC placement in young children. For example, Petrini[14] reported that primary prophylaxis can be started using a weekly infusion of factor concentrate rather than the standard 3-times-per-week prophylactic regimen as early as 1 or 2 years of age. This approach reduces the need for CVC placement in young children without increasing the occurrence of hemarthrosis. Astermark and colleagues[5] reported in a similar study that there was no difference in the occurrence of hemarthrosis or arthropathy when comparing children who received factor VIII concentrate infusions weekly during their first year of prophylaxis versus those who received prophylaxis 3 times a week.

In another study, published by van den Berg and colleagues,[15] outcomes of tailored prophylaxis were described for three cohorts according to the time at which prophylaxis was started in relationship to the number of joint bleeds. Data from this study also support the use of tailored prophylaxis to prevent hemophilic arthropathy after a first joint bleed has occurred.

A prospective, multicenter Canadian study enrolling children who have hemophilia is ongoing to evaluate frequency of infusions and dose escalation.[16] In this study, 25 children who had severe hemophilia A (ages 1 to 2.5 years) and normal joints were enrolled on a dose-escalation protocol defined by breakthrough hemarthroses. With this regimen, the dose of factor VIII concentrate increased from a weekly dose of 50 IU/kg to a twice-a week-dose of 30 IU/kg to an every-other-day dose of 25 IU/kg determined by the frequency of breakthrough musculoskeletal bleeds. An interim report of this cohort has been described after a median follow-up of 4.1 years. Of the 25 patients enrolled, 13 (52%) required a dose escalation to twice-a-week prophylaxis secondary to frequent joint bleeds (median time to escalation 3.42 years). Alternatively, dose escalation had not been required in 12 (48%) of these patients. The occurrence of a target joint, however, one in which recurrent bleeding has occurred on at least four occasions during the previous 6 months or where 20 lifetime bleeding episodes have occurred, was evident in 40% of the patients. This indicates that the long-term effect on joint outcome using this approach warrants further scrutiny.

ADJUVANT TREATMENT OPTIONS FOR PATIENTS WHO HAVE HEMOPHILIA

Desmopressin (DDAVP) has been used to control or prevent bleeding in mild hemophilia A, some cases of moderate hemophilia A, and some types of von Willebrand disease since 1977. Its mechanism of action seems multifactorial, including an increase in plasma levels of factor VIII and von Willebrand factor (VWF), stimulation of platelet adhesion, and increased expression of tissue factor.[17,18] DDAVP is not effective for the treatment of patients who have hemophilia B, as factor IX levels are not influenced by DDAVP.

For mild to moderate hemophilia and von Willebrand disease, the indications for DDAVP use are determined by the type of bleeding episode, baseline, and desired level of factor VIII and VWF. A test dose, also known as DDAVP challenge, should be performed under controlled conditions, such as in a doctor's office, where blood pressure and heart rate can be monitored. A blood sample is obtained before the test dose and approximately 2 hours after administration of the test dose. A twofold to fourfold rise in the levels of factor VIII, von Willebrand antigen, and ristocetin cofactor activity is expected. This expected rise in factor VIII levels explains why patients who have severe hemophilia A are not candidates for this type of therapy to control bleeding. The intranasal route is the administration route of choice for outpatient treatment and commonly is used before dental procedures and oral/nasal mucosal bleeding. The intravenous route also is available and typically used in the inpatient setting. One advantage of intravenous administration is that peak levels tend to be higher and achieved faster. Patients should be advised to limit water intake during DDAVP treatment and to avoid using more than three consecutive daily doses to reduce the risk for developing hyponatremia.

Antifibrinolytic agents, epsilon-aminocaproic acid and tranexamic acid, both lysine derivatives, also are useful adjuvant therapy for patients who have mild to severe hemophilia. They exert their effect by inhibiting the proteolytic activity of plasmin and, therefore, inhibiting fibrinolysis. The use of antifibrinolytic agents is indicated in the presence of mucosal bleeding, primarily oral, nasal, and menstrual blood loss. Its use is contraindicated in presence of hematuria because of increased risk for intrarenal or ureteral thrombosis, in the presence of disseminated intravascular coagulation, or thromboembolic disease. Both drugs are available for use in the United States in an intravenous form (epsilon-aminocaproic acid at 100 mg/kg/dose every 6 hours; tranexamic acid at 10 mg/kg/dose every 6–8 hours). Currently, only epsilon-aminocaproic acid is available for use in the United States in an oral form.

Topical agents, such as fibrin sealant, which is prepared by mixing two plasma-derived protein fractions (fibrinogen-rich concentrate and thrombin concentrate), are used for local bleeding control in hemophilia. There are concerns, however, regarding the use of bovine thrombin in this setting. First, there seems to be a high rate (approximately 20% or higher) of antibody formation[19] against thrombin and factor V, which may inactivate an individual's own endogenous factor V or thrombin production, thereby creating a new bleeding diathesis. Another legitimate concern is the potential risk for transmitting blood-borne pathogens, such as variant Creutzfeldt-Jakob virus.[20] When available commercially, the use of recombinant human thrombin will likely minimize these risks.

A phase 3, prospective, randomized, double-blind, comparative study evaluating the safety and efficacy of topical recombinant human thrombin and bovine thrombin in surgical hemostasis has been published.[21] The primary objective of this study was to evaluate the efficacy of both products whereas the secondary objective was to evaluate safety and antigenicity. This multicenter study enrolled more than 400 patients, who were randomized in a 1:1 ratio. The study showed that both topical agents had a comparable efficacy of 95% with similar adverse events rates. A statistically significant lower incidence of antibodies, however, was identified against recombinant human thrombin (1.5%) compared with antibovine thrombin (21.5%). Based on the results of this study, recombinant human thrombin seems the preferred option to achieve topical hemostasis.

Recombinant factor VIIa is a Food and Drug Administration–approved product used to promote hemostasis in patients who have hemophilia A or B with inhibitors. Its mechanism of action includes binding of activated factor VII to tissue factor, which activates factor X and leads to thrombin generation. Recombinant factor VIIa also binds the surface of activated platelets independent of tissue factor, activating factor X and leading to thrombin generation. The standard dose in hemophilia with inhibitors is 90 to 120 µg/kg every 2 to 3 hours until hemostasis is achieved. Subsequent dosing and interval is based on clinical judgment. At the present time, there is no validated laboratory test to monitor recombinant factor VIIa therapy. Clinical experience shows an excellent or effective response in more than 90% of patients who have hemophilia and low risk for thrombosis.[22,23]

EXPERIMENTAL ASPECTS OF SYNOVITIS AND ALTERNATIVE METHODS FOR INTERVENTION

In hemophilia, the joints are the most common site of serious bleeding.[10] Synovitis occurs after repeated episodes of bleeding into the joints and is characterized by a highly vascular synovial membrane with prominent proliferation of synovial fibroblasts and infiltration by inflammatory cells.[24] Ultimately, destruction of the cartilage and bone leads to crippling arthritis if adequate treatment is not administered in a timely manner. The exact mechanisms leading to the characteristic changes seen in synovitis are not understood fully. It is hypothesized, however, that synovial cell proliferation, immune system activation, and angiogenesis (the formation of new blood vessels from preexisting ones) occur secondary to the presence of blood components, especially iron, in the joint space. These events self-amplify each other, ultimately leading to cartilage and bone destruction (**Fig. 2**). Different therapeutic options for synovial control in hemophilia are available. For example, the synovium can be removed surgically by means of an open or arthroscopic synovectomy. Another alternative, synoviorthesis, allows for the destruction of the synovial tissue by intra-articular injection of a chemical or radioactive agent. The main indications for synoviorthesis are chronic synovitis and recurrent hemarthroses. The procedure is performed by an orthopedic surgeon or invasive radiologist/nuclear medicine specialist who has expertise in hemophilia. The majority of patients require a single injection, although a few patients may require more than one injection to the same joint at different time periods. Synoviorthesis offers several advantages over surgical synovectomy. It is less invasive and costly, requires minimal factor coverage, is associated with fewer infections and minimal pain, and does not require extensive rehabilitation. Even though this procedure may not halt joint degeneration, it may effectively reduce the frequency of joint bleeding along with a reduction in arthropathic pain.

Radioactive synovectomy (RS) using P^{32} has been used for chronic synovitis in the United States since 1988. Initial comprehensive review of its use suggested that this technique was efficient, safe, and not associated with malignancies.[25] Subsequently, however, two cases of acute lymphoblastic leukemia (ALL) after RS were reported in children who had hemophilia. The first patient was a 9-year-old boy who had severe hemophilia A who developed pre–B-cell ALL. The second was a 14-year-old boy who had severe hemophilia A who developed T-cell ALL. Both patients developed their ALL less than 1 year after treatment with RS,[26] which raises the question as to whether or not this may be too early for radiation-induced malignancy. Both patients had a history of exaggerated immunologic response or autoimmune disease.

There have been no further reports of cancer after RS in hemophilia or rheumatoid arthritis in the United States. Data from a retrospective, long-term, Canadian study evaluating the incidence of cancer in more than 2400 patients who had chronic synovitis from multiple diseases, including rheumatoid arthritis and hemophilia, and who underwent RS were presented at World Federation of Hemophilia (Georges Rivard, MD, Montreal, Canada, unpublished data, 2007). In this study, Infante-Rivard and colleagues[27] compared the incidence rates of cancer in a cohort of patients treated

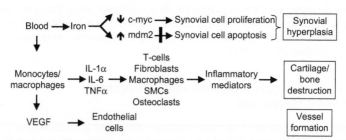

Fig. 2. Proposed mechanism in the pathogenesis of hemophilic synovitis. IL-6, interleukin 6; IL-1α, interleukin 1α; SMC, synovial mesenchymal cell; TNFα, tumor necrosis factor alpha; VEGF, vascular endothelial growth factor. (*Adapted from* Valentino LA, Hakobyan N, Rodriguez N, et al. Pathogenesis of haemophilic synovitis: experimental studies on blood-induced joint damage. Haemophilia 2007;13(3):10–3; with permission.)

with RS to the incidence rates of cancer in the general Quebec population, as documented in the Quebec Province Cancer Registry. The majority of the patients (80%) received one or two treatments using radioactive isotopes, whereas the remaining underwent three or more procedures. Most patients received yttrium[90] (70%) whereas close to 30% of the patients received P[32]. Data analysis using a Cox regression model showed no evidence of increased risk for cancer with the use of RS.[27]

Currently, the use of RS is based on defined risks versus benefits. Therefore, this approach may be recommended for patients who have no known risk factors for malignancy who have developed a target joint and continue to present recurrent hemarthrosis despite prophylactic therapy or in whom prophylaxis is not an option. Nevertheless, informed consent should describe the risks (discussed previously) clearly to parents and, when applicable, to patients.

CURRENT CHALLENGES IN HEMOPHILIA MANAGEMENT
Inhibitor Development

There is no question that the development of inhibitory antibodies in hemophilia is one of the most challenging aspects of current management. The incidence of inhibitors in patients who have hemophilia A is estimated at 30%, whereas the incidence in hemophilia B is much lower, at approximately 3%. Genetic and environmental risk factors for inhibitor development are described.[28,29] These antibodies, usually of the IgG4 subtype, occur early within the first 50 exposure days and are classified as low- or high-titer inhibitor according to measurement by the Bethesda unit (BU) laboratory assay (<5 BU is referred to as low titer, >5 BU as high titer) and the propensity of the antibody to anamnese after re-exposure to the antigen (factor VIII or IX). Patients who have low-titer inhibitors may be treated successfully with high doses of factor VIII or IX. Alternatively, patients who have high-titer inhibitors require bypassing agents, such as recombinant factor VIIa or activated prothrombin complex concentrates, for bleeding control. Ultimately, ITI to eradicate the inhibitor is desired. This intervention is effective at eradicating all inhibitors in approximately 70% of patients.

An ongoing international multicenter trial, International Immune Tolerance Study , investigates the impact of factor VIII dose on the rate of ITI success along with the time to ITI success. Patients who have severe hemophilia are randomized to receive either a high-dose factor VIII (200 U/kg daily) or a low-dose factor VIII (50 U/kg 3 times per week for 33 months). The primary endpoints of this study are to compare the success rate, time to achieve tolerance, complications, and cost of both regimens.

Whether or not the type of factor VIII concentrate to treat hemophilia A influences inhibitor development has been a subject of debate since the introduction of recombinant products in the 1990s. Although some studies suggest an increased risk for inhibitor development with the use of recombinant products compared with the experience with plasma-derived products, other studies have not confirmed such findings.[29–31] Now, with almost 2 decades of experience with the use of recombinant products, it is clear that the incidence of inhibitor development has remained stable when compared with historical data.

More recently, a possible therapeutic advantage of using VWF-containing products to achieve ITI has been proposed. Inhibitory antibodies against the factor VIII molecule are directed primarily against epitopes located at the A2, A3, and C2 domains.[28] VWF is known to bind the A3 and C2 domains of factor VIII,[32] which may result in a blockade to inhibitor binding (**Fig. 3**). Another proposed mechanism is that VWF may protect the infused factor VIII from rapid degradation by plasma proteases.[33] In vitro studies show that VWF protects factor VIII from neutralizing antibodies.[34,35] In vivo confirmation of

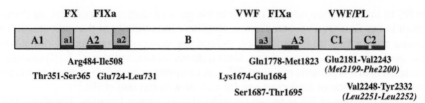

Fig. 3. Schematic model showing the domain structure of factor VIII (FVIII) and the localization of the main binding epitopes of FVIII antibodies. (*From* Astermark J. Basic aspects of inhibitors to factors VIII and IX and the influence of non-genetic risk factors. Haemophilia 2006;12(Suppl 6):8–13; with permission.)

these findings in an animal model showed that VWF-C2 binding confers protection against inhibitor development.[36]

In 2006, Gringeri and colleagues[37] reported a low incidence of inhibitors (9.8%) in patients who had severe hemophilia A who previously were untreated and received a VWF-containing factor VIII concentrate. More recently, Gringeri and colleagues[38] reported the results of the first prospective ITI study using a VWF-containing factor VIII concentrate in patients who had hemophilia A considered at high risk for a poor response to ITI. This study showed successful inhibitor eradication in 9 of the 16 (53%) patients who completed this study. The median time to inhibitor eradication was 24 months (range 4–30 months). The remaining seven patients showed partial success documented by a decreased inhibitor titer (median of 1.5 BU, range 1.1–2.8 BU), without complete disappearance. One patient was withdrawn 12 months after enrollment as a result of persistent high-titer inhibitor (70 BU). Overall, this study demonstrated a relatively high success rate of inhibitor eradication, taking into consideration that this group of patients was at high risk for a poor response and two of them previously had failed ITI.

Rituximab Experience in Hemophilia with Inhibitors

Rituximab, a human-mouse chimeric monoclonal antibody directed against the CD20 antigen, has demonstrated a therapeutic benefit in the treatment of B-cell–mediated malignancies and immune-mediated disorders, such as immune thrombocytopenic purpura and autoimmune hemolytic anemia.[39–41] The use of rituximab in acquired hemophilia versus congenital hemophilia is reported more extensively.[42,43] The standard dose for rituximab use in hemophilia has been 375 mg/m^2/dose, administered weekly for 4 weeks and then monthly (up to 5 months) until the inhibitor disappears.

Rituximab has been used in congenital hemophilia with inhibitors in only 18 documented patients (12 who had severe hemophilia A, four who had mild or moderate hemophilia A, and two who had severe hemophilia B). Thirteen of them responded favorably to rituximab, three with a complete response and 10 with a partial response, whereas the remaining five patients had no response.[42,43] The data suggest that the efficacy of rituximab may be enhanced by concomitant administration of factor VIII. The long-term success of such an approach is not clear, however, as further follow-up is needed.

CARRIER STATE AND GENETIC TESTING IN HEMOPHILIA

Carrier status in women cannot be established based solely on factor VIII or IX levels because there is a significant overlap between factor levels in carrier and noncarrier women. For this reason, genetic testing is recommended. Women who are obligate carriers (daughter of a man who has hemophilia or the mother of more than one son who has hemophilia) do not need carrier testing as it is evident that they have inherited an affected X chromosome from a father who has hemophilia (see **Fig. 1**).

In approximately 30% of patients who have hemophilia, there is no family history of the disease and it seems to occur as a result of spontaneous novel mutations.[44] In such cases, molecular testing can identify mutations in 95% to 98% of patients who have hemophilia A or B.[45]

Candidates for genetic testing include patients who have a diagnosis of hemophilia A or B, at-risk women who are related to an affected man (proband) who has a known mutation, and female carriers of hemophilia A or B seeking prenatal diagnosis.

Although in many cases the whole gene needs to be sequenced, this is not necessarily the case for patients who have severe hemophilia A, in whom intron 22 inversion is found in approximately 45%. In hemophilia A, therefore, it is recommended initially to perform intron 22 gene inversion analysis and, if not present, to proceed with full sequencing of the factor VIII gene. For patients who have mild or moderate hemophilia A, full sequencing of the factor VIII gene is recommended unless a mutation already is identified in another family member. To identify a mutation in patients who have hemophilia B, full sequencing of the factor IX gene is performed. After a mutation is identified in a proband with hemophilia A or B, carrier testing and prenatal diagnosis can be offered to at-risk family members. If a proband is not available for testing, genetic analysis can be performed on a blood sample from an obligate carrier.

POTENTIAL NEW THERAPIES IN THE HORIZON
Gene Therapy

Gene therapy involves the transfer of genes that express a particular gene product into human cells resulting in a therapeutic advantage. Particularly for hemophilia, the goal of gene transfer is aimed at the secretion of a functional factor VIII or IX protein. Different strategies for hemophilia using animal models or humans include retroviral, lentiviral, adenoviral, and adeno-associated viral vectors.

There have been several gene therapy phase I clinical trials using direct in vivo gene delivery or ex vivo plasmid transfections with hepatic reimplantation of gene-engineered cells.[46,47] Even though a therapeutic effect has been seen in some of these studies, stable production of the coagulation protein is not yet demonstrated in human subjects. These trials have failed to show long-term gene expression observed in preclinical animal models.[1]

The only active human clinical trial is in patients who have severe hemophilia B, evaluating the safety of adeno-associated viral vector in delivering human factor IX gene into the liver using immunomodulation at the time of gene transfer. Hence, gene therapy in hemophilia continues to be a topic of intense investigation and holds promise as an enduring therapy for hemophilia A and B.

Novel Bioengineering Technologies

Another novel approach aims to improve recombinant factor VIII synthesis and secretion by targeting modifications, such as increased mRNA expression, reduced interaction with endoplasmic reticulum chaperones, or increased endoplasmic reticulum–Golgi transport.[48] Strategies to improve factor VIII functional activity may be achieved by increasing molecular activation or by inducing resistance to inactivation. Targets to reduce factor VIII immunogenicity also are foci of current research. Similar strategies are being evaluated in hemophilia B, in particular modifications to increase factor IX synthesis, secretion, and activity.[49]

Another promising approach is the development of strategies that result in a longer plasma half-life for factor VIII, thereby reducing the frequency of factor infusions. Three of these strategies are described.

Polyethylene glycol conjugation

Pegylation, the modification of proteins by conjugation with polyethylene glycol (PEG) polymers, initially was described in the 1970s.[50] These polymers incorporate water molecules within their hydrophilic structure. As a result, pegylation increases the size of the conjugated protein above the renal threshold for filtration, resulting in an extended half-life. Pegylation also may result in antigenic shielding for the factor VIII molecule.[51] Animal studies show an increased half-life of pegylated factor VIII, resulting in improved hemostasis.[52]

Pegylated liposomes

Liposomes are able to encapsulate drugs within their lipid bilayer or within their aqueous phase.[53] As they may be cleared rapidly, however, structural modifications are incorporated to reduce clearance and extend half-life. Animal studies using pegylated liposomal factor VIII (PEGLip-FVIII) have shown an increased half-life and hemostatic efficacy for PEGLip-FVIII compared with standard factor VIII. Spira and colleagues[54] recently published the results of a clinical pilot study showing prolongation in the mean number of days without bleeding episodes in patients receiving PEGLip-FVIII compared with nonpegylated factor VIII. Although these early results are encouraging, concerns regarding its clearance mechanism have been raised. A phase I clinical trial using this PEGLip formulation of Kogenate has demonstrated similar pharmacokinetics as native Kogenate. Further studies are required to ascertain whether or not this is the case.

Polysialic acid polymers

Polysialic acids are polymers of N-acetylneuraminic acid. Similarly to pegylation, the hydrophilic properties of polysialic acids allow the formation of a "watery cloud" that protects the target molecule from degradation and rapid clearance. In contrast to pegylation, however, these polymers are biodegradable. Hence, concerns regarding long-term product accumulation in the body should not apply to this strategy.

SUMMARY

From a clinical perspective, the use of prophylaxis in patients who have hemophilia is strongly recommended to prevent arthropathy. Different prophylactic regimens are used to achieve this goal. The use of radionuclide synovectomy with radioisotopes, such as P^{32}, seems a safe and efficacious approach to treat arthropathy, a major complication of chronic joint bleedings. The management of patients who have inhibitory antibodies against factor VIII or IX remains challenging. Further clinical studies are necessary in this field.

Understanding the pathogenesis of hemophilic arthropathy likely begins with deciphering the biochemical and cellular response after blood-induced joint damage. Information gleaned from early in vitro models indicates a role for oxidative iron in inducing genetic alteration in proximal synovial cells of the joint that lead to their enhanced proliferation. In addition, the cytokine response to the initial iron injury creates an inflammatory milieu that incites chondrocyte dysfunction, resulting in dysfunctional cartilage matrix, and the initiation of osteoclastogenesis. When this process is repetitive, as seen in hemophilic arthropathy, accentuation of these destructive and inflammatory processes is accompanied by significant angiogenesis. In addition, the fragility of the blood vessels in these neovascularized tissues may predispose to renewed hemorrhage, a process that spirals out of control gradually until end-stage hemarthropathy is the outcome.

Much experimental work is yet to be done to demonstrate definitively each step along this evolutionary process. Some may mimic other joint disease states, such as rheumatoid arthritis. Others may be unique to hemophilic arthropathy. New investigative capacities in genomics and proteomics may provide the tools to elucidate the pathogenesis and to point to new avenues of prevention and therapy.

REFERENCES

1. Kessler CM. New perspectives in hemophilia treatment. Hematology Am Soc Hematol Educ Program 2005;429–35.
2. Berntorp E, Astermark J, Bjorkman S, et al. Consensus perspectives on prophylactic therapy for haemophilia: summary statement. Haemophilia 2003;9(Suppl 1):1–4.
3. Galiè N, Seeger W, Naeije R, et al. Comparative analysis of clinical trials and evidence-based treatment algorithm in pulmonary arterial hypertension. J Am Coll Cardiol 2004;43:81–8.
4. Manco-Johnson MJ, Abshire TC, Shapiro AD, et al. Prophylaxis versus episodic treatment to prevent joint disease in boys with severe hemophilia. N Engl J Med 2007;357(6):535–44.
5. Astermark J, Petrini P, Tengborn L, et al. Primary prophylaxis in severe haemophilia should be started at an early age but can be individualized. Br J Haematol 1999;105(4):1109–13.
6. Funk M, Schmidt H, Escuriola-Ettingshausen C, et al. Radiological and orthopedic score in pediatric hemophilic patients with early and late prophylaxis. Ann Hematol 1998;77(4):171–4.
7. Kreuz W, Escuriola-Ettingshausen C, Funk M, et al. When should prophylactic treatment in patients with haemophilia A and B start?–The German experience. Haemophilia 1998;4(4):413–7.
8. Petrini P, Lindvall N, Egberg N, et al. Prophylaxis with factor concentrates in preventing hemophilic arthropathy. Am J Pediatr Hematol Oncol 1991;13(3):280–7.
9. Fischer K, van der Bom JG, Mauser-Bunschoten EP, et al. The effects of postponing prophylactic treatment on long-term outcome in patients with severe hemophilia. Blood 2002;99(7):2337–41.
10. Aledort LM, Haschmeyer RH, Pettersson H. A longitudinal study of orthopaedic outcomes for severe factor-VIII-deficient haemophiliacs. The Orthopaedic Outcome Study Group. J Intern Med 1994;236(4):391–9.
11. Smith PS, Teutsch SM, Shaffer PA, et al. Episodic versus prophylactic infusions for hemophilia A: a cost-effectiveness analysis. J Pediatr 1996;129(3):424–31.
12. Szucs TD, Offner A, Kroner B, et al. Resource utilisation in haemophiliacs treated in Europe: results from the European Study on Socioeconomic Aspects of Haemophilia Care. The European Socioeconomic Study Group. Haemophilia 1998; 4(4):498–501.
13. Fischer K, van der Bom JG, Molho P, et al. Prophylactic versus on-demand treatment strategies for severe haemophilia: a comparison of costs and long-term outcome. Haemophilia 2002;8(6):745–52.

14. Petrini P. What factors should influence the dosage and interval of prophylactic treatment in patients with severe haemophilia A and B? Haemophilia 2001;7(1): 99–102.

15. van den Berg HM, Fischer K, Mauser-Bunschoten EP, et al. Long-term outcome of individualized prophylactic treatment of children with severe haemophilia. Br J Haematol 2001;112(3):561–5.

16. Feldman BM, Pai M, Rivard GE, et al. Tailored prophylaxis in severe hemophilia A: interim results from the first 5 years of the Canadian Hemophilia Primary Prophylaxis Study. J Thromb Haemost 2006;4(6):1228–36.

17. Villar A, Jimenez-Yuste V, Quintana M, et al. The use of haemostatic drugs in haemophilia: desmopressin and antifibrinolytic agents. Haemophilia 2002;8: 189–93.

18. Galves A, Gomez-Ortiz G, Diaz-Ricart M, et al. Desmopressin (DDAVP) enhances platelet adhesion to the extracellular matrix of cultured human endothelial cells through increased expression of tissue factor. Thromb Haemost 1997;77:975–80.

19. Winterbottom N, Kuo JM, Nguyen K, et al. Antigenic responses to bovine thrombin exposure during surgery: a prospective study of 309 patients. Journal of Applied Research 2002;2:1–11.

20. Bruce ME, Will RG, Ironside JW, et al. Transmissions to mice indicate that 'new variant' CJD is caused by the BSE agent. Nature 1997;389(6650):498–501.

21. Chapman WC, Singla N, Genyk Y, et al. A phase 3, randomized, double-blind comparative study of the efficacy and safety of topical recombinant human thrombin and bovine thrombin in surgical hemostasis. J Am Coll Surg 2007 Aug;205(2):256–65.

22. O'Connell N, Mc Mahon C, Smith J, et al. Recombinant factor VIIa in the management of surgery and acute bleeding episodes in children with haemophilia and high responding inhibitors. Br J Haematol 2002;116(3):632–5.

23. Hedner U. Treatment of patients with factor VIII and IX inhibitors with special focus on the use of recombinant factor VIIa. Thromb Haemost 1999;82(2):531–9.

24. Rodriguez-Merchan EC. Effects of hemophilia on articulations of children and adults. Clin Orthop Relat Res 1996;(328):7–13.

25. Dunn AL, Busch MT, Wyly JB, et al. Radionuclide synovectomy for hemophilic arthropathy: a comprehensive review of safety and efficacy and recommendation for a standarized treatment protocol. Thromb Haemost 2002;87:383–93.

26. Manco-Johnson MJ, Nuss R, Lear J, et al. 32P radiosynoviorthesis in children with hemophilia. J Pediatr Hematol Oncol 2002;24:534–9.

27. Infante-Rivard C, Rivard G, Winikoff R, et al. Is there an increased risk of cancer associated with radiosynoviorthesis? [abstract 18FP539]. Haemophilia 2006; 12(2).

28. Astermark J. Basic aspects of inhibitors to factors VIII and IX and the influence of non-genetic risk factors. Haemophilia 2006;12(6):8–14.

29. Scharrer I, Bray GL, Neutzling O. Incidence of inhibitors in haemophilia A patients—a review of recent studies of recombinant and plasma-derived factor VIII concentrates. Haemophilia 1999;5:145–54.

30. Goudemand J, Rothschild C, Demiguel V, et al. Influence of the type of factor VIII concentrate on the incidence of factor VIII inhibitors in previously untreated patients with severe hemophilia A. Blood 2006;107(1):46–51.

31. Gouw SC, van der Bom JG, Auerswald G, et al. Recombinant versus plasma-derived factor VIII products and the development of inhibitors in previously untreated patients with severe hemophilia A: the CANAL cohort study. Blood 2007;109(11):4693–7.

32. Scandella D, de Graaf Mahoney S, Mattingly M, et al. Epitope mapping of human FVIII inhibitor antibodies by deletion analysis of FVIII fragments expressed in Escherichia coli. Proc Natl Acad Sci U S A 1988;85:6152-6.
33. Auerswald G, Spranger T, Brackmann HH. The role of plasma-derived factor VIII/ von Willebrand factor concentrates in the treatment of hemophilia A patients. Haematologica 2003;88(9):16-20.
34. Suzuki T, Arai M, Amano K, et al. Factor VIII inhibitor antibodies with C2 domain specificity are less inhibitory to factor VIII complexed with von Willebrand factor. Thromb Haemost 1996;76:749-54.
35. Gensana M, Altisent C, Aznar JA, et al. Influence of von Willebrand factor on the reactivity of human factor VIII inhibitors with factor VIII. Haemophilia 2001;7: 369-74.
36. Behrmann M, Pasi J, Saint-Remy JM, et al. von Willebrand factor modulates factor VIII immunogenicity: comparative study of different factor VIII concentrates in a haemophilia A mouse model. Thromb Haemost 2002;88:221-9.
37. Gringeri A, Monzini M, Tagariello G, et al. Occurrence of inhibitors in previously untreated or minimally treated patients with haemophilia A after exposure to a plasma-derived solvent-detergent factor VIII concentrate. Haemophilia 2006; 12:128-32.
38. Gringeri A, Musso R, Mazzucconi G, et al. Immune tolerance induction with a high purity von Willebrand factor/VIII complex concentrate in haemophilia A patients with inhibitors at high risk of a poor response. Haemophilia 2007;13:373-9.
39. Gopal AK, Press OW. Clinical applications of anti CD 20 antibodies. J Lab Clin Med 1999;134:445-50.
40. Stasi R, Pagano A, Stipa E, et al. Rituximab chimeric anti-CD 20 monoclonal antibody treatment for adults with chronic idiopathic thrombocytopenic purpura. Blood 2001;98:952-7.
41. Zecca M, Nobili B, Ramenghi U, et al. Rituximab for the treatment of refractory autoimmune hemolytic anemia in children. Blood 2003;101:3857-61.
42. Carcao M, St. Louis J, Poon MC, et al. Rituximab for congenital haemophiliacs with inhibitors: a Canadian experience. Haemophilia 2006;12:7-18.
43. Fox RA, Neufeld EJ, Bennett CM. Rituximab for adolescents with haemophilia and high titre inhibitors. Haemophilia 2006;12:218-22.
44. Lawn RM. The molecular genetics of hemophilia: blood clotting factors VIII and IX. Cell 1985;42:405-6.
45. Goodeve AC, Peake IR. The molecular basis of hemophilia A: genotype-phenotype relationships and inhibitor development. Semin Thromb Hemost 2003; 29(1):23-30.
46. Pierce GF, Lillicrap D, Pipe SW, et al. Gene therapy, bioengineered clotting factors and novel technologies for hemophilia treatment. J Thromb Haemost 2007;5:901-6.
47. Ponder KP. Gene therapy for hemophilia. Curr Opin Hematol 2006;13(5):301-7.
48. Miao HZ, Sirachainan N, Palmer L, et al. Bioengineering of coagulation factor VIII for improved secretion. Blood 2004;103:3412-9.
49. Pipe SW. The promise and challenges of bioengineered recombinant clotting factors. J Thromb Haemost 2005;3:1692-701.
50. Abuchowski A, van Es T, Palczuk NC, et al. Alteration of immunological properties of bovine serum albumin by covalent attachment of polyethylene glycol. J Biol Chem 1977;252:3578-81.
51. Molineaux G. Pegylation: engineering improved biopharmaceuticals for oncology. Pharmacotherapy 2003;23:3S-8S.

52. Baru M, Carmel-Goren L, Barenholz Y, et al. Factor VIII efficient and specific non-covalent binding to PEGylated liposomes enables prolongation of its circulation time and haemostatic efficacy. Thromb Haemost 2005;93:1061–8.
53. Goyal P, Goyal K, Vijaya Kumar SG, et al. Liposomal drug delivery systems—clinical applications. Acta Pharm 2005;55:1–25.
54. Spira J, Ply Ushch OP, Andreeva TA, et al. Prolonged bleeding-free period following prophylactic infusion of recombinant factor VIII (Kogenate (R) FS) reconstituted with pegylated liposomes. Blood 2006;108:3668–73.

Hydroxyurea for Children with Sickle Cell Disease

Matthew M. Heeney, MD[a,b,]*, Russell E. Ware, MD, PhD[c]

KEYWORDS

- Sickle cell anemia • Antisickling agents • Hydroxyurea
- Child • Human

Sickle cell disease (SCD) refers to a group of genetic hemolytic anemias in which the erythrocytes have a predominance of sickle hemoglobin (HbS) due to inheritance of a β-globin mutation ($β^S$). The $β^S$ mutation is the result of a single amino acid substitution (HbS, *HBB Glu6Val*) in the β-globin of the hemoglobin heterotetramer, thus forming HbS. Affected individuals typically are homozygous for the sickle mutation (HbSS) or have a compound heterozygous state (eg, HbSC, HbS β-thalassemia). The $β^S$ mutation creates a hydrophobic region that, in the deoxygenated state, facilitates a noncovalent polymerization of HbS molecules that damages the erythrocyte membrane and changes the rheology of the erythrocyte in circulation, causing hemolytic anemia, vaso-occlusion, and vascular endothelial dysfunction.

SCD is the most common inherited hemolytic anemia in the United States. Approximately 70,000 to 100,000 individuals in the United States are affected, most commonly those who have ancestry from Africa, the Indian subcontinent, the Arabian Peninsula, or the Mediterranean Basin. Worldwide, millions of persons are affected with SCD, especially in regions with endemic malaria, such as Africa, the Middle East, and India. SCD is characterized by a lifelong hemolytic anemia with an ongoing risk for acute medical complications and inexorable accrual of organ damage in most affected individuals.

There is wide variability in the phenotypic severity of SCD that is not well understood. This variation can be explained partly by differences in the total hemoglobin concentration, the mean corpuscular hemoglobin concentration, erythrocyte

A version of this article was previously published in the *Pediatric Clinics of North America*, 55:2.
Dr. Heeney is supported by NIH K12 HL087164 and U54 HL070819. Dr. Ware is supported by U54 HL070590, U01 HL078787, N01 HB 07155, and American Syrian Lebanese Associated Charities.
[a] Department of Pediatrics, Harvard Medical School, Boston, MA, USA
[b] Division of Hematology/Oncology, Children's Hospital Boston, 300 Longwood Avenue, Boston, MA 02115, USA
[c] Department of Hematology, St. Jude Children's Research Hospital, 262 Danny Thomas Place, MS 355, Memphis, TN 38105, USA
* Corresponding author. Division of Hematology/Oncology, Department of Medicine, Children's Hospital, Boston, 300 Longwood Avenue, Boston, MA 02115.
E-mail address: matthew.heeney@childrens.harvard.edu (M.M. Heeney).

rheology, the percentage of adhesive cells, the proportion of dense cells, the presence or absence of α-thalassemia, and the β-globin haplotype.[1–5] The percentage of fetal hemoglobin (HbF), however, is perhaps the most important laboratory parameter influencing clinical severity in SCD.[6,7] In unaffected individuals, HbF comprises only 5% of the total hemoglobin by age 3 to 6 months and falls to below 1% in adults.[8] In contrast, patients with SCD typically have HbF levels ranging from 1% to 20%[9] and those with genetic mutations leading to hereditary persistence of HbF (HPFH) can have HbF levels that reach 30% to 40% of the total hemoglobin.[10]

Based on the observation that infants with SCD have few complications early in life, it was hypothesized that HbF, the predominant hemoglobin in fetal and infant stages of life, might ameliorate the phenotypic expression of SCD.[11] In addition, compound heterozygotes for the sickle mutation and HPFH are relatively protected from severe clinical symptoms.[12] Subsequently, it was shown that increased HbF percentage is associated with decreased clinical severity in SCD, using endpoints, such as the number of vaso-occlusive painful events, transfusions, and hospitalizations.[1,13] HbF does not, however, seem to protect from some complications,[14] perhaps because the HbF levels were inadequate to provide protection.[3,15] A potential threshold of 20% HbF is suggested, above which patients experience fewer clinical events.[16] The % HbF also has emerged as the most important predictor of early mortality in patients with SCD.[6,17]

Although the genetic and molecular pathophysiology of SCD are well described and understood in considerable detail, there has been disappointing progress toward definitive, curative therapy. Bone marrow transplantation offers a cure but currently requires an HLA-matched sibling donor for best results. This requirement limits the number of patients who can benefit from this approach. Moreover, even using a matched sibling donor, bone marrow transplantation remains associated with considerable morbidity (primarily graft-versus-host disease) and low, but not negligible, mortality.

In lieu of curative therapy, one approach given considerable effort over the past 25 years has been the pharmacologic induction of HbF beyond the fetal and newborn period. Several pharmacologic agents have shown promise, including demethylating agents, such as 5-azacytidine[18] and decitabine,[19–21] and short-chain fatty acids, such as butyrate,[22–25] but each has limitations in route of administration, safety, or sustained efficacy. Hydroxyurea, in contrast, has a long and growing track record in inducing HbF in patients with SCD. In addition, hydroxyurea has a variety of salutary effects on other aspects of the pathophysiology of SCD, such as increased erythrocyte hydration, improved rheology, and reduced adhesiveness. Hydroxyurea also decreases leukocyte count, and releases nitric oxide. This article reviews the usefulness of hydroxyurea for children with SCD but is not intended to be an exhaustive review of the drug's biochemistry, its therapeutic rationale, or previously published data. Interested readers may read more thorough reviews of hydroxyurea for the management of SCD.[26,27] This article is intended as a practical user's guide for clinicians who wish to know how and why treatment with hydroxyurea should be considered for children with SCD.

AN IDEAL DRUG FOR SICKLE CELL DISEASE?

Hydroxyurea may be an ideal therapeutic agent for use in children with SCD. It has excellent bioavailability after oral administration; requires only once-daily dosing, which improves medication adherence; has few if any immediate side effects; has predictable hematologic toxicities that are dose dependent, transient, and reversible;

and has potential benefits against multiple pathophysiologic mechanisms of SCD. Although several therapeutic agents currently under development address specific aspects of the pathophysiology of SCD, only hydroxyurea offers a broad range of beneficial effects that collectively can ameliorate the overall clinical severity of disease.

The drug is classified as an antimetabolite and antineoplastic agent. The exact mechanism of its antineoplastic activity is not elucidated fully but believed to be S-phase specific. Hydroxyurea is converted in vivo to a free radical nitroxide that quenches the tyrosyl free radical at the active site of the M2 subunit of ribonucleotide reductase. As a potent ribonucleotide reductase inhibitor, hydroxyurea blocks the conversion of ribonucleotides to deoxyribonucleotides, which interferes with the synthesis of DNA without any effects on RNA or protein synthesis. The drug is used widely in oral doses (ranging from 20 to 80 mg/kg/d) for the long-term treatment of chronic myeloproliferative disorders, such as polycythemia vera and essential thrombocythemia. In combination with reverse transcriptase inhibitors (eg, didanosine), hydroxyurea is finding a role within HIV therapy as a virostatic agent that produces potent and sustained viral suppression.[28]

In patients with hemoglobinopathies, the myelosuppressive and cytotoxic effects of hydroxyurea seem to induce erythroid regeneration and the premature commitment of erythroid precursors, with resulting increased production of HbF-containing reticulocytes and total HbF.[29] Additional pharmacologic effects of hydroxyurea that may contribute to its beneficial effects in SCD include increasing erythrocyte HbF through nitric oxide dependent pathways, decreasing the neutrophil count, increasing erythrocyte volume and hydration, increasing deformability of sickle erythrocytes, and altering the adhesion of sickle erythrocytes to the endothelium.[29–33] The release of nitric oxide directly from the hydroxyurea molecule[34,35] should allow beneficial local effects on the endothelium, thereby ameliorating the vaso-occlusive process and limiting vascular dysfunction.

CLINICAL EXPERIENCE

Preclinical studies in anemic cynomolgus monkeys showed that hydroxyurea increased HbF levels.[33] Pilot trials in patients with SCD demonstrated that hydroxyurea also increased HbF in humans and caused little short-term toxicity.[29–32] These proof-of-principle experiments were critical first steps toward an important multicenter phase I/II trial involving adults with HbSS, which identified the short-term efficacy and toxicities of hydroxyurea used at maximum tolerated dose (MTD).[32]

Developed on the basis of favorable results from the phase I/II trial, the National Heart, Lung, and Blood Institute (NHLBI) sponsored the pivotal Multicenter Study of Hydroxyurea (MSH), a double-blinded, placebo-controlled, randomized control trial conducted from 1992 to 1995 in 21 centers in the United States. and Canada.[36] Two hundred and ninety-nine adult patients with HbSS were randomized (152 on hydroxyurea and 147 received placebo) but because of the beneficial effects observed, the trial was stopped early and only 134 subjects completed the planned 24 months of treatment. The hydroxyurea-treated subjects had a 44% reduction in painful crises per year (2.5 events per year versus 4.5 events per year) and a 58% reduction in median annual hospitalization rate for painful crisis (1.0 versus 2.4). In addition there were significantly fewer hydroxyurea-treated subjects who developed acute chest syndrome (ACS) (25 versus 51) and who received blood transfusions (48 versus 73); the number of units of blood transfused also was significantly less (336 versus 586). The incidence of death and stroke did not differ between the two treatment arms; there were no deaths related to hydroxyurea treatment and none of the patients who had received hydroxyurea developed cancer during the trial. The study did not address long-term safety or potential reversibility or prevention of chronic organ damage.[36]

The results of this study led the Food and Drug Administration in 1998 to add to the indications for hydroxyurea, "to reduce the frequency of painful crises and to reduce the need for blood transfusions in adult patients with sickle cell anemia with recurrent moderate to severe painful crises." This additional labeling refers only to adults severely affected by painful events rather than the broader spectrum of patients with SCD. Now, 10 years later, there is no change in the manufacturer's drug labeling for hydroxyurea. Therefore, at this time, all children or patients with mild-to-moderate disease severity or those who do not have painful events but who have ACS or end-organ damage require off-label usage.

The initial success of hydroxyurea in adults led to the first pediatric multicenter phase I/II trial, known as HUG-KIDS, from 1994 to 1996.[37] Eighty-four children ages 5 to 15 years with severe HbSS disease (defined as three or more painful events within the year before entry, three episodes of ACS within 2 years of entry, or three episodes of ACS or pain within 1 year of entry) were enrolled. Sixty-eight reached MTD and 52 were treated at MTD for 12 months. Similar hematologic effects were seen as in the MSH trial with decreased hemolysis (increased Hb and decreased reticulocytosis, decreased lactate dehydrogenase, and decreased total bilirubin), macrocytosis, improved erythrocyte hydration, myelosuppression, and increased HbF and F cells (**Table 1**). Laboratory toxicities were mild and reversible with temporary interruption of the medication, and no life-threatening clinical adverse events were observed. Subsequent evaluation of this cohort revealed no adverse effect on height or weight gain or pubertal development.[38] Predictors of HbF response were complex, but a higher treatment HbF was associated with higher baseline HbF, Hb, white blood cell count (WBC), and reticulocytes and compliance.[39]

Short-term clinical efficacy in children initially was reported in small open-label studies.[40,41] In a small, randomized study from Belgium, children with HbSS treated with hydroxyurea had significantly fewer hospitalizations for pain, with shorter lengths of stay, compared with those receiving placebo.[42] Additional European data showed improved laboratory and clinical response without significant toxicity and no growth or pubertal delay.[43] Follow-up studies have revealed continued efficacy in association

Table 1
Children with homozygous sickle cell anemia have similar laboratory efficacy using hydroxyurea at maximum tolerated dose as adults

	Adults	Children
MTD (mg/kg/d)	21.3	25.6
Δ Hb (g/dL)	+1.2	+1.2
Δ MCV (fL)	+23	+14
Δ HbF (%)	+11.2	+9.6
Δ Reticulocytes (10^9/L)	−158	−146
Δ WBC (10^9/L)	−5.0	−4.2
Δ ANC (10^9/L)	−2.8	−2.2
Δ Bilirubin (mg/dL)	−2.0	−1.0

Data from published phase I/II trials for adults[32] and children[37] with HbSS.

with long-term hydroxyurea use in children,[44] including a sustained HbF response greater than 20% using hydroxyurea at MTD.[45]

The role of hydroxyurea in preserving organ function in SCD is not yet determined. From a practical standpoint, these beneficial effects are difficult to assess prospectively because organ damage develops broadly over the whole pediatric age range, beginning with splenic and renal changes in infancy and evolving to pulmonary and neurologic deficits with vasculopathy among older children. In the Hydroxyurea Safety and Organ Toxicity (HUSOFT) study, infants with HbSS tolerated open-label liquid hydroxyurea and had preserved splenic filtrative function compared with historical controls.[46] A follow-up study on this cohort identified preservation of splenic function and apparent gain of function in some cases.[47] In a recent retrospective study, 43 children with HbSS had splenic function measured before and during treatment with hydroxyurea for a median duration of 2.6 years; six patients (14%) completely recovered splenic function and two (5%) had preserved splenic function, suggesting that hydroxyurea might help preserve or recover splenic function.[48] Similar beneficial effects of hydroxyurea are reported anecdotally for children who have proteinuria,[49] priapism,[50,51] or hypoxemia.[52]

The role of hydroxyurea in the prevention of stroke in SCD is an area of active investigation. In a retrospective study, hydroxyurea therapy was associated with lower transcranial Doppler (TCD) flow velocities.[53] In a recent prospective single institution study, hydroxyurea was shown to decrease elevated TCD velocities significantly, often into the normal range,[54] suggesting that hydroxyurea might serve as an alternative to chronic erythrocyte transfusions for primary stroke prophylaxis. Hydroxyurea also is reported as an alternative to chronic transfusions for secondary stroke prophylaxis in children for whom transfusions cannot be continued safely (eg, erythrocyte allosensitization).[55,56] Hydroxyurea in combination with serial phlebotomy effectively prevented secondary stroke and led to resolution of transfusional iron overload in 35 children from a single institution.[57] Based on these encouraging preliminary results, the NHLBI-sponsored Stroke With Transfusions Changing to Hydroxyurea (SWiTCH) trial is underway[58]; this study randomizes children with previous stroke to standard therapy (transfusions and chelation) or alternative therapy (hydroxyurea and phlebotomy) for the prevention of secondary stroke and management of iron overload.

There are limited data regarding the prolonged use of hydroxyurea in SCD, particularly with regard to its long-term risks and benefits, but current clinical experience has not identified any clear detrimental effects or safety concerns. The possibility of hydroxyurea having negative effects on growth and development in children has not been realized.[45,47] Similarly, concerns about DNA damage and leukemogenesis are not validated, with more than 15 years of exposure among adults and more than 12 years of exposure among children; continued vigilance is warranted but current data are encouraging regarding the long-term safety of this therapy. A 9-year observational follow-up study suggests that adults taking hydroxyurea had a significant 40% reduction in overall mortality.[59] During the MSH Patients' Follow-up study, there was little risk associated with the careful use of hydroxyurea; however, it was stated that hydroxyurea must be taken indefinitely to be effective and concerns remain over long-term safety. The teratogenicity of hydroxyurea for SCD is not elucidated fully. Anecdotes of normal offspring of women taking hydroxyurea during pregnancy[60,61] are supported by the lack of birth defects observed in the MSH cohort (Abdullah Kutlar, personal communication, December 2007). Recent reports, however, document abnormal spermatogenesis in men taking hydroxyurea,[62,63] so further investigation in this area is needed. A recently opened study at St Jude Children's Research Hospital, entitled Long Term Effects of Hydroxyurea Therapy in Children with Sickle Cell Disease,[64] should provide important data regarding long-term risks and benefits of hydroxyurea in this young patient population.

PRACTICAL CONSIDERATIONS

Hydroxyurea therapy cannot be prescribed, monitored, and adjusted properly according to exact and specific written guidelines. Instead, optimal treatment with hydroxyurea (as with many other medications) requires careful attention to the details of each patient's treatment response; such individualized therapy often involves as much art as science. The following sections represent the distillation of a combined 25 years of experience with hydroxyurea (>300 treated children), but none of the text should be considered dogma. Instead, these recommendations and suggestions represent a workable and historically successful approach that can serve as a good starting point for health care teams.

Beginning Hydroxyurea Therapy

The decision to initiate hydroxyurea therapy in a child who has SCD should be made deliberately and thoughtfully. The medical history of a patient should be reviewed carefully to document the number and severity of acute vaso-occlusive events plus any evidence of clinical or laboratory evidence of chronic organ damage, such as hypoxemia, proteinuria, or elevated TCD velocities. Indications for hydroxyurea therapy are not universally agreed upon and each health care team must determine their own threshold; a proposed list is in **Table 2**. In addition to the laboratory and clinical profile, previous compliance with outpatient clinic visits should be reviewed and the neurocognitive status and psychosocial milieu for the child considered. There

Table 2
Potential indications for hydroxyurea therapy in children with homozygous sickle cell anemia

Acute vaso-occlusive complications	Painful events	
	Dactylitis	
	Acute chest syndrome	
Laboratory markers of severity	Low hemoglobin	
	Low HbF	
	Elevated WBC	
	Elevated LDH	
Organ dysfunction	Brain	Elevated TCD velocities
		Silent MRI or MRA changes
		Stroke prophylaxis
	Lungs	Hypoxemia
	Kidney	Proteinuria
Miscellaneous	Sibling on hydroxyurea	
	Parental request	

Most pediatric hematologists have accepted clinical severity with acute vaso-occlusive complications as an indication for hydroxyurea therapy, but there is little agreement about indications for children with laboratory abnormalities or organ dysfunction. Similarly, the appropriate age for hydroxyurea initiation has not been determined, although clinical trials have demonstrated safety and efficacy for infants, young children, and school-aged children with SCD.

are many nonpharmacologic reasons that hydroxyurea therapy can fail in children with SCD, and anticipation of problems with development of creative solutions represents the best way to promote adherence and obtain the optimal drug effects for a child receiving treatment.

Healthcare providers never should make the decision to start hydroxyurea unilaterally; team members must discuss the recommendation openly with patients and families. Ideally, all of a patient's caregivers who might dispense the medication should be present during the initial pretreatment discussions, to ensure that all questions are answered and all concerns addressed. Only if all of the parties involved (patient, parents/guardians, extended family members providing care, and the health care team) are in agreement should hydroxyurea therapy be started. Treatment is likely to fail due to medication nonadherence if any key family member (including the child) is not fully supportive of the decision to begin treatment. Families are told that 6 to 12 months of therapy with monthly clinic visits for examination and blood draw are needed to establish an optimal dose and dosing regimen, so they should make a commitment to this duration before commencing treatment. This verbal contract emphasizes the importance of the commitment to therapy, which is being made by all involved parties. Two to three pretreatment visits also are advised, to explain the nuances of therapy and answer questions, because the decision to begin an indefinite treatment with monthly visits should not be made quickly by a single person at a single visit. Occasionally, an apparently motivated family member fails to return for a follow-up informational visit with an additional parent/guardian or other family member. This kind of missed visit may reflect some unspoken reluctance to begin treatment by parent or patient, unforeseen psychosocial obstacles, or unidentified financial or transportation barriers but allows an early appraisal of the likelihood of treatment success.

Explaining the Rationale

The recommendation to begin hydroxyurea therapy and a description of the potential risks and benefits of taking the drug should be communicated to patients and family members in a straightforward and honest way, using age-appropriate and culturally sensitive language and vocabulary. Some families have access to the Internet and already have acquired detailed information and formed specific questions, whereas others have little knowledge of the drug beyond what is provided by the health care team. Providing a rationale that includes mechanisms of HbF induction or nitric oxide metabolism generally is not helpful or persuasive in the majority of cases. Instead, a general review of the pathophysiology of sickle cell vaso-occlusion typically is sufficient, indicating where hydroxyurea might be beneficial. Most children recognize that sickled erythrocytes have an elongated shape; hence, comments like, "hydroxyurea helps your blood cells stay round" can help motivate even young patients to stay on therapy and serve as easy reminders of the benefits of treatment during subsequent visits. Many families realize that their children were generally healthy during the first few months of life, so the benefits of HbF can be put into this context. The importance of daily medication adherence cannot be overemphasized. To help children understand this principle, hydroxyurea can be likened to a powerful vitamin to be taken daily. Families are reminded that a child will not feel better or worse immediately after each dose, and the beneficial effects occur in the blood cells over time and leading eventually to overall improvement.

Describing Risks and Benefits

The potential benefits of hydroxyurea therapy are best discussed with patients and families not only in terms of preventing acute clinical complications, such as pain and ACS, but also as helping avoid hospitalizations and transfusions, enhancing growth, and possibly preventing chronic organ damage. Adverse short-term side effects of taking hydroxyurea are described as usually minimal and often none, except for occasional mild gastrointestinal discomfort. The treatment effects of lowering the blood counts to modest neutropenia are described as predictable and actually desired but requiring periodic dose escalation with monthly monitoring to achieve a stable MTD. Potential deleterious effects on hair or skin are mentioned but minimized, except for occasional (<5%) hyperpigmentation and melanonychia; hepatic and renal drug-related toxicity is described as rare, probably no more than approximately 1 in 1000.

The long-term risks for hydroxyurea therapy are discussed as largely unknown, although accumulating evidence of the drug's long-term safety and efficacy (currently >15 years in adults and >12 years in children) makes this particular point easier to discuss with each passing year. The risks of hydroxyurea for fertility and offspring are discussed; the potential of hydroxyurea as a teratogen in animals provides the strongest rationale for contraception, but the absence of teratogenicity or sterility observed to date among humans, including adult patients from the MSH study, is emphasized. Among the most important discussion points with families are those related to the potential of long-term hydroxyurea exposure to cause cancer in their child. First, it is noted that hydroxyurea initially was developed as an *anticancer* agent and still is used to treat certain forms of cancer. Next, it is noted that children with SCD, just like other children, can develop leukemia and other pediatric cancers.[65] Third, it is noted that adult patients who have preleukemic conditions, such as myeloproliferative disorders, may have an increased risk for developing cancer after 10 to 20 years of hydroxyurea therapy, but this has not yet been observed in children or adults with SCD. Finally, the theoretic risk of developing cancer in 20 years should be compared with the known natural history of untreated children with SCD and clinical severity, and to the high likelihood of acute and chronic clinical complications, poor quality of life, and increased risk for early death.[6,66] With this approach, the long-term risks of malignancy are not trivialized but are placed into context. A recent National Institutes of Health Consensus Conference concluded that the risk for cancer associated with hydroxyurea therapy in SCD does not appear to be higher than the baseline rate for this patient population.[67]

Dose Initiation

Before initiating hydroxyurea therapy, baseline laboratory studies should be obtained (**Fig. 1**). Based on data from the HUG-KIDS,[37] HUSOFT,[46] Toddler HUG,[68] and other studies,[45,54] the vast majority of children with HbSS tolerate an initial hydroxyurea dose of 20 mg/kg/d given as a single dose. Earlier studies used a lower initial starting dose of 15 mg/kg/d,[32,37] but almost every pediatric patient tolerates hydroxyurea at 20 mg/kg/d unless there is concomitant renal dysfunction. The dose of hydroxyurea does not need to be adjusted for ideal body weight, because obesity is rare among untreated children with SCD. Hydroxyurea capsules are available commercially (200 mg, 300 mg, 400 mg, and 500 mg capsules), allowing fairly precise dosing regimens with accuracy within 2 mg/kg/d. At some centers, dosing is achieved with only 500 mg capsules, using doses such as: one capsule per day (500 mg/d), one capsule alternating with two capsules per day (750 mg/d), two capsules per day (1000 mg/d), and so forth. Adherence is improved, however, when the same dose is administered every day. Giving the entire daily dose at once, as opposed to a twice or three times daily dosing, improves adherence and offers some pharmacokinetic advantages.[69]

For young children or those who cannot tolerate swallowing capsules, a liquid hydroxyurea formulation often can be prepared by a local or institutional pharmacy.

Laboratory Studies Before Initiation
Complete blood count with WBC differential and reticulocyte count
Hemoglobin electrophoresis with quantitative % HbF
Chemistry profile (eg, LDH, total & direct bilirubin, AST / ALT, BUN / Cr)
Pregnancy test for post-menarchal females
*Serum B-12 and RBC Folate, serum Iron, TIBC, Ferritin
    (to help interpret Hydroxyurea related-macrocytosis)
*Viral serologies (Hepatitis A, B, C; Parvovirus, HIV)
    (to help interpret transaminitis or unexpected cytopenia)

Initiation Dose
Approximately 20 mg/kg/d in a single daily oral dose
Timing of administration to be convenient for patient and family
Ideally use single formulation (eg, 500 mg capsules)

Dose Escalation to MTD
Increase dose by approximately 5 mg/kg/d q8weeks until MTD reached
    Typical MTD dose 25 - 30 mg/kg/d
    Target ANC 2000 - 4000 / µL or other hematologic toxicity
    Maximum dose 35 mg/kg/d or 2000 mg/d

Laboratory Monitoring during Dose Escalation
Monthly visits with review of toxicities and medication adherence
Monthly complete blood count with WBC differential and reticulocyte count
Bimonthly chemistry profile (LDH, total & direct bilirubin, AST / ALT, BUN / Cr)
Periodic hemoglobin electrophoresis

Subsequent Dose Modification
Hematologic toxicity:

Neutrophils	ANC < 1.0 x 10^9/L (1000 per µL)
Hemoglobin	< 7.0 gm/dL with low reticulocytes
	eg ARC < 100 x 10^9/L (100K per µL)
	Decrease > 20% from baseline with low reticulocytes
Reticulocytes	< 80 x 10^9/L (80K per µL)
	unless the hemoglobin >8.0 gm/dL
Platelets	< 80 x 10^9/L (80K per µL)

If hematologic toxicity occurs
    Discontinue medication until counts recover (usually within 1 week)
    Restart at previous dose or reduce dose by 2.5 – 5.0 mg/kg/d

Monitoring After Reaching MTD
Monthly visits can extend to bimonthly if:
    a stable MTD has been reached and
    adherence is judged unlikely to suffer with decreased visit frequency

Each visit: Complete blood count with WBC differential and reticulocyte count
            Assessment of clinical toxicity
            Reinforcement of adherence using peripheral smear or lab trends

Alternate visits: Chemistry profile (LDH, total & direct bilirubin, AST / ALT, BUN / Cr)
                   Hemoglobin electrophoresis

Fig. 1. Guideline for initiating, modifying, and monitoring hydroxyurea therapy (see text for further details). Asterisk indicates prehydroxyurea laboratory studies that are performed to help determine the etiology of potential treatment related laboratory changes or toxicities (eg, transaminitis, macrocytosis, and reticulocytopenia).

Hydroxyurea capsule contents or bulk hydroxyurea powder can be dissolved in water with vigorous stirring and sweetener can be added for flavoring palatability; such liquid formulations are stable for weeks to months with refrigeration or at room temperature.[70] The initial hydroxyurea slurry should not be heated to speed up dissolution, however, because structural and functional activity is diminished. Liquid hydroxyurea formulations are easy to dose (usually to 0.2 mL precision), allowing fine tuning of daily doses before and after MTD is achieved.

It is recommended that the hydroxyurea dose be administered at a time of day that is most convenient for patients and families. In many instances, this is in the morning or before school or the workday but can be in the afternoon, early evening, or before bedtime. The exact timing should not be regimented or overly emphasized; the critical feature is reliable dosing once each day. Families may worry about "missing a dose" by several hours but this is not a problem; it should be emphasized, however, that the daily dose just needs to be swallowed at some time during each day. Occasional patients (approximately 5%) mention gastrointestinal symptoms, such as stomachache or nausea, after taking hydroxyurea in the morning; in these instances, changing to evening dosing almost always leads to resolution of symptoms.

Dose Escalation to Maximum Tolerated Dose

Beneficial effects of hydroxyurea can begin in the first few weeks after commencing therapy,[71] which can lead to some reluctance by medical providers to increase the dose beyond that needed for subjective clinical improvement. Because the salutary laboratory effects of hydroxyurea, especially induction of HbF and diminution of WBC and absolute neutrophil count (ANC), are dose dependent,[32,45] however, it seems logical and advisable to increase the daily hydroxyurea dose to achieve the MTD. Based on comparative data documenting superior laboratory effects when hydroxyurea is prescribed at MTD,[45] the goal of hydroxyurea should be to achieve modest marrow suppression without undue hematologic toxicity.

After initiating hydroxyurea therapy (approximately 20 mg/kg/d), the child is seen in the outpatient clinic setting approximately every 4 weeks. At each interval visit, medical history is obtained and physical examination performed along with a discussion of dosing issues and emphasis on daily adherence. A complete blood cell count with WBC differential and reticulocyte count should be performed at each interval visit, and the next month's dose should not be ordered or dispensed until that day's weight and blood counts are available. The daily dose should be increased by approximately 5 mg/kg/d every 8 weeks if no toxicity occurs. The 4-week interval is too short for most dose adjustments, because hematologic toxicity can accumulate and not manifest fully until 8 weeks after a dose increase. It is critical to examine the trends in peripheral blood counts at each visit—sometimes toxicity is slowly cumulative and can be anticipated based on changes identified over 8 to 16 weeks.

Hydroxyurea is titrated most easily according to the peripheral blood counts and typically is limited by neutropenia, occasionally by reticulocytopenia, and more rarely by thrombocytopenia. The target ANC for MTD should be approximately 2 to 4 × 10^9/L (2000–4000 per μL), although other hematologic toxicity may limit dose escalation. Based on published data,[45,55,57] most children with HbSS require a dose of 25 to 30 mg/kg/d to reach this MTD. The maximum daily dose of hydroxyurea should not exceed 35 mg/kg/d or 2000 mg/d; failure to achieve marrow suppression at these doses strongly suggests medication nonadherence. The MTD, measured in mg/kg/d, typically is established within 4 to 8 months of initiating hydroxyurea therapy but should be assigned only after a child tolerates a particular dose for at least 8 weeks. The MTD then usually remains relatively stable unless there is substantial weight gain, development of splenomegaly, or change in renal function. Once a child reaches MTD, the dose in mg/kg/d, should not be modified frequently, because multiple dose changes and blood count checks are unnecessary and may incorrectly suggest a narrow therapeutic window. Periodic increases in absolute daily dose due to weight gain are appropriate. When a stable MTD is reached, it may be appropriate to decrease the frequency of clinic visits to bimonthly, depending on patient response and family reliability. Extension to quarterly visits usually is associated, however, with a decline in adherence, likely because of lack of frequent reminders from medical providers.

Dose Modification

Hematologic toxicity is by far the most common reason to modify the hydroxyurea dose, usually before reaching the MTD. Although early studies on children with SCD used conservative thresholds for medication stoppage and subsequent dose modifications (eg, ANC <2000 in HUG-KIDS),[37] a more liberal approach can be used safely in the majority of children. Practical toxicity definitions and thresholds for erythrocytes, reticulocytes, neutrophils, and platelets are listed in **Table 3**. Traditionally, hydroxyurea toxicity guidelines also include thresholds for hepatic or renal toxicity (eg, alanine aminotransferase increase >3–5 × the upper limit of normal or a doubling of creatinine) but such organ toxicity almost never is associated with hydroxyurea treatment. An increase in alanine aminotransferase or creatinine should never be assumed to be drug related, and additional investigations with ultrasonography or other tests should be strongly considered.

When a hematologic toxicity occurs on hydroxyurea therapy, the medication should be discontinued to allow the counts to recover. Almost all hematologic toxicities are transient, reversible, and dose dependent and recover within 1 week of drug interruption, although severe toxicities may feature pancytopenia and take 2 to 3 weeks until recovery. If the counts recover in 1 week, then the dose can either be resumed at the previous amount or decreased modestly (eg, reduced by 2.5–5 mg/kg/d). Conversely, if laboratory values suggest that a dose increase would be tolerated after 2 months at a stable dose, the MTD dose can be increased by a small amount (such as 2.5 mg/kg/d). Before increasing a hydroxyurea dose beyond a previously established stable MTD, however, the likelihood of diminished medication adherence should be strongly considered.

Increasing Adherence

Medication adherence is "perhaps the best documented but least understood health-related behavior".[72] Children and their family members are much more likely to be adherent to hydroxyurea therapy and the frequent clinic visits if they believe that treatment will be beneficial. At each clinic visit, the importance of daily medication should be emphasized; specific questions should be asked regarding who gives the dose,

Table 3
Hematologic toxicity thresholds requiring hydroxyurea dose modifications
Neutrophils   ANC <1.0 × 10^9/L (1000 per μL)
Hemoglobin   <7.0 g/dL with low reticulocytes (eg, absolute reticulocyte count <100 × 10^9/L [100 K per μL])   Decrease by >20% from previous value, with low reticulocytes (as previously)
Reticulocytes   <80 × 10^9/L (80 K per μL) unless the hemoglobin concentration is >8.0 g/dL
Platelets   <80 × 10^9/L (80 K per μL)

what time it is administered, how many doses are missed per week, and so forth. Visualization of the peripheral blood smear is an effective way to illustrate the benefits of hydroxyurea therapy. The de-identified peripheral blood smears of several patients, which were obtained pre- and post-treatment MTD, can be shown to children and family members. The authors use a multiheaded microscope before initiating hydroxyurea therapy to demonstrate the obvious changes that occur with good adherence and a good treatment response (**Fig. 2**), including anisocytosis, macrocytosis, decreased polychromasia, and fewer sickled forms. This viewing and explanation should be performed by an experienced medical provider who can emphasize that adherence also can be monitored by review of the blood counts and the peripheral blood smear.

When explanations of risks and benefits of hydroxyurea therapy are given to patients and family members, it is emphasized that a parent must be in charge of ensuring that the medication actually is swallowed each day. It is imperative to anticipate that occasionally children miss a dose of hydroxyurea without any ill effect, and therefore be tempted to miss several days, wondering if they somehow have been cured. Explaining that blood cells are produced every day, hence the medication must be taken every day, is logical even for young patients. Parents must be reminded at each interval visit that they must be sure to give the medication; teenagers are especially notorious for embellishing adherence. In some instances, patients can be remarkably adherent and even remind parents about dosing.

The use of a "medication score card" can be helpful for improving hydroxyurea adherence. Serial listing of monthly blood counts according to various blood count parameters can be used to show beneficial changes, such as increased hemoglobin concentration, mean corpuscular volume (MCV), and HbF; concomitant decreases in WBC and ANC also easily can be seen. Additional strategies to improving

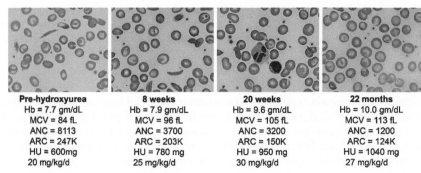

Pre-hydroxyurea	8 weeks	20 weeks	22 months
Hb = 7.7 gm/dL	Hb = 7.9 gm/dL	Hb = 9.6 gm/dL	Hb = 10.0 gm/dL
MCV = 84 fL	MCV = 96 fL	MCV = 105 fL	MCV = 113 fL
ANC = 8113	ANC = 3700	ANC = 3200	ANC = 1200
ARC = 247K	ARC = 203K	ARC = 150K	ARC = 124K
HU = 600mg	HU = 780 mg	HU = 950 mg	HU = 1040 mg
20 mg/kg/d	25 mg/kg/d	30 mg/kg/d	27 mg/kg/d

Fig. 2. Changes in complete blood cell count parameters and erythrocyte morphology in association with hydroxyurea therapy, from dose initiation through escalation to MTD. The initial panel shows blood counts and the peripheral blood smear at dose initiation, with hemolytic anemia and leukocytosis evident along with sickled forms. The second panel is after 8 weeks of hydroxyurea therapy (at approximately 20 mg/kg/d) with some macrocytes and anisocytosis present, along with reductions in the ANC and ARC; the dose was escalated (to approximately 25 mg/kg/d). The third panel is after 20 weeks of hydroxyurea therapy, with less anemia and sickling, more macrocytosis, and modest myelosuppression; the dose was escalated (to approximately 30 mg/kg/d). The fourth panel is after 22 months of hydroxyurea therapy (at MTD of 27 mg/kg/d); there is improved Hb with pronounced macrocytosis and no sickled forms, along with modest neutropenia and reticulocytopenia. ARC, absolute reticulocyte count; Hb, hemoglobin; HU, hydroxyurea.

hydroxyurea adherence include providing a calendar to mark off days after medicine has been swallowed, preloading a weekly/biweekly/monthly pill container with prescribed capsules, keeping the pill bottle in plain sight (eg, the kitchen table) to minimize forgotten doses, and counting leftover or unused pills. Whatever the mnemonic devices used, among the best strategies for successful treatment are a thorough understanding of the rationale for treatment, a limited number of health care providers for continuity to patients and family, and regular clinic visits on a 1 to 2 month basis, to engender trust and loyalty with emphasis on the beneficial treatment effects and the need for daily adherence.

SUMMARY

Hydroxyurea is a powerful therapeutic agent with proved laboratory and clinical efficacy for children with SCD. Although there are important questions regarding its long-term efficacy and safety, hydroxyurea has the potential to ameliorate many of the signs and symptoms of the disease. Ongoing clinical trials will help answer questions about the proper clinical indications for its use and, in particular, its ability to prevent organ damage and preserve organ function and long-term safety.

ACKNOWLEDGMENTS

The authors thank Nicole A. Mortier, MHS PA-C, and William H. Schultz, MHS PA-C, for years of experience and dedication to treating children with SCD. We appreciate their insights and advice regarding the optimal use of hydroxyurea in this patient population.

REFERENCES

1. Platt OS, Thorington BD, Brambilla DJ, et al. Pain in sickle cell disease. Rates and risk factors. N Engl J Med 1991;325(1):11–6.
2. Steinberg MH, Rosenstock W, Coleman MB, et al. Effects of thalassemia and microcytosis on the hematologic and vasoocclusive severity of sickle cell anemia. Blood 1984;63(6):1353–60.
3. Baum KF, Dunn DT, Maude GH, et al. The painful crisis of homozygous sickle cell disease. A study of the risk factors. Arch Intern Med 1987;147(7):1231–4.
4. Phillips G Jr, Coffey B, Tran-Son-Tay R, et al. Relationship of clinical severity to packed cell rheology in sickle cell anemia. Blood 1991;78(10):2735–9.
5. Powars DR. Sickle cell anemia: beta s-gene-cluster haplotypes as prognostic indicators of vital organ failure. Semin Hematol 1991;28(3):202–8.
6. Platt OS, Brambilla DJ, Rosse WF, et al. Mortality in sickle cell disease. Life expectancy and risk factors for early death. N Engl J Med 1994;330(23):1639–44.
7. Charache S. Fetal hemoglobin, sickling, and sickle cell disease. Adv Pediatr 1990;37:1–31.
8. Wood WG. Increased HbF in adult life. Baillieres Clin Haematol 1993;6(1):177–213.
9. Serjeant GR. Fetal haemoglobin in homozygous sickle cell disease. Clin Haematol 1975;4(1):109–22.
10. Wood WG, Stamatoyannopoulos G, Lim G, et al. F-cells in the adult: normal values and levels in individuals with hereditary and acquired elevations of Hb F. Blood 1975;46(5):671–82.
11. Watson J, Stahman AW, Bilello FP. Significance of paucity of sickle cells in newborn negro infants. Am J Med Sci 1948;215:419–23.

12. Steinberg MH. Compound heterozygous and other hemoglobinopathies. In: Steinberg MH, Forget BG, Higgs DR, editors. Disorders of hemoglobin: genetics, pathophysiology, and clinical management. Cambridge (UK): Cambridge University Press; 2001. p. 786–810.

13. Odenheimer DJ, Sarnaik SA, Whitten CF, et al. The relationship between fetal hemoglobin and disease severity in children with sickle cell anemia. Am J Med Genet 1987;27(3):525–35.

14. Gladwin MT, Sachdev V, Jison ML, et al. Pulmonary hypertension as a risk factor for death in patients with sickle cell disease. N Engl J Med 2004;350(9):886–95.

15. Powars DR, Schroeder WA, Weiss JN, et al. Lack of influence of fetal hemoglobin levels or erythrocyte indices on the severity of sickle cell anemia. J Clin Invest 1980;65(3):732–40.

16. Powars DR, Weiss JN, Chan LS, et al. Is there a threshold level of fetal hemoglobin that ameliorates morbidity in sickle cell anemia? Blood 1984;63(4):921–6.

17. Leikin SL, Gallagher D, Kinney TR, et al. Mortality in children and adolescents with sickle cell disease. Cooperative Study of Sickle Cell Disease. Pediatrics 1989;84(3):500–8.

18. Ley TJ, DeSimone J, Noguchi CT, et al. 5-Azacytidine increases gamma-globin synthesis and reduces the proportion of dense cells in patients with sickle cell anemia. Blood 1983;62(2):370–80.

19. DeSimone J, Koshy M, Dorn L, et al. Maintenance of elevated fetal hemoglobin levels by decitabine during dose interval treatment of sickle cell anemia. Blood 2002;99(11):3905–8.

20. Koshy M, Dorn L, Bressler L, et al. 2-Deoxy 5-azacytidine and fetal hemoglobin induction in sickle cell anemia. Blood 2000;96(7):2379–84.

21. Saunthararajah Y, Hillery CA, Lavelle D, et al. Effects of 5-aza-2'-deoxycytidine on fetal hemoglobin levels, red cell adhesion, and hematopoietic differentiation in patients with sickle cell disease. Blood 2003;102(12):3865–70.

22. Atweh GF, Sutton M, Nassif I, et al. Sustained induction of fetal hemoglobin by pulse butyrate therapy in sickle cell disease. Blood 1999;93(6):1790–7.

23. Dover GJ, Brusilow S, Charache S. Induction of fetal hemoglobin production in subjects with sickle cell anemia by oral sodium phenylbutyrate. Blood 1994;84(1):339–43.

24. Resar LM, Segal JB, Fitzpatric LK, et al. Induction of fetal hemoglobin synthesis in children with sickle cell anemia on low-dose oral sodium phenylbutyrate therapy. J Pediatr Hematol Oncol 2002;24(9):737–41.

25. Sher GD, Ginder GD, Little J, et al. Extended therapy with intravenous arginine butyrate in patients with beta-hemoglobinopathies. N Engl J Med 1995;332(24):1606–10.

26. Davies SC, Gilmore A. The role of hydroxyurea in the management of sickle cell disease. Blood Rev 2003;17(2):99–109.

27. Halsey C, Roberts IA. The role of hydroxyurea in sickle cell disease. Br J Haematol 2003;120(2):177–86.

28. Lori F, Foli A, Groff A, et al. Optimal suppression of HIV replication by low-dose hydroxyurea through the combination of antiviral and cytostatic ('virostatic') mechanisms. AIDS 2005;19(11):1173–81.

29. Dover GJ, Humphries RK, Moore JG, et al. Hydroxyurea induction of hemoglobin F production in sickle cell disease: relationship between cytotoxicity and F cell production. Blood 1986;67(3):735–8.

30. Platt OS, Orkin SH, Dover G, et al. Hydroxyurea enhances fetal hemoglobin production in sickle cell anemia. J Clin Invest 1984;74(2):652–6.

31. Charache S, Dover GJ, Moyer MA, et al. Hydroxyurea-induced augmentation of fetal hemoglobin production in patients with sickle cell anemia. Blood 1987;69(1):109–16.

32. Charache S, Dover GJ, Moore RD, et al. Hydroxyurea: effects on hemoglobin F production in patients with sickle cell anemia. Blood 1992;79(10):2555–65.

33. Letvin NL, Linch DC, Beardsley GP, et al. Augmentation of fetal-hemoglobin production in anemic monkeys by hydroxyurea. N Engl J Med 1984;310(14):869–73.

34. Gladwin MT, Shelhamer JH, Ognibene FP, et al. Nitric oxide donor properties of hydroxyurea in patients with sickle cell disease. Br J Haematol 2002;116(2):436–44.

35. Huang J, Yakubu M, Kim-Shapiro DB, et al. Rat liver-mediated metabolism of hydroxyurea to nitric oxide. Free Radic Biol Med 2006;40(9):1675–81.

36. Charache S, Terrin ML, Moore RD, et al. Effect of hydroxyurea on the frequency of painful crises in sickle cell anemia. Investigators of the Multicenter Study of Hydroxyurea in Sickle Cell Anemia. N Engl J Med 1995;332(20):1317–22.

37. Kinney TR, Helms RW, O'Branski EE, et al. Safety of hydroxyurea in children with sickle cell anemia: results of the HUG-KIDS study, a phase I/II trial. Pediatric Hydroxyurea Group. Blood 1999;94(5):1550–4.

38. Wang WC, Helms RW, Lynn HS, et al. Effect of hydroxyurea on growth in children with sickle cell anemia: results of the HUG-KIDS Study. J Pediatr 2002;140(2): 225–9.

39. Ware RE, Eggleston B, Redding-Lallinger R, et al. Predictors of fetal hemoglobin response in children with sickle cell anemia receiving hydroxyurea therapy. Blood 2002;99(1):10–4.

40. Scott JP, Hillery CA, Brown ER, et al. Hydroxyurea therapy in children severely affected with sickle cell disease. J Pediatr 1996;128(6):820–8.

41. Jayabose S, Tugal O, Sandoval C, et al. Clinical and hematologic effects of hydroxyurea in children with sickle cell anemia. J Pediatr 1996;129(4):559–65.

42. Ferster A, Vermylen C, Cornu G, et al. Hydroxyurea for treatment of severe sickle cell anemia: a pediatric clinical trial. Blood 1996;88(6):1960–4.

43. de Montalembert M, Belloy M, Bernaudin F, et al. Three-year follow-up of hydroxyurea treatment in severely ill children with sickle cell disease. The French Study Group on Sickle Cell Disease. J Pediatr Hematol Oncol 1997;19(4):313–8.

44. Ferster A, Tahriri P, Vermylen C, et al. Five years of experience with hydroxyurea in children and young adults with sickle cell disease. Blood 2001;97(11):3628–32.

45. Zimmerman SA, Schultz WH, Davis JS, et al. Sustained long-term hematologic efficacy of hydroxyurea at maximum tolerated dose in children with sickle cell disease. Blood 2004;103(6):2039–45.

46. Wang WC, Wynn LW, Rogers ZR, et al. A two-year pilot trial of hydroxyurea in very young children with sickle-cell anemia. J Pediatr 2001;139(6):790–6.

47. Hankins JS, Ware RE, Rogers ZR, et al. Long-term hydroxyurea therapy for infants with sickle cell anemia: the HUSOFT extension study. Blood 2005; 106(7):2269–75.

48. Hankins JS, Helton KJ, McCarville MB, et al. Preservation of spleen and brain function in children with sickle cell anemia treated with hydroxyurea. Pediatr Blood Cancer 2008;50(2):293–7.

49. Fitzhugh CD, Wigfall DR, Ware RE. Enalapril and hydroxyurea therapy for children with sickle nephropathy. Pediatr Blood Cancer 2005;45(7):982–5.

50. Saad ST, Lajolo C, Gilli S, et al. Follow-up of sickle cell disease patients with priapism treated by hydroxyurea. Am J Hematol 2004;77(1):45–9.

51. Maples BL, Hagemann TM. Treatment of priapism in pediatric patients with sickle cell disease. Am J Health Syst Pharm 2004;61(4):355–63.

52. Singh S, Koumbourlis A, Aygun B. Resolution of chronic hypoxemia in pediatric sickle cell patients after treatment with hydroxyurea. Pediatr Blood Cancer. [Epub ahead of print].

53. Kratovil T, Bulas D, Driscoll MC, et al. Hydroxyurea therapy lowers TCD velocities in children with sickle cell disease. Pediatr Blood Cancer 2006;47(7):894–900.

54. Zimmerman SA, Schultz WH, Burgett S, et al. Hydroxyurea therapy lowers transcranial Doppler flow velocities in children with sickle cell anemia. Blood 2007; 110(3):1043–7.

55. Ware RE, Zimmerman SA, Schultz WH. Hydroxyurea as an alternative to blood transfusions for the prevention of recurrent stroke in children with sickle cell disease. Blood 1999;94(9):3022–6.

56. Sumoza A, de Bisotti R, Sumoza D, et al. Hydroxyurea (HU) for prevention of recurrent stroke in sickle cell anemia (SCA). Am J Hematol 2002;71(3):161–5.

57. Ware RE, Zimmerman SA, Sylvestre PB, et al. Prevention of secondary stroke and resolution of transfusional iron overload in children with sickle cell anemia using hydroxyurea and phlebotomy. J Pediatr 2004;145(3):346–52.

58. ClinicalTrials.gov. Stroke with transfusions changing to hydroxyurea (SWiTCH). Available at: http://clinicaltrials.gov/ct2/show/NCT00122980.

59. Steinberg MH, Barton F, Castro O, et al. Effect of hydroxyurea on mortality and morbidity in adult sickle cell anemia: risks and benefits up to 9 years of treatment. JAMA 2003;289(13):1645–51.

60. Pata O, Tok CE, Yazici G, et al. Polycythemia vera and pregnancy: a case report with the use of hydroxyurea in the first trimester. Am J Perinatol 2004;21(3): 135–7.

61. Byrd DC, Pitts SR, Alexander CK. Hydroxyurea in two pregnant women with sickle cell anemia. Pharmacotherapy 1999;19(12):1459–62.

62. Grigg A. Effect of hydroxyurea on sperm count, motility and morphology in adult men with sickle cell or myeloproliferative disease. Intern Med J 2007;37(3):190–2.

63. Masood J, Hafeez A, Hughes A, et al. Hydroxyurea therapy: a rare cause of reversible azoospermia. Int Urol Nephrol 2007;39(3):905–7.

64. ClinicalTrials.gov. Long term effects of hydroxyurea therapy in children with sickle cell disease. Available at: http://clinicaltrials.gov/ct2/show/NCT00305175.

65. Schultz WH, Ware RE. Malignancy in patients with sickle cell disease. Am J Hematol 2003;74(4):249–53.

66. Miller ST, Sleeper LA, Pegelow CH, et al. Prediction of adverse outcomes in children with sickle cell disease. N Engl J Med 2000;342(2):83–9.

67. NIH. National Institutes of Health Consensus Development Conference statement: hydroxyurea treatment for sickle cell disease; 2008. Available at: http://consensus.nih.gov/2008/Sickle%20Cell%20Draft%20Statement%2002-27-08.pdf.

68. Thornburg CD, Dixon N, Burgett S, et al. Efficacy of hydroxyurea to prevent organ damage in young children with sickle cell anemia. Blood 2007;110(11):3386.

69. Yan JH, Ataga K, Kaul S, et al. The influence of renal function on hydroxyurea pharmacokinetics in adults with sickle cell disease. J Clin Pharmacol 2005; 45(4):434–45.

70. Heeney MM, Whorton MR, Howard TA, et al. Chemical and functional analysis of hydroxyurea oral solutions. J Pediatr Hematol Oncol 2004;26(3):179–84.

71. Bridges KR, Barabino GD, Brugnara C, et al. A multiparameter analysis of sickle erythrocytes in patients undergoing hydroxyurea therapy. Blood 1996;88(12): 4701–10.

72. Becker MH, Maiman LA. Sociobehavioral determinants of compliance with health and medical care recommendations. Med Care 1975;13(1):10–24.

Update on Thalassemia: Clinical Care and Complications

Melody J. Cunningham, MD

- Thalassemia • Hemoglobinopathy • Iron-overload

β-Thalassemia, originally named Cooley anemia, initially was described by Dr Cooley in 1925 in Detroit as an inherited blood disease.[1] It is speculated that thalassemia was first recognized in the United States and not in its area of highest prevalence (the Mediterranean) because its presentation as a distinct clinical entity was masked by the fact that malaria, with its similar clinical picture of hemolysis, anemia, and splenomegaly, was ubiquitous in that region.[1] Thus, patients who had this clinical triad were assumed to have malaria, not thalassemia.[1] Now it is recognized that various types of thalassemia are inherited anemias caused by mutations at the globin gene loci on chromosomes 16 and 11, affecting the production of α- or β-globin protein, respectively.[2,3]

The thalassemia syndromes are named according to the globin chain affected or the abnormal hemoglobin produced. Thus, β-globin gene mutations give rise to β-thalassemia and α-globin mutations cause α-thalassemia. In addition, the thalassemias are characterized by their clinical severity (phenotype). Thalassemia major (TM) refers to disease requiring more than eight red blood cell (RBC) transfusions per year and thalassemia intermedia (TI) to disease that requires no or infrequent transfusions.[4] Thalassemia trait refers to carriers of mutations; such individuals have microcytosis and hypochromia but no or only mild anemia.[5,6] Untreated TM uniformly is fatal in the first few years of life.[1] In addition, TM and severe TI can lead to considerable morbidity affecting nearly all organ systems.[7–9] The combination of early diagnosis, improvements in monitoring for organ complications, and advances in supportive care, however, have enabled many patients who have severe thalassemia syndromes to live productive, active lives well into adulthood.[9–11]

EPIDEMIOLOGY

Similar to sickle cell disease and G6PD deficiency, the high prevalence of α- and β-thalassemia genotypes is believed a consequence of an evolutionary protection of

Hematol Oncol Clin N Am 24 (2010) 215–227
doi:10.1016/j.hoc.2009.11.006
0889-8588/10/$ – see front matter © 2010 Elsevier Inc. All rights reserved.

heterozygotes against death from *Plasmodium falciparum* malaria.[11,12] Before the twentieth century, thalassemia tracked with areas of malarial prevalence. β-Thalassemia arose in the Mediterranean, Middle East, South and Southeast Asia, and southern China. α-Thalassemia originated in Africa, the Middle East, China, India, and Southeast Asia.[13–15] Immigration and emigration, however, have led to changing demographics, and patients who have thalassemia syndromes and heterozygote carriers now reside in all parts of the world.[16,17] Thus, it is important for pediatricians, obstetrician, and hematologists to be aware of a possible diagnosis of thalassemia wherever they practice and for any patients they evaluate who have anemia. Consideration of the diagnosis allows proper diagnosis and management of individual patients and identification of carriers and ensures necessary testing and counseling to the population at risk for having children who have thalassemia.

DIAGNOSIS

Understanding how thalassemia can be diagnosed requires a review of the structure of hemoglobin and the genetics of the thalassemia syndromes. Normal human hemoglobin is comprised of two α-like and two β-like globin chains. Adult hemoglobin consists of hemoglobin A ($\alpha_2\beta_2$) plus small amounts of hemoglobin A_2 ($\alpha_2\delta_2$) and hemoglobin F ($\alpha_2\gamma_2$). Genetic mutations in one of the globin genes (α or β) result in decreased or absent production of that globin chain and a relative excess of the other. These mutations can result in no globin production (β° or α°) or decreased globin production (β^+ or α^+).

The α-globin gene is duplicated on chromosome 16; thus, each diploid cell carries four copies. The clinical syndromes of α-thalassemia reflect the number of inherited genes that are mutated. The α-thalassemia syndromes are silent carrier, α-thalassemia trait, hemoglobin H disease, and hydrops fetalis and reflect inheritance of 1, 2, 3, or 4 α-globin gene mutations, respectively. In contrast, a single β-globin gene resides on each chromosome 11. The four clinical syndromes of β-thalassemia, namely silent carrier, thalassemia trait, TI, and TM, correspond to the degree of expression of the two β-globin genes that encode β-globin and not the number of mutated genes.

α-Thalassemia has a wide spectrum of syndromes due to the possibility of one, two, three, or four allelic mutations. Mutation in one of the four alleles results in the silent carrier, with no clinical symptoms, normal complete blood cell count, and hemoglobin electrophoresis results past infancy. If two of the four α-globin alleles are mutated, affected individuals have α-thalassemia trait, with no clinical symptoms, but microcytosis and hypochromia and only mild anemia. The newborn screen often reports hemoglobin Bart, a fast-migrating hemoglobin that appears only in cord and neonatal blood when there is a deletion of one or more of the four α-globin alleles. Hemoglobin Bart is a γ_4 homotetramer that disappears rapidly in the neonatal period; its amount at birth corresponds to the number of affected alleles.[18] Three α-gene mutations cause hemoglobin H disease with anemia characterized by microcytosis and hypochromia. Complete absence of α-globin chain production (all four alleles affected) leads to hydrops fetalis, which usually results in death in utero if intrauterine transfusions are not available.[6,18]

β-Thalassemia has a similar spectrum of clinical phenotypes that reflect the underlying allelic mutations in the β-globin genes. If only a single β-globin gene is affected, then the resulting β-thalassemia silent carrier or trait results from partial (β^+) or absent (β°) gene expression, respectively. Similar to α-thalassemia trait, patients who have β-thalassemia trait typically have mild anemia, microcytosis, and hypochromia.

When both β-globin genes are affected, then the resulting phenotype is more severe, depending on the degree of gene expression and relative imbalance of globin chains. For example, β⁺/β⁺ genotypes typically are associated with an intermediate pheno-type (TI), whereas the β°/β° genotype leads to the more severe TM.

Specific mutations in the α or β genes may lead to production of unique hemoglo-bins on electrophoresis, two of which have unusual features worth discussing in the context of thalassemia. Hemoglobin Constant Spring (Hb CS) is an α-globin gene variant caused by a mutation in the normal stop codon. The resulting elongated α-globin chain forms an unstable hemoglobin tetramer. Hb CS often occurs in conjunction with α-thalassemia so is associated with the more severe α-thalassemia phenotypes. Hemoglobin E (HbE) is caused by a nucleotide change in the β-globin gene, which leads to a single amino acid substitution (Glu26Lys) and diminished expression with a β⁺ phenotype. HbE thus is an unusual "thalassemic hemoglobinop-athy" that can lead to clinically severe phenotypes when paired with other forms of β-thalassemia.

PATHOPHYSIOLOGY

The thalassemia syndromes were among the first genetic diseases to be understood at the molecular level. More than 200 β-globin and 30 α-globin mutations deletions have been identified; these mutations result in decreased or absent production of one globin chain (α or β) and a relative excess of the other. The resulting imbalance leads to unpaired globin chains, which precipitate and cause premature death (apoptosis) of the red cell precursors within the marrow, termed ineffective erythropoi-esis. Of the damaged but viable RBCs that are released from the bone marrow, many are removed by the spleen or hemolyzed directly in the circulation due to the hemo-globin precipitants. Combined RBC destruction in the bone marrow, spleen, and periphery causes anemia and, ultimately, an escalating cycle of pathology resulting in the clinical syndrome of severe thalassemia.

Damaged erythrocytes enter the spleen and are trapped in this low pH and low oxygen environment; subsequent splenomegaly exacerbates the trapping of cells and worsens the anemia. Anemia and poor tissue oxygenation stimulate increased kidney erythropoietin production that further drives marrow erythropoiesis, resulting in increased ineffective marrow activity and the classic bony deformities associated with poorly managed TM and severe TI.[19] Anemia in the severe thalassemia pheno-types necessitates multiple RBC transfusions and, over time, without proper chela-tion, results in transfusion-associated iron overload. In addition, ineffective erythropoiesis enhances gastrointestinal iron absorption and can result in iron over-load, even in untransfused patients who have TI.[20–22] It has long been recognized that the severity of ineffective erythropoiesis affects the degree of iron loading, but until the recent discovery of hepcidin and understanding, its role in iron metabolism the link was not understood.

Hepcidin, an antimicrobial hormone, is recognized as playing a major role in iron deficiency and overload.[23] Hepcidin initially was discovered due to its role in the etiology of anemia of chronic inflammation or chronic disease.[24] Elevated levels, asso-ciated with increased inflammatory markers, maintain low levels of circulating bioavail-able iron in two important ways: (1) by preventing iron absorption and transport from the gut and (2) by preventing release and recycling of iron from macrophages and the reticuloendothelial system.[23] Conversely, inadequate hepcidin allows increased gastrointestinal absorption of iron and ultimately may lead to excess iron sufficient to result in organ toxicity.[22,25,26]

Iron not bound to transferrin, also referred to as nontransferrin-bound iron, damages the endocrine organs, liver, and heart.[27] Nontransferrin-bound iron can result in myocyte damage leading to arrhythmias and congestive heart failure, the primary causes of death in patients who have thalassemia.[9,10,28] Appropriate chelation therapy and close monitoring of cardiac siderosis can avoid this devastating complication (see the article by Kwiatkowski elsewhere in this issue for discussion of iron chelators).

CHANGING DEMOGRAPHICS AND CARRIER SCREENING

The clinical spectrum of thalassemia in the developed world has changed dramatically in the 3 decades since the introduction of deferoxamine chelation.[9,10] In addition, new treatment options and prevention strategies to avoid complications of the disease and its compulsory treatments, coupled with immigration changes, have altered the demography of thalassemia in North America.[16,17] Younger patients are now predominantly of Asian descent, whereas the aging population of patients who have thalassemia are of Mediterranean descent (**Fig. 1**). According to the United States Census Bureau, the number of Asians increased significantly from 1980 to a total of 6.9 million in the census count in 1990. Coupled with other changes that have occurred over the past few decades, it is estimated that up to 100 million people of African, Hispanic, Southern and Eastern European, Middle Eastern, and Asian ethnic backgrounds reside in the United States. Similarly, it is estimated that approximately one sixth of the Canadian population is foreign born. This includes a considerable influx of Asians: in the 1990s more than 2 million people immigrated to Canada, approximately half from Asia. Many of the ethnic immigrants who relocated to North America are carriers of globin gene mutations, which have important implications for carrier screening.

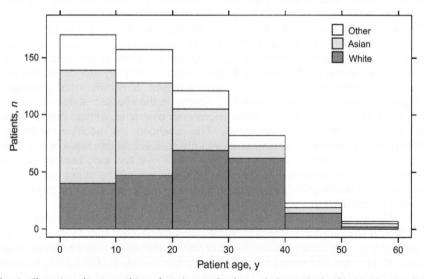

Fig. 1. Changing demographics of patients who have thalassemia in the North American Thalassemia Clinical Research Network. Patients of Asian descent predominate in the younger population. (*From* Vichinsky EP, Macklin EA, Waye JS, et al. Changes in the epidemiology of thalassemia in North America: a new minority disease. Pediatrics 2005;116(6):e818–25; with permission.)

Recent reports reveal births of children who have severe α- or β-thalassemia in which appropriate screening and counseling was not offered to the parents.[18]

Screening is inexpensive and simple but requires clinicians to be astutely attentive and aware of potential carriers. A complete blood cell count identifies microcytosis and hypochromia, which are present in nearly all thalassemia carriers at risk for having babies who have a severe thalassemia syndrome. In an adult, a mean corpuscular volume of less than 80 fL and mean corpuscular hemoglobin of less than 27 pg should alert a clinician to perform further screening, specifically hemoglobin electrophoresis and, in some cases, globin genotype testing. In addition, β-thalassemia carriers have elevated hemoglobin A_2 on adult electrophoresis unless there is concomitant iron deficiency, which may falsely normalize the hemoglobin A2 (HbA_2) level.[29] Once confirmed, genetic counseling should be offered to parents or potential parents.[18]

A newborn hemoglobinopathy screen can be helpful in the recognition and diagnosis of potential thalassemia syndromes. Severe β-thalassemia with absent β production due to two $\beta°$ mutations has only fetal hemoglobin (HbF) as there is no hemoglobin A ($\alpha_2\beta_2$) produced. This abnormal "HbF only" result should prompt a clinician to follow the baby's hemoglobin and growth to determine at what age the baby will need to initiate transfusions to prevent the complications of severe anemia. The anticipated severity of the α-thalassemia syndromes not always is determined easily by the results of a newborn screen. These babies all have an elevated percentage of hemoglobin Bart (γ_4) at birth but the level does not always correspond directly to the number of affected genes. This should alert pediatricians, however, to counsel parents to receive personal testing to determine the number of abnormal α-globin genes in each parent. If each parent has only one mutated α-globin gene, the most clinically significant outcome results in the birth of a baby who has a two-gene α-thalassemia (α-thalassemia trait), which has no clinical consequences. Conversely, if each parent has a two-gene mutation on the same chromosome, termed a *cis* mutation, there exists a risk for the most severe form of α-thalassemia, four-gene deletion, leading to hydrops fetalis, which often results in fetal demise without in utero transfusion.[30,31]

CLINICAL COMPLICATIONS
Transfusion-associated Issues

Iron overload
The primary long-term complication of chronic RBC transfusions for thalassemia is iron loading and the resultant parenchymal organ toxicity. Cardiac iron-overload leading to cardiac failure or arrhythmias is the most common fatal complication seen in chronically transfused patients who have thalassemia.[9] Adherence to chelation can prevent cardiac damage and death from cardiac injury. Patients who present with cardiac arrythmias or failure due to iron injury often can be rescued by continuous infusion deferoxamine although adherence to the regimen of subcutaneous deferoxamine delivered 24 hours per day, 7 days per week, is difficult.[32]

In addition, the endocrine organs are exquisitely sensitive to the toxic effects of iron and this may result in hypogonadotropic hypogonadism, pituitary damage, diabetes,[4,8,33] osteopenia, and osteoporosis. Hypogonadotrophic hypogonadism is common in young adults who have TM and is believed to contribute to low fertility in this population.[34,35] Additionally, cardiac complications of iron overload may exacerbate pregnancy and delivery complications in women who have thalassemia. Case reports and small published series reveal, however, that successful pregnancy and delivery of healthy babies is possible in women who have TM.[33,35,36] Spontaneous pregnancy without hormonal assistance is reported.[33,35] Recent literature on hypogo-nadotrophic hypogonadism suggests that early intervention with hormonal therapy and aggressive iron chelation therapy to prevent permanent damage may help preserve innate fertility. The effect of chelation on preservation of gonadal function currently is being investigated. For example, deferasirox, which provides extended blood chelator levels, may have a protective effect against toxicity to the endocrino-logic organs, but further research remains necessary.

Alloimmunization

Chronic transfusions may result in the development of anti-RBC antibodies, alloanti-bodies and autoantibodies, in a variety of diseases.[37] Although several studies have investigated the rates of alloimmunization in patients who had sickle cell disease,[37,38] the thalassemia population is less well studied. Small retrospective analyses have suggested alloimmunization rates of 2.7% to 37% in patients who had thalas-semia.[39,40] Rates of alloimmunization are suggested as higher for transfusions with donor/recipient ethnic disparity [41] and in splenectomized patients.[42] Because of the risk for alloimmunization and autoimmunization, it is recommended that extended RBC antigen phenotyping be performed before initiation of RBC transfusions, so that patients can be transfused safely in the event of anti-RBC autoantibody or alloan-tibody formation. If a patient then develops autoantibodies directed against ubiquitous RBC antigens or multiple alloantibodies, blood that is matched more fully can be transfused more safely. For sickle cell patients requiring chronic transfusions, Rh and Kell antigen matching is considered standard of care and performed by many, but not all, care centers. For patients who have thalassemia, this matching strategy is not performed routinely. One recent study suggests, however, that matching for Rh and Kell in this population can decrease the alloantibody rate by 53%.[42] Unlike most patients who have sickle cell disease, patients who have thalassemia usually initiate chronic transfusions at 6 months to 2 years of age. Many clinicians believe that chronic transfusions early in life may allow development of tolerance to foreign RBC antigens and prevent development of alloimmunization. Further prospective studies in this area are required to determine the appropriate transfusion strategy in patients who have thalassemia.

Viral infection

The transmission of infections, in particular HIV, hepatitis B, and hepatitis C, remains a serious complication and a significant problem in some developing countries.[43] For now the sole use of volunteer donors who have no financial incentive to donate and thus are likely to answer a detailed donor questionnaire honestly provides the greatest protection against transfusion transmission of infections. Additionally, serologic and nucleic acid testing, used in the developed world, augment the safety of blood prod-ucts.[44] When these safety measures are in place, the risk for transfusion-transmission of known infections is extraordinarily low.[45]

The development of the hepatitis B vaccine, identification of the hepatitis C virus (HCV), and a serologic test to screen donors has greatly minimized the risk for trans-fusion-transmitted hepatitis B virus and HCV. The prevalence of HCV in patients who have thalassemia is disparate and depends on the screening procedures and donor pool. In the developing world, the prevalence is 20% to 64%,[46] with recent data demonstrating continued exposure and infection to patients who have thalassemia receiving transfusions, including many pediatric patients.[46] In the North American population studied in the National Heart, Lung, and Blood Institute–sponsored

Thalassemia Clinical Research Network, the prevalence of exposure was 70% in patients over 25 years of age but only 5% in patients under 15 years of age.[4]

Chronic active hepatitis can lead to fibrosis, cirrhosis, and hepatocellular carcinoma (HCC) if untreated.[9] Treatment with interferon-α and ribavirin is the standard of care for patients who have chronic hepatitis C. Because ribavirin causes hemolysis and thus increases transfusion requirements and concomitant iron exposure, the package guidelines for ribavirin still recommend that it not be used to treat chronic hepatitis in patients who are chronically transfused. Small studies have demonstrated, however, that ribavirin can be given safely and effectively to patients who have thalassemia.[47–50] Because hepatic cirrhosis, liver failure, and HCC all are potential consequences of chronic active hepatitis, the majority of clinicians who care for these patients recommend treatment with interferon and ribavirin.

HCV-infected patients who have thalassemia are living long enough to develop prolonged chronic active hepatitis and be at risk for developing HCC. A multicenter retrospective review by Borgna-Pignatti and colleagues reported 22 patients who had HCC from a cohort of approximately 5000 patients who had thalassemia followed in 52 Italian centers.[51] These numbers likely underestimate, however, the true risk for cirrhosis and HCC to patients who have thalassemia and are infected with hepatitis C, because many succumbed to cardiac complications before living long enough to develop frank cirrhosis or HCC.[9] Patients who do not have evidence of hepatitis C exposure should have annual screening for HCV. Patients who have chronic hepatitis and are at risk for HCC should undergo routine screening with serum α-fetoprotein and liver ultrasound because survival in patients who have HCC is inversely proportional to the size of the tumor.[52]

Thrombosis and Hypercoagulable State

Data compiled from many series present compelling clinical evidence for increased risk for thrombosis in patients who have β-TI, β-TM, α-thalassemia syndromes, or hemoglobin E/β-thalassemia.[53–55] The risk for thromboses is increased in patients who are nontransfused or infrequently transfused and in patients who are splenectomized. This is believed to result in part from increased proportion of defective, innate RBCs.[56] Defective RBCs have disrupted membranes resulting in exposure of negatively charged lipids, including phosphatidylserine, on the external cell surface, which are believed thrombogenic. In the absence of the splenic removal of senescent cells, more of these defective cells are circulating, which increases the risk for thrombosis. In addition, markers studied show increased platelet activation, which also is believed to increase thrombotic risk.[57] The difficulty in ascertaining absolute clinical risk and determining appropriate preventive strategies is that many patients reported in the literature do not have exact transfusion regimens known.[55] More frequent transfusions result in an increased ratio of normal transfused RBCs to disrupted innate RBCs, thus decreasing the clinical risk for thrombosis based on current knowledge of risk factors.

Data in hemolytic states, including sickle cell disease and thalassemia, suggest depletion of nitric oxide resulting from chronic hemolysis and increased plasma levels of free hemoglobin.[58] Nitric oxide is a smooth muscle relaxant and decreased levels are believed to cause increased peripheral vascular resistance and ultimately pulmonary hypertension. Nitric oxide scavenging by free hemoglobin is implicated in the pulmonary arterial disease of sickle cell anemia and data suggest that this is a possible factor in thalassemia. Studies aimed at increasing the levels of nitric oxide and decreasing pulmonary hypertension[59] are ongoing and will be critical in determining clinical approaches to this problem in the aging thalassemia population.

IMPROVEMENTS IN PROGNOSIS AND SURVIVAL
Survival

Historically, patients who had thalassemia had a poor prognosis. In a United States cohort born between 1960 and 1976, the median survival was 17 years.[32] In an Italian cohort born in the mid-1960s, the median survival was 12 years.[9] Remarkable and promising improvement in survival of patients who have thalassemia has been made, however, as demonstrated in two reports by Pearson and collagues.[60,61] In the first 1973 manuscript, before the era of deferoxamine chelation, they reported the ages of 243 patients who had thalassemia in 12 North American centers. In this cohort, 22% were younger than 5 years of age and 2.1% older than 25. The precipitous decrease in number of living patients who had thalassemia began at 15 years of age. Just over a decade later, in 1985, the same centers were surveyed and of the 303 patients, 11% were younger than 5 years and the population of patients older than 25 years had increased to 11% ($P<.01\%$).

More recently, Borgna-Pignatti and colleagues[28] published cohort survival data for nearly 1100 patients who had TM from seven centers in Italy. Kaplan-Meier survival curves were evaluated for 5-year birth cohorts (**Fig. 2**). The curves demonstrated a statistically significant difference in survival in patients in the later birth cohorts. Patients born between 1960 and 1964 had a greater than 60% mortality rate at 30 years of age as compared with the rate of 10% at 25 years of age in the cohort born from 1975 to 1979. The majority of the deaths resulted from cardiac hemosiderosis.

Curative Therapies

Bone marrow transplantation

Successful cure of β-thalassemia by bone marrow transplantation first was reported by Thomas and associates in 1982.[62] Subsequently, several centers have explored the use of this modality as definitive therapy.[63–65] The most extensive published experience with bone marrow transplantation in β-thalassemia is that of Lucarelli and coworkers in Italy.[65] Early on they reported thalassemia-free survival of only 53% in

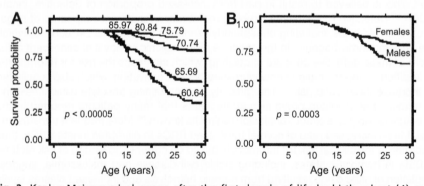

Fig. 2. Kaplan-Meier survival curves after the first decade of life by birth cohort (*A*) and gender (*B*) of 977 patients who had thalassemia in Italy. This demonstrates the dramatic improvement in the younger cohort born between 1985 and 1997. Because they have not had sufficient time to age into the fourth and fifth decades, it makes it difficult to determine the life expectancy of patients treated in developed countries who have access to appropriate chelation therapy and adequate medical care. (*From* Borgna-Pignatti C, Rugolotto S, De SP, et al. Survival and complications in patients with thalassemia major treated with transfusion and deferoxamine. Haematologica 2004;89(10):1187–93; with permission.)

the older patients who had thalassemia with hepatomegaly, liver fibrosis, and inadequate pretransplant chelation.[65] More recent data, however, even in patients considered at high-risk for transplant, demonstrate significant improvements.[66] Survival for the most recently transplanted 33 pediatric patients was 93% and the rate of graft rejection decreased from 30% to 8%.[66] Adults treated with this protocol demonstrated improved thalassemia-free survival, from 62% to 67%, and transplant-related mortality decreased from 37% but still was significant at 27%.

On the basis of available data, bone marrow transplantation may be recommended to patients receiving adequate chelation without evidence of liver disease who have an HLA-matched sibling donor. Many of these patients can be cured.[67–69] Chronic graft-versus-host disease still is a potential long-term complication of successful allogeneic transplantation. A current limitation to the general applicability of this therapy is the availability of a related HLA-matched donor. Only one in four siblings on average is HLA identical. Improved management of graft-versus-host disease and the development of technologies for bone marrow transplantation from unrelated donors may expand the pool of potential donors in the near future. The use of cord blood stem cells and unrelated donors is extending the donor pool and number of patients who may receive bone marrow transplantation.[70–72]

Gene therapy

Treatment of hematologic and other diseases through gene therapy is actively studied in murine and primate models.[73,74] The obstacles to success of this therapeutic modality and the availability of this therapy for humans include the need for improved efficiency of gene delivery, regulated and sustained expression of introduced genes, and insertion of the gene into non-oncogenic sites. Although gene therapy is an area of active clinical investigation, the aforementioned obstacles currently preclude its use in the management of thalassemia or sickle cell anemia. Nonetheless, the successful transfer of globin genes into hematopoietic cells of primates and humans has been demonstrated and is encouraging.[75] A phase I human gene therapy trial for thalassemia and sickle cell disease has been initiated in France but clinical data are not yet available.

REFERENCES

1. Weatherall DJ, Clegg JB. Historical perspectives: the many and diverse routes to our current understanding of the thalassaemias. In: Weatherall DJ, Clegg JB, editors. The thalassaemia syndromes. 4th edition. Oxford (England): Blackwell Science; 2001. p. 3–62.
2. Deisseroth A, Nienhuis A, Turner P, et al. Localization of the human alpha-globin structural gene to chromosome 16 in somatic cell hybrids by molecular hybridization assay. Cell 1977;12(1):205–18.
3. Deisseroth A, Nienhuis A, Lawrence J, et al. Chromosomal localization of human beta globin gene on human chromosome 11 in somatic cell hybrids. Proc Natl Acad Sci U S A 1978;75(3):1456–60.
4. Cunningham MJ, Macklin EA, Neufeld EJ, et al. Complications of beta-thalassemia major in North America. Blood 2004;104(1):34–9.
5. Cao A. Carrier screening and genetic counselling in beta-thalassemia. Int J Hematol 2002;76(Suppl 2):105–13.
6. Galanello R, Sanna MA, Maccioni L, et al. Fetal hydrops in Sardinia: implications for genetic counselling. Clin Genet 1990;38(5):327–31.

7. Calleja EM, Shen JY, Lesser M, et al. Survival and morbidity in transfusion-dependent thalassemic patients on subcutaneous desferrioxamine chelation. Nearly two decades of experience. Ann N Y Acad Sci 1998;850:469–70.

8. Mohammadian S, Bazrafshan HR, Sadeghi-Nejad A. Endocrine gland abnormalities in thalassemia major: a brief review. J Pediatr Endocrinol Metab 2003;16(7): 957–64.

9. Borgna-Pignatti C, Cappellini MD, De SP, et al. Survival and complications in thalassemia. Ann N Y Acad Sci 2005;1054:40–7.

10. Olivieri NF, Nathan DG, MacMillan JH, et al. Survival in medically treated patients with homozygous beta-thalassemia. N Engl J Med 1994;331(9):574–8.

11. Clegg JB, Weatherall DJ. Thalassemia and malaria: new insights into an old problem. Proc Assoc Am Physicians 1999;111(4):278–82.

12. Weatherall DJ. Thalassaemia and malaria, revisited. Ann Trop Med Parasitol 1997;91(7):885–90.

13. Flint J, Hill AV, Bowden DK, et al. High frequencies of alpha-thalassaemia are the result of natural selection by malaria. Nature 1986;321(6072):744–50.

14. Kanavakis E, Tzotzos S, Liapaki K, et al. Molecular basis and prevalence of alpha-thalassemia in Greece. Birth Defects Orig Artic Ser 1988;23(5B):377–80.

15. Falusi AG, Esan GJ, Ayyub H, et al. Alpha-thalassaemia in Nigeria: its interaction with sickle-cell disease. Eur J Haematol 1987;38(4):370–5.

16. Vichinsky EP. Changing patterns of thalassemia worldwide. Ann N Y Acad Sci 2005;1054:18–24.

17. Vichinsky EP, Macklin EA, Waye JS, et al. Changes in the epidemiology of thalassemia in North America: a new minority disease. Pediatrics 2005;116(6):e818–25.

18. Lorey F, Cunningham G, Vichinsky EP, et al. Universal newborn screening for Hb H disease in California. Genet Test 2001;5(2):93–100.

19. Logothetis J, Economidou J, Constantoulakis M, et al. Cephalofacial deformities in thalassemia major (Cooley's anemia). A correlative study among 138 cases. Am J Dis Child 1971;121(4):300–6.

20. Kearney SL, Nemeth E, Neufeld EJ, et al. Urinary hepcidin in congenital chronic anemias. Pediatr Blood Cancer 2007;48(1):57–63.

21. Detivaud L, Nemeth E, Boudjema K, et al. Hepcidin levels in humans are correlated with hepatic iron stores, hemoglobin levels, and hepatic function. Blood 2005;106(2):746–8.

22. Gardenghi S, Marongiu MF, Ramos P, et al. Ineffective erythropoiesis in beta-thalassemia is characterized by increased iron absorption mediated by down-regulation of hepcidin and up-regulation of ferroportin. Blood 2007;109(11):5027–35.

23. Ganz T. Hepcidin, a key regulator of iron metabolism and mediator of anemia of inflammation. Blood 2003;102(3):783–8.

24. Weinstein DA, Roy CN, Fleming MD, et al. Inappropriate expression of hepcidin is associated with iron refractory anemia: implications for the anemia of chronic disease. Blood 2002;100(10):3776–81.

25. Breda L, Gardenghi S, Guy E, et al. Exploring the role of hepcidin, an antimicrobial and iron regulatory peptide, in increased iron absorption in beta-thalassemia. Ann N Y Acad Sci 2005;1054:417–22.

26. De FL, Daraio F, Filippini A, et al. Liver expression of hepcidin and other iron genes in two mouse models of beta-thalassemia. Haematologica 2006;91(10): 1336–42.

27. Porter JB, Abeysinghe RD, Marshall L, et al. Kinetics of removal and reappearance of non-transferrin-bound plasma iron with deferoxamine therapy. Blood 1996;88(2):705–13.

28. Borgna-Pignatti C, Rugolotto S, De SP, et al. Survival and complications in patients with thalassemia major treated with transfusion and deferoxamine. Haematologica 2004;89(10):1187–93.
29. Aghai E, Shabbad E, Quitt M, et al. Discrimination between iron deficiency and heterozygous beta-thalassemia in children. Am J Clin Pathol 1986;85(6):710–2.
30. Lie-Injo LE, Jo BH. A fast-moving haemoglobin in hydrops foetalis. Nature 1960; 185:698.
31. Kan YW, Allen A, Lowenstein L. Hydrops fetalis with alpha thalassemia. N Engl J Med 1967;276(1):18–23.
32. Ehlers KH, Giardina PJ, Lesser ML, et al. Prolonged survival in patients with beta-thalassemia major treated with deferoxamine. J Pediatr 1991;118(4 Pt 1):540–5.
33. Karagiorga-Lagana M. Fertility in thalassemia: the Greek experience. J Pediatr Endocrinol Metab 1998;11(Suppl 3):945–51.
34. Skordis N, Petrikkos L, Toumba M, et al. Update on fertility in thalassaemia major. Pediatr Endocrinol Rev 2004;2(Suppl 2):296–302.
35. Skordis N, Christou S, Koliou M, et al. Fertility in female patients with thalassemia. J Pediatr Endocrinol Metab 1998;11(Suppl 3):935–43.
36. Pafumi C, Farina M, Pernicone G, et al. At term pregnancies in transfusion-dependent beta-thalassemic women. Clin Exp Obstet Gynecol 2000;27(3–4):185–7.
37. Hmida S, Mojaat N, Maamar M, et al. Red cell alloantibodies in patients with haemoglobinopathies. Nouv Rev Fr Hematol 1994;36(5):363–6.
38. Olujohungbe A, Hambleton I, Stephens L, et al. Red cell antibodies in patients with homozygous sickle cell disease: a comparison of patients in Jamaica and the United Kingdom. Br J Haematol 2001;113(3):661–5.
39. Economidou J, Constantoulakis M, Augoustaki O, et al. Frequency of antibodies to various antigenic determinants in polytransfused patients with homozygous thalassaemia in Greece. Vox Sang 1971;20(3):252–8.
40. Wang LY, Liang DC, Liu HC, et al. Alloimmunization among patients with transfusion-dependent thalassemia in Taiwan. Transfus Med 2006;16(3):200–3.
41. Vichinsky EP, Earles A, Johnson RA, et al. Alloimmunization in sickle cell anemia and transfusion of racially unmatched blood. N Engl J Med 1990;322(23): 1617–21.
42. Singer ST, Wu V, Mignacca R, et al. Alloimmunization and erythrocyte autoimmunization in transfusion-dependent thalassemia patients of predominantly asian descent. Blood 2000;96(10):3369–73.
43. Moroni GA, Piacentini G, Terzoli S, et al. Hepatitis B or non-A, non-B virus infection in multitransfused thalassaemic patients. Arch Dis Child 1984;59(12): 1127–30.
44. Allain JP, Thomas I, Sauleda S. Nucleic acid testing for emerging viral infections. Transfus Med 2002;12(4):275–83.
45. O'Brien SF, Yi QL, Fan W, et al. Current incidence and estimated residual risk of transfusion-transmitted infections in donations made to Canadian Blood Services. Transfusion 2007;47(2):316–25.
46. Ansar MM, Kooloobandi A. Prevalence of hepatitis C virus infection in thalassemia and haemodialysis patients in north Iran-Rasht. J Viral Hepat 2002;9(5): 390–2.
47. Butensky E, Pakbaz Z, Foote D, et al. Treatment of hepatitis C virus infection in thalassemia. Ann N Y Acad Sci 2005;1054:290–9.
48. Inati A, Taher A, Ghorra S, et al. Efficacy and tolerability of peginterferon alpha-2a with or without ribavirin in thalassaemia major patients with chronic hepatitis C virus infection. Br J Haematol 2005;130(4):644–6.

49. Telfer PT, Garson JA, Whitby K, et al. Combination therapy with interferon alpha and ribavirin for chronic hepatitis C virus infection in thalassaemic patients. Br J Haematol 1997;98(4):850–5.

50. Wonke B, Hoffbrand AV, Bouloux P, et al. New approaches to the management of hepatitis and endocrine disorders in Cooley's anemia. Ann N Y Acad Sci 1998; 850:232–41.

51. Borgna-Pignatti C, Vergine G, Lombardo T, et al. Hepatocellular carcinoma in the thalassaemia syndromes. Br J Haematol 2004;124(1):114–7.

52. Ren FY, Piao XX, Jin AL. Efficacy of ultrasonography and alpha-fetoprotein on early detection of hepatocellular carcinoma. World J Gastroenterol 2006;12(29): 4656–9.

53. Borgna PC, Carnelli V, Caruso V, et al. Thromboembolic events in beta thalassemia major: an Italian multicenter study. Acta Haematol 1998;99(2):76–9.

54. Cappellini MD. Coagulation in the pathophysiology of hemolytic anemias. Hematology Am Soc Hematol Educ Program 2007;2007:74–8.

55. Eldor A, Rachmilewitz EA. The hypercoagulable state in thalassemia. Blood 2002; 99(1):36–43.

56. Borenstain-Ben YV, Barenholz Y, Hy-Am E, et al. Phosphatidylserine in the outer leaflet of red blood cells from beta-thalassemia patients may explain the chronic hypercoagulable state and thrombotic episodes. Am J Hematol 1993;44(1):63–5.

57. Eldor A, Krausz Y, Atlan H, et al. Platelet survival in patients with beta-thalassemia. Am J Hematol 1989;32(2):94–9.

58. Reiter CD, Gladwin MT. An emerging role for nitric oxide in sickle cell disease vascular homeostasis and therapy. Curr Opin Hematol 2003;10(2):99–107.

59. Machado RF, Martyr S, Kato GJ, et al. Sildenafil therapy in patients with sickle cell disease and pulmonary hypertension. Br J Haematol 2005;130(3):445–53.

60. Pearson HA, Rink L, Guiliotis DK. Thalassemia major in Connecticut: a 20-year study of changing age distribution and survival. Conn Med 1994;85(5):259–60.

61. Pearson HA, Guiliotis DK, Rink L, et al. Patient age distribution in thalassemia major: changes from 1973 to 1985. Pediatrics 1987;80(1):53–7.

62. Thomas ED, Buckner CD, Sanders JE, et al. Marrow transplantation for thalassaemia. Lancet 1982;2(8292):227–9.

63. Hongeng S, Pakakasama S, Chuansumrit A, et al. Reduced intensity stem cell transplantation for treatment of class 3 Lucarelli severe thalassemia patients. Am J Hematol 2007;82(12):1095–8.

64. La NG, Argiolu F, Giardini C, et al. Unrelated bone marrow transplantation for beta-thalassemia patients: the experience of the Italian Bone Marrow Transplant Group. Ann N Y Acad Sci 2005;1054:186–95.

65. Lucarelli G, Galimberti M, Polchi P, et al. Bone marrow transplantation in patients with thalassemia. N Engl J Med 1990;322(7):417–21.

66. Sodani P, Gaziev D, Polchi P, et al. New approach for bone marrow transplantation in patients with class 3 thalassemia aged younger than 17 years. Blood 2004; 104(4):1201–3.

67. Lucarelli G, Andreani M, Angelucci E. The cure of the thalassemia with bone marrow transplantation. Bone Marrow Transplant 2001;28(Suppl 1):S11–3.

68. Walters MC, Quirolo L, Trachtenberg ET, et al. Sibling donor cord blood transplantation for thalassemia major: experience of the Sibling Donor Cord Blood Program. Ann N Y Acad Sci 2005;1054:206–13.

69. Bhatia M, Walters MC. Hematopoietic cell transplantation for thalassemia and sickle cell disease: past, present and future. Bone Marrow Transplant 2008; 41(2):109–17.

70. Adamkiewicz TV, Szabolcs P, Haight A, et al. Unrelated cord blood transplantation in children with sickle cell disease: review of four-center experience. Pediatr Transplant 2007;11(6):641–4.

71. Adamkiewicz TV, Boyer MW, Bray R, et al. Identification of unrelated cord blood units for hematopoietic stem cell transplantation in children with sickle cell disease. J Pediatr Hematol Oncol 2006;28(1):29–32.

72. Walters MC. Cord blood transplantation for sickle cell anemia: bust or boom? Pediatr Transplant 2007;11(6):582–3.

73. Nishino T, Tubb J, Emery DW. Partial correction of murine beta-thalassemia with a gammaretrovirus vector for human gamma-globin. Blood Cells Mol Dis 2006; 37(1):1–7.

74. Rivella S, May C, Chadburn A, et al. A novel murine model of Cooley anemia and its rescue by lentiviral-mediated human beta-globin gene transfer. Blood 2003; 101(8):2932–9.

75. Sadelain M, Lisowski L, Samakoglu S, et al. Progress toward the genetic treatment of the beta-thalassemias. Ann N Y Acad Sci 2005;1054:78–91.

Oral Iron Chelators

Janet L. Kwiatkowski, MD, MSCE[a,b,*]

KEYWORDS

- Transfusion • Iron overload • Chelation
- Sickle cell disease • Thalassemia

TRANSFUSION-RELATED IRON OVERLOAD

Regular red cell transfusions are used in the management of many hematologic disorders in children. In β-thalassemia major, transfusions relieve severe anemia, suppress compensatory bone marrow hyperplasia, and prolong survival. Regular red cell transfusions also are used frequently in children who have sickle cell disease, primarily to prevent and treat devastating complications, such as stroke.[1] Other conditions that may be treated with transfusion therapy include Diamond-Blackfan anemia that is poorly responsive to steroids; Fanconi anemia; hemolytic anemias, such as pyruvate kinase deficiency; sideroblastic anemias; congenital dyserythropoietic anemias; and myelodysplastic syndromes.

In humans, iron is required for many essential functions, including oxygen transport, oxidative energy production, mitochondrial respiration, and DNA synthesis.[2] Iron loss is limited to small amounts in the stool, urine, desquamated nail and skin cells, and menstrual losses in women, and humans lack physiologic mechanisms to excrete excess iron. Chronic red cell transfusion therapy leads to progressive iron accumulation in the absence of chelation therapy because the iron contained in the transfused red cells is not excreted efficiently.

Each milliliter of packed red cells contains approximately 1.1 mg of iron. A regular transfusion regimen usually consists of 10 to 15 mL/kg of packed red cells administered every 3 to 4 weeks to maintain a trough hemoglobin level of 9 to 10 g/dL in patients who have thalassemia and other congenital anemias and to maintain the hemoglobin S percentage at less than 30% in children who have sickle cell disease. This leads to an average iron accumulation of approximately 0.3 to 0.5 mg/kg per day, although there is considerable interpatient variability in iron loading. In addition, gastrointestinal iron absorption is increased greatly in patients who have ineffective erythropoiesis, such as thalassemia, and in some red cell enzyme deficiencies, in

A version of this article was previously published in the *Pediatric Clinics of North America*, 55:2.
[a] University of Pennsylvania School of Medicine, 34th Street and Civic Center Boulevard, Philadelphia, PA 19104, USA
[b] Division of Hematology, The Children's Hospital of Philadelphia, 34th Street and Civic Center Boulevard, Children's Seashore House, 4th Floor, Hematology, Philadelphia, PA 19104, USA
* Division of Hematology, The Children's Hospital of Philadelphia, 34th Street and Civic Center Boulevard, Children's Seashore House, 4th Floor, Hematology, Philadelphia, PA 19104.
E-mail address: kwiatkowski@email.chop.edu

particular pyruvate kinase deficiency. The increased absorption of dietary iron can cause iron overload even in the absence of transfusions, although at a slower rate than that associated with chronic transfusions. Serial phlebotomy may be used to treat iron overload in some patients who have congenital anemia, but chelation therapy is needed to remove iron for those who have more severe anemia or transfusion dependence.

HEREDITARY HEMOCHROMATOSIS

Iron overload can result from hereditary causes that lead to increased intestinal absorption of dietary iron. Hepcidin, a small peptide produced by the liver in response to high iron levels and inflammation, inhibits iron absorption.[3] Dysregulation of hepcidin now seems central in many of the hereditary forms of hemochromatosis. The most common form of hereditary hemochromatosis is caused by mutations in the HFE gene, which prevent the appropriate up-regulation of hepcidin expression in response to increased iron levels.[4] A mutation causing a cysteine-to-tyrosine substitution (C282Y) in the HFE protein is common in those of Northern European ancestry and a second mutation causing a histidine-to-aspartic acid substitution (H63D) is distributed worldwide. Homozygosity for the C282Y mutation or compound heterozygosity for C282Y/H63D is associated with the development of iron overload, although clinical penetrance is variable. Clinical manifestations, including bronzing of the skin, cirrhosis, arthropathies, diabetes mellitus, and endocrinopathies, usually do not develop until middle age. Cardiac disease also can occur, although less commonly than with transfusional iron overload (discussed later). Mutations in the hepcidin gene or in another protein involved in hepcidin regulation, hemojuvelin, lead to a juvenile form of hemochromatosis with symptoms presenting by the third decade of life.[5] The standard treatment for hereditary hemochromatosis is phlebotomy to reduce iron stores, although iron chelation therapy may be used in patients who are unable to tolerate the procedure.

ORGAN TOXICITY RELATED TO IRON OVERLOAD

Free iron is toxic to cells and, therefore, iron normally is shielded by forming tight complexes with proteins. In plasma, iron is bound to transferrin, which transports iron to the cells. The main storage form of iron is ferritin, whereas hemosiderin is another iron storage protein, consisting of large iron-salt aggregates. Both are found principally in the liver, reticuloendothelial cells, and red cell precursors, but ferritin also is found in the blood, where it can be measured readily. In iron overload states, high levels of iron exceed the iron-carrying capacity of transferrin within the plasma, leading to accumulation of nontransferrin-bound iron.[6] The nontransferrin-bound iron is taken up into cells, including liver, heart, and endocrine cells. Within the cells, the iron storage proteins become saturated, and instead, iron is bound only weakly to various low molecular weight proteins, known as labile iron.[7] Iron that is not tightly bound can participate in the generation of free radicals that damage the cells leading to organ toxicity.

Most knowledge of the complications of iron overload comes from patients who have thalassemia who require lifelong red blood cell transfusions. Whether or not patients who have different diseases requiring chronic transfusions, in particular sickle cell disease, develop the same complications remains to be determined.[8,9] Given the lack of substantial information about disease-specific responses to iron overload, data from the thalassemia population continue to guide monitoring and treatment for other transfused patient populations.

Iron overload leads to many clinical complications. Cardiac toxicity, including congestive heart failure and arrhythmias, is the leading cause of death related to iron overload in patients who have thalassemia major.[10] Excess iron deposition in the liver leads to inflammation, fibrosis, and cirrhosis,[11] which may be exacerbated by concomitant transfusion-acquired viral hepatitis. Iron is toxic to the endocrine organs, leading to growth failure, delayed puberty,[12] diabetes mellitus, hypothyroidism, and hypoparathyroidism.[13] In a report of 342 North American patients who had thalassemia major, 38% of subjects had at least one endocrinopathy, most commonly hypogonadism, and 13% had more than one endocrinopathy.[13] Moreover, in that study, the prevalence of endocrine abnormalities increased with age, likely reflecting an accumulating iron burden. The goal of chelation therapy is to maintain the body iron at levels low enough to prevent the development of these organ toxicities. Once organ toxicity has developed, chelation therapy can reverse some of the complications, such as the cardiac complications (discussed later), although the endocrinopathies usually are not reversible.

MEASUREMENT OF IRON LEVELS

There are several methods of assessing the degree of iron overload and each method has benefits and limitations (**Table 1**). Thus, combinations of measurements, including serial measurements, are used in clinical practice to determine individual iron burden and response to iron chelation therapy over time.

The serum ferritin level is the test that is available most widely and easiest to perform. Because it is a simple blood test, many measurements can be performed without difficulty to establish trends in iron burden over time. In transfusional iron overload, the ferritin level correlates with total body iron burden, although the correlation is not precise, especially at higher values.[14] Changes in the serum ferritin level in response to chelation have been shown to parallel changes in liver iron concentration measured by liver biopsy and noninvasive means.[15,16] Thus, trends in serum ferritin levels may be useful for monitoring adequacy of chelation therapy. In addition, the ferritin level has prognostic significance for patients who have thalassemia major receiving chelation therapy with deferoxamine. Sustained levels of over 2500 μg/L are associated with an increased risk for organ toxicity and death.[17,18] Thus, optimal chelation regimens should maintain the ferritin level at least lower than this value.

A limitation of the ferritin level is that a variety of disease states, including infection, inflammation, and ascorbate deficiency, can raise or lower serum ferritin levels. The limitation of ferritin in predicting iron stores is relevant particularly for patients who have sickle cell disease. In an analysis of 50 children who had sickle cell disease and were receiving regular red cell transfusions for primary stroke prevention in the Stroke Prevention Trial in Sickle Cell Anemia (STOP), great variability in the rate of rise of serum ferritin despite similar transfusion regimens was found among patients.[19] Serum ferritin levels also underestimate liver iron concentration in patients who have thalassemia-intermedia and nontransfusion-associated iron overload.[20]

Given that the liver is the major target organ for iron accumulation after multiple transfusions, the liver iron concentration is a good indicator of total iron burden.[21] Various methods are available to estimate liver iron concentration, but liver biopsy generally is considered the gold standard for accurate iron measurement. In addition, this procedure allows direct assessment of liver inflammation and fibrosis. Liver iron concentration is a useful predictor of prognosis in patients who have thalassemia: levels in excess of 15 mg/g dry weight are associated with an increased risk for cardiac complications and death.[22] Maintenance of the liver iron concentration

Table 1
Comparison of techniques to measure iron burden

Method	Advantages	Disadvantages
Serum ferritin	Inexpensive Widely available Repeated measurements possible	Imprecise correlation with total body iron Value altered by inflammation, infection, ascorbate deficiency Less reliable in sickle cell disease and nontransfusional secondary iron overload disease states
Liver iron concentration by biopsy	Correlates well with total body iron burden Allows for assessment of liver histology High levels predict risk for cardiac disease, endocrine complications, and death	Invasive Accuracy affected by sample size (>1 mg dry weight is best) Sampling errors due to fibrosis and uneven distribution of iron Cardiac disease may be present when liver iron is low
Liver iron concentration by SQUID	Noninvasive Well tolerated Correlates well with liver iron concentration	Expensive Complex equipment Very limited availability Cardiac disease may be present when liver iron is low
Liver iron concentration by MRI	Noninvasive More widely available Correlates well with liver iron concentration by biopsy	Expensive Variety of techniques and analytic programs may limit comparability among sites Cardiac disease may be present when liver iron is low
Cardiac iron loading by MRI	Noninvasive Correlates with risk for cardiac disease	Expensive Difficult to validate with biopsy specimen

between 3 and 7 mg/g dry weight in those receiving chelation therapy is considered ideal.[23] Several limitations to liver biopsy exist, however. First, it is an invasive procedure, which restricts the acceptability to patients and its frequent use to monitor trends over time. In addition, liver fibrosis and cirrhosis cause an uneven distribution of iron, which may lead to an underestimation of liver iron in patients who have advanced liver disease.[24] Finally, although high levels of liver iron predict an increased risk for cardiac disease, the converse not always is true: low levels do not always predict a low risk for cardiac disease.[25] This may reflect the different organ-specific rates of iron accumulation and iron removal in response to chelation therapy. In patients who have a history of poor chelation and high iron levels in the past who subsequently use chelation, hepatic iron may be removed more rapidly then cardiac iron, so liver iron levels can fall before cardiac iron levels improve.[26]

The superconducting quantum interference device (SQUID) technique uses magnetometers to measure very small magnetic fields and can be used as a noninvasive technique to measure ferritin and hemosiderin in the liver.[27] Estimation of liver iron concentration by SQUID correlates linearly with concentrations measured by liver biopsy.[27] Because this is a noninvasive technique, repetitive iron concentration measurements by SQUID have been used to monitor the efficacy of chelation in several studies.[16,28–30] A major limitation to using SQUID is that it is a highly specialized and expensive approach. In addition, in recent clinical trials of the oral chelator, deferasirox, SQUID measurements underestimated liver iron concentrations obtained by biopsy by approximately 50%.[15] Currently, only four sites worldwide offer the technology, limiting accessibility to patients.

MRI increasingly is used to monitor iron overload. This technique takes advantage of local inhomogeneities of the magnetic field caused by iron deposition in tissues.[31] Magnetic resonance scanners are more widely available than SQUID, which should allow greater accessibility to patients. Differences in the type of machine, the strength of the magnetic field, and the analytic measurements, however, can limit accuracy and comparability among different sites. Although MRI may be used to estimate iron levels in a variety of organs, including the pituitary, pancreas, and bone marrow, it is used most commonly to measure hepatic[32] and cardiac iron.[25,33] MRI images darken at a rate proportional to the iron concentration. The darkening can be measured by two different techniques, spin-echo imaging and gradient-echo imaging. T2 refers to the time constant (half-life) of darkening for spin echo and T2* for gradient echo, with values inversely proportional to the amount of iron accumulation. The reciprocals of T2 and T2*, known as R2 and R2*, respectively, refer to rates of signal decay and are directly proportional to iron concentration.[34] Studies using R2 to estimate liver iron show good correlation with iron levels determined by liver biopsy and reproducibility across different scanners.[32,35] Other approaches using T2* or R2* also are promising for determining liver iron content.[25,36] Cardiac iron levels also can be assessed using MRI, most commonly with T2* measurements. Determination of cardiac iron may be of greater clinical relevance than liver iron measurements because cardiac disease is the leading cause of death in patients who have thalassemia and transfusional iron overload.[10] Cardiac T2* values below 20 ms indicate cardiac iron overload, whereas levels below 10 ms are associated with an increased risk for cardiac disease, including ventricular dysfunction and arrhythmias.[25,33] Thus, patients who have very low cardiac T2* values may benefit from intensification of chelation therapy.

HISTORY OF IRON CHELATION

Deferoxamine, a naturally occurring iron chelator produced by *Streptomyces pilosus*, was the first iron chelator approved for human use.[37] It is a hexadentate iron chelator that binds iron stably in a 1:1 ratio (**Table 2**). Deferoxamine is absorbed poorly from the gastrointestinal tract and has an extremely short half-life.[38] Thus, it must be administered parenterally, usually as a continuous subcutaneous infusion (25 to 50 mg/kg given over 8 to 12 hours, 5 to 7 days per week). Iron bound to deferoxamine is excreted in urine and feces.

The efficacy of deferoxamine is well established. In the 1960s, the ability of deferoxamine to induce substantial iron excretion and a net negative iron balance was demonstrated.[39] Subsequently, in the 1970s, deferoxamine therapy was shown to reduce hepatic iron content and prevent progression of fibrosis.[40] Most importantly, the use of deferoxamine is associated with a reduced incidence of cardiac complications and death.[17,37,41] In addition, cardiac disease secondary to iron overload can be

Table 2
Comparison of iron chelators

Property	Deferoxamine	Deferiprone	Deferasirox
Chelator:iron binding	1:1	3:1	2:1
Route of administration	Subcutaneous or intravenous	Oral	Oral
Usual dosage	25–50 mg/kg per day	75 mg/kg per day	20–30 mg/kg per day
Schedule	Administered over 8–24 hours, 5–7 days per week	Three times a day	Daily
Primary route(s) of excretion	Urine/feces	Urine	Feces
Adverse effects	Local reactions Ophthalmologic Auditory Bone abnormalities Pulmonary Neurologic Allergic reactions	Agranuloctyosis/ neutropenia Gastrointestinal disturbances Transminase elevations Arthralgia	Gastrointestinal disturbances Transaminase elevations Rise in serum creatinine Proteinuria Rash
Advantages	Long-term data available	May be superior in removal of cardiac iron	The only oral chelator licensed for use in United States
Disadvantages	Compliance problems may be greater	Not licensed for use in United States Variable efficacy in removal of hepatic iron	Long-term data lacking Efficacy at cardiac iron removal not known
Special monitoring considerations	Long bone films in growing children Annual ophthalmology exam Annual audiology exam	Weekly complete blood count with differential	Monthly blood urea nitrogen, creatinine, hepatic transaminases, and urinalysis

Adapted from Kwiatkowski JL, Cohen AR. Iron chelation therapy in sickle cell disease and other transfusion-dependent anemias. Hematol Oncol Clin N Am 2004;18(6):1355–77; with permission.

reversed with the use of deferoxamine, typically administered as a 24-hour infusion.[42] Chelation therapy with deferoxamine prevents other organ toxicities, such as diabetes.[37]

Local infusion site reactions, including induration and erythema, commonly are seen with administration of deferoxamine. Low zinc levels also can develop with deferoxamine use. Other adverse effects, including high frequency hearing loss, ophthalmologic toxicity,[43] growth retardation, and skeletal changes, including rickets-like lesions and genu valgum,[44] are more common when patients receive high doses of deferoxamine relative to their total body iron burden and can be minimized by maintaining an optimal chelator dose.[45] Acute pulmonary toxicity with respiratory distress and hypoxemia and a diffuse interstitial pattern on chest roentgenogram is reported with the administration of high doses of deferoxamine (10 to 20 mg/kg per hour).[46]

The major limitation to deferoxamine is the need to administer the drug parenterally, which is painful and time consuming. As a result, poor compliance remains a significant problem with administration of this drug, and preventable, premature deaths related to iron overload continue to occur.[47,48]

CHARACTERISTICS OF AN IDEAL CHELATOR

The limitations of treatment with deferoxamine have led investigators to search for more acceptable iron chelators to be used in the management of iron overload. An optimal chelator should have adequate gastrointestinal absorption to allow oral administration, a long half-life permitting once or twice daily dosing, and a high affinity for iron with lesser affinities for other metals. The chelator should be able to induce iron excretion at a rate of at least 0.5 mg/kg per day to offset the amount of transfusional iron loading, and should be able to remove excess cardiac iron. Finally, toxicities associated with the drug should be minimal and manageable.

DEFERIPRONE
Pharmacology

Deferiprone, or 1,2 dimethyl-3-hydroxypyrid-4-1 (Ferriprox), was the first orally active chelator studied extensively for the treatment of transfusional iron overload, introduced into clinical trials 20 years ago (see **Table 2**). Most studies have been open-label, noncomparative studies, often including patients who had a history of inadequate iron chelation, but a few randomized trials comparing deferiprone to deferoxamine are reported. A substantial amount of data on the safety and efficacy of the drug has been acquired, but considerable controversy surrounding the drug exists. In the European Union, deferiprone is approved for use for patients in whom deferoxamine therapy is contraindicated or inadequate, but the drug is not approved for use in North America and currently is available only to a limited number of patients through expanded access programs or research trials.

Deferiprone is a bidentate chelator, which forms a 3:1 chelator:iron complex. Given its short plasma half-life of 1.5 to 2.5 hours,[49,50] the drug usually is dosed 3 times daily, although regimens of 2 or 4 times daily have been explored.[51] The usual daily dose is 75 mg/kg per day, but higher doses have been studied.[51] Deferiprone induces iron excretion almost exclusively in the urine, with minimal contribution from fecal elimination.[52,53]

Efficacy

Urinary iron excretion with deferiprone at 75 mg/kg is comparable to that induced by deferoxamine at a dose of 50 mg/kg.[52,53] Given that deferoxamine induces fecal iron excretion, total iron excretion with deferiprone is approximately 60% of that with deferoxamine at these doses.[52] The mean urinary iron excretion with deferiprone at 75 mg/kg was 0.48 mg/kg per day in one study, a level predicted to maintain or decrease iron stores in most patients.[52] Significant interpatient variability exists, however, so not all patients can achieve a negative iron balance at this dose. For example, in one study, urinary iron excretion ranged from 11.2 to 74.9 mg per day at a 75 mg/kg dosing level.[54] Higher doses of deferiprone, 90 to 119 mg/kg, induced greater urinary iron excretion and may be beneficial for patients who have inadequate responses at lower doses.[51,54,55]

Short-term studies of deferiprone generally show a reduction[51,56–58] or stabilization[59] in serum ferritin levels over a treatment period of 1 year or less. Similarly, studies that assessed the response to deferiprone over longer treatment periods, of 3 to 4 years, show reduced[30,54,60,61] or stable[62,63] mean serum ferritin levels. Similar responses are shown across different disease states, including sickle cell disease and thalassemia.

A small proportion of patients demonstrated a significant increase in serum ferritin levels while receiving long-term deferiprone.[30,61–63] In a group of 151 Italian patients who received deferiprone for 3 years or more, 20% of subjects had clinically significant rises in ferritin levels during the first year of treatment.[61] In general, patients who had higher baseline ferritin levels showed a greater reduction in serum ferritin than those who had lower pretreatment ferritin levels. In a long-term, multicenter study, 84 patients received deferiprone for 4 years at a mean daily dosage of 73 mg/kg. Mean serum ferritin levels declined significantly from 3661 to 2630 µg/L in the group whose baseline serum ferritin was above 2500 µg/L, whereas ferritin levels remained stable in those with baseline values less than 2500 µg/L.[63]

Studies on the effect of chelation with deferiprone on liver iron content have mixed results.[30,57,62,64,65] In a report of 21 patients who received deferiprone (75 mg/kg per day), mean liver iron concentration assessed by biopsy or SQUID decreased from 15 to 8.7 mg/g dry weight after an average of 3.1 years of treatment.[30] Eight of 10 patients who had initial liver iron concentrations associated with a high risk for cardiotoxicity (>15 mg/g dry weight) had levels that fell to below that threshold with deferiprone treatment, and no patient who had lower initial hepatic iron concentrations rose above this threshold. With longer follow-up of a mean of 4.6 years in 18 patients, although there was an overall reduction in liver iron concentration from baseline (16.5 to 12.1 mg/g dry weight, $P = .07$), in seven patients, the liver iron concentration remained above 15 mg/g liver dry weight.[65] In another report of 20 patients who received deferiprone (70 mg/kg daily) for 1 year or more, the mean liver iron content increased from 16 to 21 mg/g dry weight, although this change did not reach statistical significance.[64] Liver iron content decreased in seven patients, rose in 12 patients, and remained the same in one patient. Thus, the data suggest that chelation with deferiprone (at a dose of 75 mg/kg per day) does not reduce liver iron concentration effectively in some patients.

Few randomized clinical trials have compared the efficacy of deferiprone directly to deferoxamine for the treatment of iron overload. In one study of 144 patients randomized to receive deferiprone (75 mg/kg per day) or deferoxamine (50 mg/kg per day), the reduction in serum ferritin levels after 1 year was similar between the two treatment groups.[57] In a subset of 36 patients who underwent liver biopsy at the beginning and end of treatment, the mean reduction in liver iron content also was not significantly different between the two groups. In a more recent study, 61 Italian and Greek patients were randomized to receive deferoxamine (50 mg/kg daily for 5 days a week) or deferiprone (75 mg/kg per day initially, increasing to 100 mg/kg per day).[66] The changes over a 1-year period in serum ferritin level and liver iron content assessed by SQUID did not differ significantly between the two treatment groups. In contrast, in a third study, in which 30 children were randomized into three groups to receive deferoxamine (40 mg/kg per day, 5 days per week), deferiprone (75 mg/kg daily), or combination treatment with deferiprone (75 mg/kg daily) and deferoxamine (40 mg/kg per day, twice weekly), after 6 months of treatment, those receiving deferoxamine alone had a significant reduction in serum ferritin, whereas the other two groups had a slight rise in ferritin levels.[67]

The lack of reduction in serum ferritin or liver iron concentration in some patients receiving deferiprone may be explained by a variety of reasons, including poor compliance, variability in drug metabolism rate, or higher transfusional iron burden. The latter two problems potentially might be overcome by treating with a higher dosage of deferiprone. In one study, increasing the daily dose of deferiprone (from 75 mg/kg to 83 to 100 mg/kg) resulted in a fall in serum ferritin level in nine patients who had had inadequate chelation at the lower dose.[55] Although no significant increased toxicity has been found in small studies using higher doses of deferiprone (up to 100 mg/kg daily),[66,68] larger studies are needed to determine the long-term safety and efficacy of doses greater than 75 mg/kg per day.

Cardiac Iron Removal

A growing body of evidence supports the theory that deferiprone may be more effective than deferoxamine at removing iron from the heart and reducing iron-related cardiotoxicity.[66,69–71] In one retrospective study, cardiac T2* and cardiac function were compared between 15 patients who had thalassemia and were receiving long-term deferiprone and 30 matched controls receiving long-term deferoxamine.[69] Patients receiving deferiprone had significantly less cardiac iron (median T2* 34 ms versus 11.4 ms, $P = .02$). Furthermore, T2* values less than 20 ms, a level associated with excess cardiac iron, were found in only 27% of patients receiving deferiprone compared with 67% of those receiving deferoxamine ($P = .025$), despite a significantly greater liver iron concentration in those receiving deferiprone. Left ventricular ejection fraction also was significantly higher in the deferiprone-treated group. Moreover, in a multicenter, retrospective study of patients who had thalassemia major, the risk for cardiac complications (cardiac failure or arrhythmia requiring drug treatment) was compared between 359 subjects who received only deferoxamine and 157 patients who received deferiprone.[70] Fifty-two patients (14.5%) developed cardiac events, including 10 deaths from cardiac causes, during therapy with deferoxamine whereas no patients developed cardiac events during treatment with deferiprone or within 18 months of discontinuing therapy.

A few prospective trials have compared the effect of deferiprone to deferoxamine on cardiac iron removal and cardiac function.[57,66,72,73] Two studies comparing deferiprone (75 mg/kg per day) to deferoxamine (50 mg/kg per day, 5–6 days per week) showed no significant difference in the reduction in cardiac iron between treatment groups after 1 year of therapy.[57,72] A third study using similar dosing, however, showed a significantly greater reduction in cardiac iron and improvement in left ventricular ejection fraction with deferiprone than with deferoxamine after 3 years of therapy.[73]

More recently, a multicenter, randomized, controlled clinical trial compared deferiprone (average dose 92 mg/kg per day) to deferoxamine (average dose 35 mg/kg per day, 7 days a week) for the treatment of 61 patients who had thalassemia major and abnormal cardiac T2* (<20 ms).[66] Patients who had severe cardiac iron loading, T2* values less than 8 ms, or left ventricular ejection fraction less than 56% were excluded. A significantly greater improvement in T2* values was seen with deferiprone compared with deferoxamine after 1 year of treatment (27% versus 13%, $P = .023$). Similarly, left ventricular ejection fraction increased more in those treated with deferiprone (3.1% versus 0.3%, $P = .003$).

Adverse Effects

The most serious adverse event associated with deferiprone is agranulocytosis. In a multicenter study of 187 patients who had thalassemia major treated with deferiprone in which weekly blood counts were monitored, the incidence of agranulocytosis (absolute neutrophil count <500 $\times$ 10^9/L) was 0.6 per 100 patient-years and the incidence of milder neutropenia (absolute neutrophil count 500 to 1500 × 10⁹/L) was 5.4 per 100 patient-years.[59] In the largest study reported to date, similar rates for agranulocytosis (0.4 per 100 patient years) and for neutropenia (2.1 per 100 patient years) were reported.[61] Neutropenia usually is reversible with discontinuation of the drug but often recurs with reinstitution of therapy.[61,74] In clinical practice, blood counts should be obtained at least weekly and with all febrile illnesses or significant infections to monitor for this potentially life-threatening side effect. Treatment with deferiprone may not be appropriate for patients who have underlying bone marrow failure syndromes, such as Diamond-Blackfan anemia, who may be more likely to develop agranulocytosis or neutropenia.[75,76] Similarly, caution should be exercised when using this drug in combination with hydroxyurea, interferon, or other drugs that can cause neutropenia.

Gastrointestinal symptoms, including nausea, vomiting, diarrhea, and abdominal pain, are common side effects reported with deferiprone, occurring in 33% of subjects in one large study.[63] These symptoms usually occur in the first few weeks of treatment and rarely require discontinuation of therapy.[59,61] Arthropathy with pain or swelling of the knees and other large joints is another common complication and can occur early or late in treatment.[60,61,63] In a large study of 532 patients, the prevalence of this complication was only 4%,[61] but other studies have reported higher rates of up to 38.5%.[54,60,63] The arthropathy usually is reversible with discontinuation of the drug.[54,59] Low plasma zinc levels developed in a minority of patients receiving deferiprone; thus, periodic monitoring of zinc levels is warranted.[54,59]

Elevations in serum alanine aminotransferase (ALT) levels are observed in patients receiving deferiprone. This abnormality often is transient and resolves even if the drug continues to be administered at the same or reduced dose.[60,61] Patients who have a higher iron burden[61] and those who have hepatitis C infection[59,61] may be more likely to develop ALT elevations. In addition, concerns have been raised regarding a possible progression of hepatic fibrosis with deferiprone therapy.[65] In a retrospective study, five of 14 patients receiving deferiprone developed progression of liver fibrosis compared with none of 12 patients receiving deferoxamine.[65] Four of the five patients who had worsening liver fibrosis also had antibodies to hepatitis C compared with only two of the nine subjects who did not have progression. In addition, the patients receiving deferiprone had higher baseline hepatic iron concentrations than the group receiving deferoxamine. Given that chronic viral hepatitis and iron overload may result in liver fibrosis, it is difficult to assess the contribution of deferiprone to progression of fibrosis. Other studies fail to show significant hepatic fibrosis attributable to deferiprone.[62,77,78] In the largest study to date, no significant progression of fibrosis was observed in 56 patients (11 seronegative for hepatitis C), with liver biopsy specimens obtained before and after treatment with deferiprone at a mean interval of 3.1 years.[78]

DEFERIPRONE AND DEFEROXAMINE COMBINATION THERAPY

Several studies that explored the use of deferiprone in combination with deferoxamine, using a variety of dose regimens, have been published.[55,79,80] Such an approach could allow deferoxamine to be infused less frequently, which might improve compliance and could overcome the potential inability of deferiprone to induce sufficient hepatic iron clearance in some patients. In addition, combination therapy might remove cardiac iron more rapidly than either drug given alone, thereby improving the treatment of patients who have iron-related cardiac disease. Iron balance studies show an additive or possibly synergistic effect when the two drugs are administered together, possibly because deferiprone, a smaller molecule, can enter cardiac cells, bind iron, and then transfer it to deferoxamine for excretion.[81,82] Significant reduction in serum ferritin levels[79,80] and in cardiac iron stores measured by MRI[80] and significant improvement in left ventricular shortening fraction[79,80] are reported using combination therapy, without unexpected toxicities.

A recently reported randomized, placebo-controlled clinical trial comparing the use of deferoxamine alone or in combination with deferiprone in the treatment of 65 patients who had mild to moderate cardiac iron loading (cardiac T2* 8–20 ms) confirmed the beneficial effect of combination therapy on cardiac iron removal.[83] After a 12-month treatment period, those receiving combination therapy had significantly greater improvement in cardiac T2* and in left ventricular ejection fraction than those receiving deferoxamine alone.

DEFERASIROX
Pharmacology

Deferasirox (ICL670, Exjade) is the first oral iron chelator approved for use in the United States and it is approved in several other countries (see **Table 2**). Deferasirox is a triazole compound, designed using computer-aided molecular modeling.[84] Two molecules of deferasirox are needed to bind one molecule of iron fully (tridentate chelator). Deferasirox has a high specificity for iron, with minimal binding to copper and zinc. The drug is supplied as orally dispersible tablets that are dissolved in water or juice and administered best on an empty stomach. Deferasirox is absorbed rapidly, achieving peak plasma levels within 1 to 3 hours after administration. Its plasma half-life with repeated doses ranges from 7 to 16 hours[29] and is longer with higher drug doses.[84] The drug's long half-life supports a once-daily dosing regimen. The deferasirox-iron complex is excreted almost exclusively in the feces, with minimal urinary excretion.[84]

Efficacy

An early, short-term treatment study in which 24 adult patients who had thalassemia and transfusional iron overload were treated with deferasirox at doses of 10, 20, or 40 mg/kg daily for a 12-day period showed that mean iron excretion rose linearly related to drug dose.[85] Mean iron excretion was 0.3 mg/kg per day with the 20-mg/kg dose and 0.5 mg/kg per day with the 40-mg/kg dose, suggesting that these doses are sufficient to at least maintain iron balance in many patients receiving chronic transfusions.

The safety and efficacy of deferasirox have been investigated in several phase 2 trials and a pivotal phase 3 study. In an initial phase 2 study, 71 adult patients who had thalassemia were randomized to receive deferasirox (10 mg/kg daily or 20 mg/kg daily) or deferoxamine (40 mg/kg for 5 days per week).[29] Dose increases or reductions were allowed during the course of the study for rising or very low liver iron concentrations, respectively. Deferasirox (20 mg/kg) had similar efficacy to deferoxamine: the liver iron concentration measured by SQUID was reduced by an average of 2.1 and 2.0 mg/g dry weight, respectively, after 48 weeks of treatment. In contrast, only a minimal reduction of liver iron of 0.4 mg/g dry weight was seen with the 10 mg/kg deferasirox dose group, and more than half of the subjects in this group required dose increases to 20 mg/kg during the course of the study. A phase 2 study of 40 children who had β-thalassemia major, ages 2 to 17 years, treated with deferasirox (10 mg/kg per day), showed that this dose is unlikely to achieve negative iron balance in most patients.[28] In this study, there was an overall rise in liver iron concentration measured by SQUID during the 48 weeks of treatment, and the rise was proportional to the amount of transfusional iron loading.

A single large phase 3 clinical trial compared the efficacy of deferasirox to deferoxamine.[15] In this study, 586 patients who had β-thalassemia major were randomized to receive deferasirox or deferoxamine, and the primary endpoint was change in liver iron concentration by liver biopsy (SQUID was used in 16% of patients). More than half of the patients were under 16 years old, including children as young as 2. The dosing algorithm was based on the baseline liver iron concentration: with deferasirox dosing of 5 to 30 mg/kg daily and deferoxamine dosing of 20 to ≥50 mg/kg, 5 days per week. Patients randomized to receive deferoxamine with lower baseline liver iron concentrations were allowed to remain on their prestudy deferoxamine dose, even if higher than the protocol recommended, resulting in patients receiving proportionately higher deferoxamine than deferasirox doses in the lowest two liver iron concentration groups. The primary objective of noninferiority of deferasirox to deferoxamine across all treatment groups was not attained, likely related to this relative underdosing of deferasirox compared with deferoxamine in the lowest 2 dose groups. Noninferiority of deferasirox, however, was demonstrated at the 20- and 30-mg/kg dose groups. The average reduction in liver iron concentration over the 1-year treatment period with deferasirox at 20 or 30 mg/kg was 5.3 ± 8.0 mg/g dry weight, compared with a reduction of 4.3 ± 5.8 mg/g dry weight, with deferoxamine ($P = .367$). With deferasirox at 20 mg/kg, liver iron concentration remained relatively stable for the 1-year period, whereas with 30 mg/kg, average liver iron concentration fell. Trends in serum ferritin levels over the course of the study paralleled the changes in liver iron concentration, with stable values in those receiving deferasirox at 20 mg/kg and declining values at the 30 mg/kg dose.

Phase 2 studies in patients who had other transfusion-dependent anemias have demonstrated similar results. In a multicenter study, 195 patients who had sickle cell disease were randomized to receive deferasirox (10 to 30 mg/kg daily) or deferoxamine (20 to ≥50 mg/kg 5 days per week) with dosing based on the pretreatment liver iron content, measured by SQUID.[16] More than half of the patients studied were younger than 16 years old. With deferasirox, a mean reduction in liver iron concentration of 3 mg/g dry weight was seen after 1 year of treatment, which was similar to the decrease in liver iron concentration seen with deferoxamine (2.8 mg/g dry weight). Similarly, an overall significant reduction in liver iron concentration, measured by SQUID, was seen in a phase 2 study of 184 patients who had myelodysplasia, thalassemia, Diamond-Blackfan anemia, or other rare, transfusion-dependent anemias who received deferasirox at 20 to 30 mg/kg per day for 1 year.[86]

Subsequent analyses have shown that the response to deferasirox is dependent on ongoing tranfusional requirements. For most patients who had lower transfusional iron intake (averaging <0.3 mg/kg per day), a dose of 20 mg/kg of deferasirox was effective in reducing liver iron concentration, whereas in over half of patients with the highest iron intake (>0.5 mg/kg per day), the 20 mg/kg dose did not reduce liver iron content effectively.[87] Some patients who had higher transfusional iron loading did not have adequate reduction in iron stores with deferasirox at doses of 30 mg/kg; thus, higher doses of up to 40 mg/kg are being investigated in the ongoing extension studies. Dosing of deferasirox should be guided by the goal of maintenance or reduction of body iron stores, ongoing transfusional requirements, and trends in ferritin and liver iron content during treatment.

Cardiac Iron Removal

The ability of deferasirox to chelate cardiac iron and to prevent or reverse cardiac disease is not yet known. Preliminary data suggest, however, that deferasirox may be effective in removing cardiac iron. In cultured heart muscle cells, deferasirox was able to extract intracellular iron and restore iron-impaired contractility.[88] Similarly, in iron-overloaded gerbils, deferasirox was as effective as deferiprone in reducing cardiac iron content.[89] Furthermore, in a preliminary report of 23 patients receiving deferasirox at doses of 10 to 30 mg/kg per day, cardiac iron content measured by T2* MRI improved from an average of 18 ms to 23 ms over a treatment period of 13 months.[90] Further studies are needed to confirm the effect of deferasirox on cardiac iron and cardiac disease.

Adverse Effects

The toxicity profile of deferasirox is similar across disease states and seems tolerable. Gastrointestinal disturbances, including nausea, vomiting, and abdominal pain, are common.[15] Although usually transient and dose related, these symptoms have led to discontinuation of the drug in some patients in clinical trials and in actual practice. The gastrointestinal side effects may be related to lactose intolerance as lactose is present in the drug preparation.[16] Diffuse, maculopapular skin rashes are reported in approximately 10% of subjects receiving deferasirox.[15,16,28] The rash often improves, even if the drug is continued. More than one third of patients experience mild elevations in serum creatinine levels, but few patients experience elevations beyond the normal range.[15,16] In some patients, the creatinine returned to baseline without dose modification, whereas in others, elevated or fluctuating levels persisted. Elevations in hepatic transaminases to more than 5 times baseline values also are reported.[15,16] The abnormalities are transient in some, even with continued administration of drug, whereas in others the abnormalities resolved with discontinuation of drug and recurred with drug reinstitution, suggesting causality. Fulminant hepatic failure is reported in rare cases, often in patients who have comorbidities. Cataracts or lenticular opacities and audiotoxicity are reported at low rates, similar to deferoxamine.[15,16] To date, the use of deferasirox is reported for more than 350 pediatric patients and the toxicity profile is similar to that seen in adults.[15,16,28,86,91] In addition, no adverse effects on growth or sexual development have been found, although longer followup is needed to assess fully for this potential complication. Agranulocytosis is not seen with deferasirox administration and the rare reports of neutropenia with deferasirox all are believed related to the underlying hematologic disorder and unlikely a drug effect.

Long-term data on treatment with deferasirox are lacking, and less common side effects may become evident only when larger numbers of patients are treated with the drug for a longer duration. Ongoing extension studies and postmarketing surveillance will help better define the long-term efficacy and safety profile of this drug. In addition, the use of deferasirox in combination with other chelators is not yet tested, and studies are needed to evaluate the efficacy and safety of such an approach before combination therapy can be recommended for clinical use.

OTHER ORAL CHELATORS IN DEVELOPMENT

Deferitrin (GT56-252) is an orally active tridentate iron chelator. It is a derivative of desferrithiocin, an oral chelator that showed good iron excretion in animal studies but had unacceptable renal toxicity, so the structure of deferitrin was modified to limit this toxicity.[92] In a phase 1 study, 26 adult patients who had thalassemia were treated with at least one dose of deferitrin, ranging from 3 to 15 mg/kg.[93] The drug's half-life was 2 to 4 hours and similar at all dose levels. Thus, once-daily dosing is not adequate with this medication. One serious adverse event occurred: hypoglycemic coma believed unrelated to deferitrin in a patient who had pre-existing diabetes. No significant laboratory abnormalities or electrocardiogram changes occurred. Further early phase clinical trials are ongoing.

Pyridoxal isonicotinoyl hydraxone (PIH) is a tridentate iron chelator introduced in 1979. When orally administered to iron-overloaded rats, PIH analogs were 2.6 to 2.8 times more effective at removing hepatic iron than deferoxamine, but deferoxamine was more effective at removing iron from cultured myocytes.[94] When given in combination with deferoxamine, the PIH analogs had a synergistic effect, suggesting that there may be a future role of this drug in combination chelation therapy.[94] A study in which 30 mg/kg per day of PIH was administered to patients who had thalassemia resulted in mean iron excretion of only 0.12 mg/kg per day, which is lower than the amount required to maintain negative iron balance in most regular transfused patients.[95,96] It is possible, however, that higher doses might increase efficacy. Further studies are needed to evaluate this drug's potential.

MANAGING CHELATION THERAPY

Children who have iron overload who require chelation therapy generally should be managed in conjunction with an experienced hematologist. Special considerations for children include the potential for adverse effects on growth and bone development with excess chelation, and these risks must be balanced against the risk for organ damage with prolonged iron accumulation. A variety of measurements can be used to determine when chelation therapy should be initiated for transfusional iron overload, including a cumulative transfusional iron burden of 120 mL/kg or greater, liver iron concentration of at least 7 mg/g dry weight,[97] and serum ferritin levels persistently elevated above 1000 μg/L. Typically, chelation therapy is not administered to children younger than 2 years of age, and often it is deferred until at least 3 or 4 years of age. When administering chelation to children younger than 5 years old, lower doses of chelation usually are used to avoid toxicity.[97] The available chelator options and their toxicities should be discussed with patients and their families. Oral chelation often is used first line in children given that subcutaneous administration is painful, which limits compliance. Serial ferritin and liver and cardiac iron measurements and testing for organ dysfunction are used to monitor efficacy and make dose adjustments. Patient interviews and examinations, serial measurements of growth and pubertal development, appropriate laboratory studies (see **Table 2**), and annual ophthalmologic examination and audiologic testing are used to monitor for toxicity.

SUMMARY

Effective chelation therapy can prevent or reverse organ toxicity related to iron overload, yet cardiac complications and premature death continue to occur, largely related to difficulties with compliance that may occur in patients who receive parenteral therapy. The use of oral chelators may be able to overcome these difficulties and improve patient outcomes. Two oral agents, deferiprone and deferasirox, have been studied extensively and are in clinical use worldwide, although in North America, deferasirox currently is the only approved oral chelator. Newer oral agents are under study. The chelator's efficacy at cardiac and liver iron removal and side effect profile should be considered in tailoring individual chelation regimens. Broader options for chelation therapy, including possible combination therapy, should improve clinical efficacy and enhance patient care.

REFERENCES

1. Adams RJ, McKie VC, Hsu L, et al. Prevention of a first stroke by transfusions in children with sickle cell anemia and abnormal results on transcranial doppler ultrasonography. N Engl J Med 1998;339:5–11.
2. Lieu PT, Heiskala M, Peterson PA, et al. The roles of iron in health and disease. Mol Aspects Med 2001;22(1–2):1–87.
3. Hugman A. Hepcidin: an important new regulator of iron homeostasis. Clin Lab Haematol 2006;28(2):75–83.
4. Bridle KR, Frazer DM, Wilkins SJ, et al. Disrupted hepcidin regulation in HFE-associated haemochromatosis and the liver as a regulator of body iron homoeostasis. Lancet 2003;361(9358):669–73.
5. Wallace DF, Subramaniam VN. Non-HFE haemochromatosis. World J Gastroenterol 2007;13(35):4690–8.
6. Breuer W, Hershko C, Cabantchik ZI. The importance of non-transferrin bound iron in disorders of iron metabolism. Transfus Sci 2000;23:185–92.
7. Kushner JP, Porter JP, Olivieri NF. Secondary iron overload. Hematology Am Soc Hematol Educ Program 2001;47–61.
8. Fung EB, Harmatz PR, Lee PD, et al. Increased prevalence of iron-overload associated endocrinopathy in thalassaemia versus sickle-cell disease. Br J Haematol 2006;135(4):574–82.
9. Wood JC, Tyszka M, Carson S, et al. Myocardial iron loading in transfusion-dependent thalassemia and sickle cell disease. Blood 2004;103(5):1934–6.
10. Zurlo MG, De Stefano P, Borgna-Pignatti C, et al. Survival and causes of death in thalassaemia major. Lancet 1989;2:27–30.
11. Jean G, Terzoli S, Mauri R, et al. Cirrhosis associated with multiple transfusions in thalassaemia. Arch Dis Child 1984;59(1):67–70.
12. Borgna-Pignatti C, De Stefano P, Zonta L, et al. Growth and sexual maturation in thalassemia major. J Pediatr 1985;106:150–5.
13. Cunningham MJ, Macklin EA, Neufeld EJ, et al. Complications of beta-thalassemia major in North America. Blood 2004;104(1):34–9.
14. Brittenham GM, Cohen AR, McLaren CE, et al. Hepatic iron stores and plasma ferritin concentration in patients with sickle cell anemia and thalassemia major. Am J Hematol 1993;42:81–5.
15. Cappellini MD, Cohen A, Piga A, et al. A phase 3 study of deferasirox (ICL670), a once-daily oral iron chelator, in patients with beta-thalassemia. Blood 2006;107(9):3455–62.
16. Vichinsky E, Onyekwere O, Porter J, et al. A randomised comparison of deferasirox versus deferoxamine for the treatment of transfusional iron overload in sickle cell disease. Br J Haematol 2007;136(3):501–8.
17. Olivieri NF, Nathan DG, MacMillan JH, et al. Survival in medically treated patients with homozygous beta-thalassemia. N Engl J Med 1994;331(9):574–8.
18. Telfer PT, Prestcott E, Holden S, et al. Hepatic iron concentration combined with long-term monitoring of serum ferritin to predict complications of iron overload in thalassaemia major. Br J Haematol 2000;110(4):971–7.
19. Files B, Brambilla D, Kutlar A, et al. Longitudinal changes in ferritin during chronic transfusion: a report from the Stroke Prevention Trial in Sickle Cell Anemia (STOP). J Pediatr Hematol Oncol 2002;24(4):284–90.
20. Pakbaz Z, Fischer R, Fung E, et al. Serum ferritin underestimates liver iron concentration in transfusion independent thalassemia patients as compared to

regularly transfused thalassemia and sickle cell patients. Pediatr Blood Cancer 2007;49(3):329–32.

21. Angelucci E, Brittenham GM, McLaren CE, et al. Hepatic iron concentration and total body iron stores in thalassemia major. N Engl J Med 2000;343(5):327–31.

22. Olivieri NF, Brittenham GM. Iron-chelating therapy and the treatment of thalassemia. Blood 1997;89(3):739–61.

23. Olivieri NF. The beta-thalassemias. N Engl J Med 1999;341(2):99–109.

24. Villeneuve JP, Bilodeau M, Lepage R, et al. Variability in hepatic iron concentration measurement from needle-biopsy specimens. J Hepatol 1996;25(2):172–7.

25. Anderson LJ, Holden S, Davis B, et al. Cardiovascular T2-star (T2*) magnetic resonance for the early diagnosis of myocardial iron overload. Eur Heart J 2001;22(23):2171–9.

26. Anderson LJ, Westwood MA, Holden S, et al. Myocardial iron clearance during reversal of siderotic cardiomyopathy with intravenous desferrioxamine: a prospective study using T2* cardiovascular magnetic resonance. Br J Haematol 2004;127(3):348–55.

27. Brittenham GM, Farrell DE, Harris JW, et al. Magnetic-susceptibility measurement of human iron stores. N Engl J Med 1982;307(27):1671–5.

28. Galanello R, Piga A, Forni GL, et al. Phase II clinical evaluation of deferasirox, a once-daily oral chelating agent, in pediatric patients with beta-thalassemia major. Haematologica 2006;91(10):1343–51.

29. Piga A, Galanello R, Forni GL, et al. Randomized phase II trial of deferasirox (Exjade, ICL670), a once-daily, orally-administered iron chelator, in comparison to deferoxamine in thalassemia patients with transfusional iron overload. Haematologica 2006;91(7):873–80.

30. Olivieri NF, Brittenham GM, Matsui D, et al. Iron-chelation therapy with oral deferiprone in patients with thalassemia major. N Engl J Med 1995;332(14):918–22.

31. Brittenham GM, Badman DG. Noninvasive measurement of iron: report of an NIDDK workshop. Blood 2003;101(1):15–9.

32. St. Pierre TG, Clark PR, Chua-Anusorn W, et al. Noninvasive measurement and imaging of liver iron concentrations using proton magnetic resonance. Blood 2005;105(2):855–61.

33. Westwood MA, Wonke B, Maceira AM, et al. Left ventricular diastolic function compared with T2* cardiovascular magnetic resonance for early detection of myocardial iron overload in thalassemia major. J Magn Reson Imaging 2005; 22(2):229–33.

34. Wood JC. Magnetic resonance imaging measurement of iron overload. Curr Opin Hematol 2007;14(3):183–90.

35. Clark PR, Chua-Anusorn W, St. Pierre TG. Proton transverse relaxation rate (R2) images of iron-loaded liver tissue; mapping local tissue iron concentrations with MRI. Magnet Reson Med 2003;49:572–5.

36. Wood JC, Enriquez C, Ghugre N, et al. MRI R2 and R2* mapping accurately estimates hepatic iron concentration in transfusion-dependent thalassemia and sickle cell disease patients. Blood 2005;106(4):1460–5.

37. Brittenham GM, Griffith PM, Nienhuis AW, et al. Efficacy of deferoxamine in preventing complications of iron overload in patients with thalassemia major. N Engl J Med 1994;331(9):567–73.

38. Lee P, Mohammed N, Marshall L, et al. Intravenous infusion pharmacokinetics of desferrioxamine in thalassaemic patients. Drug Metab Disp 1993;21:640–4.

39. Pippard MJ, Letsky EA, Callender ST, et al. Prevention of iron loading in transfusion-dependent thalassaemia. Lancet 1978;1(8075):1178–81.

40. Barry M, Flynn DM, Letsky EA, et al. Long-term chelation therapy in thalassaemia major: effect on liver iron concentration, liver histology, and clinical progress. Br Med J 1974;2:16–20.

41. Wolfe L, Oliveri N, Sallan D, et al. Prevention of cardiac disease by sucutaneous deferoxamine in patients with thalassemia major. N Engl J Med 1985;312(25): 1600–3.

42. Davis BA, Porter JB. Long-term outcome of continuous 24-hour deferoxamine infusion via indwelling intravenous catheters in high-risk beta-thalassemia. Blood 2000;95(4):1229–36.

43. Olivieri NF, Buncic JR, Chew E, et al. Visual and auditory neurotoxicity in patients receiving subcutaneous deferoxamine infusions. N Engl J Med 1986;314(14): 869–73.

44. De Sanctis V, Pinamonti A, DiPalma A, et al. Growth and development in thalassemia major patients with severe bone lesions due to desferrioxamine. Eur J Pediatr 1996;155:368–72.

45. Porter JB, Jaswon MS, Huehns ER, et al. Desferrioxamine ototoxicity: evaluation of risk factors in thalassaemic patients and guidelines for safe dosage. Br J Haematol 1989;73(73):403–9.

46. Freedman MH, Grisaru D, Oliveri N, et al. Pulmonary syndrome in patients with thalassemia major receiving intravenous deferoxamine infusions. Am J Dis Child 1990;144:565–9.

47. Borgna-Pignatti C, Rugolotto S, DeStefano P, et al. Survival and disease complications in thalassemia major. Ann N Y Acad Sci 1998;850:227–31.

48. Ceci A, Baiardi P, Catapano M, et al. Risk factors for death in patients with beta-thalassemia major: results of a case-control study. Haematologica 2006;91(10): 1420–1.

49. Al-Refaie FN, Sheppard LN, Nortey P, et al. Pharmacokinetics of the oral iron chelator deferiprone (L1) in patients with iron overload. Br J Haematol 1995; 89(2):403–8.

50. Matsui D, Klein J, Hermann C. Relationship between the pharmacokinetics and iron excretion of the new oral iron chelator 1,2-dimethyl-3-hydroxypyrid-4-1 in patients with thalassemia. Clin Pharmacol Ther 1991;50:294–8.

51. Al-Refaie FN, Wonke B, Hoffbrand AV, et al. Efficacy and possible adverse effects of the oral iron chelator 1,2-dimethyl-3-hydroxypyrid-4-one (L1) in thalassemia major. Blood 1992;80(3):593–9.

52. Collins AF, Fassos FF, Stobie S, et al. Iron-balance and dose-response studies of the oral iron chelator 1,2-dimethyl-3-hydroxypyrid-4-one (L1) in iron-loaded patients with sickle cell disease. Blood 1994;83(8):2329–33.

53. Olivieri NF, Koren G, Hermann C, et al. Comparison of oral iron chelator L1 and desferrioxamine in iron-loaded patients. Lancet 1990;336(8726):1275–9.

54. Agarwal MB, Gupte SS, Viswanathan C, et al. Long-term assessment of efficacy and safety of L1, an oral iron chelator, in transfusion dependent thalassaemia: Indian trial. Br J Haematol 1992;82(2):460–6.

55. Wonke B, Wright C, Hoffbrand AV. Combined therapy with deferiprone and desferrioxamine. Br J Haematol 1998;103(4):361–4.

56. Kersten MJ, Lange R, Smeets ME, et al. Long-term treatment of transfusional iron overload with the oral iron chelator deferiprone (L1): a Dutch multicenter trial. Ann Hematol 1996;73(5):247–52.

57. Maggio A, D'Amico G, Morabito A, et al. Deferiprone versus deferoxamine in patients with thalassemia major: a randomized clinical trial. Blood Cells Mol Dis 2002;28(2):196–208.

58. Voskaridou E, Douskou M, Terpos E, et al. Deferiprone as an oral iron chelator in sickle cell disease. Ann Hematol 2005;84(7):434–40.
59. Cohen AR, Galanello R, Piga A, et al. Safety profile of the oral iron chelator deferiprone: a multicentre study. Br J Haematol 2000;108(2):305–12.
60. Al-Refaie FN, Hershko C, Hoffbrand AV, et al. Results of long-term deferiprone (L1) therapy: a report by the International Study Group on oral iron chelators. Br Haematol 1995;91(1):224–9.
61. Ceci A, Baiardi P, Felisi M, et al. The safety and effectiveness of deferiprone in a large-scale, 3-year study in Italian patients. Br J Haematol 2002;118(1):330–6.
62. Hoffbrand AV, Al-Refaie F, Davis B, et al. Long-term trial of deferiprone in 51 transfusion-dependent iron overloaded patients. Blood 1998;91(1):295–300.
63. Cohen AR, Galanello R, Piga A, et al. Safety and effectiveness of long-term therapy with the oral iron chelator deferiprone. Blood 2003;102(5):1583–7.
64. Mazza P, Amurri B, Lazzari G, et al. Oral iron chelating therapy. A single center interim report on deferiprone (L1) in thalassemia. Haematologica 1998;83(6):496–501.
65. Olivieri NF, Brittenham GM, McLaren CE, et al. Long-term safety and effectiveness of iron-chelation therapy with deferiprone for thalassemia major. N Engl J Med 1998;339(7):417–23.
66. Pennell DJ, Berdoukas V, Karagiorga M, et al. Randomized controlled trial of deferiprone or deferoxamine in beta-thalassemia major patients with asymptomatic myocardial siderosis. Blood 2006;107(9):3738–44.
67. Gomber S, Saxena R, Madan N. Comparative efficacy of desferrioxamine, deferiprone and in combination on iron chelation in thalassemic children. Indian Pediatr 2004;41(1):21–7.
68. Taher A, Sheikh-Taha M, Sharara A, et al. Safety and effectiveness of 100 mg/kg/day deferiprone in patients with thalassemia major: a two-year study. Acta Haematol 2005;114(3):146–9.
69. Anderson LJ, Wonke B, Prescott E, et al. Comparison of effects of oral deferiprone and subcutaneous desferrioxamine on myocardial iron concentrations and ventricular function in beta-thalassaemia. Lancet 2002;360(9332):516–20.
70. Borgna-Pignatti C, Cappellini MD, De Stefano P, et al. Cardiac morbidity and mortality in deferoxamine- or deferiprone-treated patients with thalassemia major. Blood 2006;107(9):3733–7.
71. Piga A, Gaglioti C, Fogliacco E, et al. Comparative effects of deferiprone and deferoxamine on survival and cardiac disease in patients with thalassemia major: a retrospective analysis. Haematologica 2003;88(5):489–96.
72. Galia M, Midiri M, Bartolotta V, et al. Potential myocardial iron content evaluation by magnetic resonance imaging in thalassemia major patients treated with Deferoxamine or Deferiprone during a randomized multicenter prospective clinical study. Hemoglobin 2003;27(2):63–76.
73. Peng CT, Chow KC, Chen JH, et al. Safety monitoring of cardiac and hepatic systems in beta-thalassemia patients with chelating treatment in Taiwan. Eur J Haematol 2003;70(6):392–7.
74. Al-Refaie FN, Wonke B, Hoffbrand AV. Deferiprone-associated myelotoxicity. Eur J Haematol 1994;53(5):298–301.
75. Henter JI, Karlen J. Fatal agranulocytosis after deferiprone therapy in a child with Diamond-Blackfan anemia. Blood 2007;109(12):5157–9.
76. Hoffbrand AV, Bartlett AN, Veys PA, et al. Agranulocytosis and thrombocytopenia in patient with Blackfan-Diamond anaemia during oral chelator trial. Lancet 1989;2(8660):457.

77. Tondury P, Zimmerman A, Nielsen P, et al. Liver iron and fibrosis during long-term treatment with deferiprone in Swiss thalassaemic patients. Br J Haematol 1998; 101(3):413–5.
78. Wanless IR, Sweeney G, Dhillon AP, et al. Lack of progressive hepatic fibrosis during long-term therapy with deferiprone in subjects with transfusion-dependent beta-thalassemia. Blood 2002;100(5):1566–9.
79. Origa R, Bina P, Agus A, et al. Combined therapy with deferiprone and desferrioxamine in thalassemia major. Haematologica 2005;90(10):1309–14.
80. Kattamis A, Ladis V, Berdousi H, et al. Iron chelation treatment with combined therapy with deferiprone and deferioxamine: a 12-month trial. Blood Cells Mol Dis 2006;36(1):21–5.
81. Breuer W, Ermers MJJ, Pootrakul P, et al. Desferrioxamine-chelatable iron, a component of serum non-transferrin-bound iron, used for assessing chelation therapy. Blood 2001;97(3):792–8.
82. Link G, Konijn AM, Breuer W, et al. Exploring the "iron shuttle" hypothesis in chelation therapy: effects of combined deferoxamine and deferiprone treatment in hypertransfused rats with labeled iron stores and in iron-loaded rat heart cells in culture. J Lab Clin Med 2001;138(2):130–8.
83. Tanner MA, Galanello R, Dessi C, et al. A randomized, placebo-controlled, double-blind trial of the effect of combined therapy with deferoxamine and deferiprone on myocardial iron in thalassemia major using cardiovascular magnetic resonance. Circulation 2007;115(14):1876–84.
84. Galanello R, Piga A, Alberti D, et al. Safety, tolerability, and pharmacokinetics of ICL670, a new orally active iron-chelating agent in patients with transfusion-dependent iron overload due to beta-thalassemia. J Clin Pharmacol 2003; 43(6):565–72.
85. Nisbet-Brown E, Olivieri NF, Giardina PJ, et al. Effectiveness and safety of ICL670 in iron-loaded patients with thalassaemia: a randomised, double-blind, placebo-controlled, dose-escalation trial. Lancet 2003;361(9369):1597–602.
86. Porter J, Galanello R, Saglio G, et al. Relative response of patients with myelodysplastic syndromes and other transfusion-dependent anaemias to deferasirox (ICL670): a 1-year prospective study. Eur J Haematol 2008;80(2):168–76.
87. Cohen AR, Glimm E, Porter JB. Effect of transfusional iron intake on response to chelation therapy in beta-thalassemia major. Blood 2008;111(2):583–7.
88. Glickstein H, El RB, Link G, et al. Action of chelators in iron-loaded cardiac cells: Accessibility to intracellular labile iron and functional consequences. Blood 2006; 108(9):3195–203.
89. Wood JC, Otto-Duessel M, Gonzalez I, et al. Deferasirox and deferiprone remove cardiac iron in the iron-overloaded gerbil. Transl Res 2006;148(5):272–80.
90. Porter JB, Tanner MA, Pennell DJ, et al. Improved myocardial T2* in transfusion dependent anemias receiving ICL670 (deferasirox). Blood 2005;106(11):1003a.
91. Cappellini MD, Bejaoui M, Agaoglu L, et al. Prospective evaluation of patient-reported outcomes during treatment with deferasirox or deferoxamine for iron overload in patients with beta-thalassemia. Clin Ther 2007;29(5):909–17.
92. Barton JC. Drug evaluation: Deferitrin for iron overload disorders. IDrugs 2007; 10(7):480–90.
93. Donovan JM, Yardumian A, Gunawardena KA, et al. The safety and pharmacokinetics of deferitrin, a novel orally available iron chelator. Blood 2004;104(11):146a.
94. Link G, Ponka P, Konijn AM, et al. Effects of combined chelation treatment with pyridoxal isonicotinoyl hydrazone analogs and deferoxamine in hypertransfused rats and in iron-loaded rat heart cells. Blood 2003;101(10):4172–9.

95. Brittenham GM. Pyridoxal isonicotinoyl hydrazone: an effective iron-chelator after oral administration. Semin Hematol 1990;27(2):112–6.
96. Cohen AR, Galanello R, Pennell DJ, et al. Thalassemia. Hematology Am Soc Hematol Educ Program 2004;14–34.
97. Vichinsky E. Consensus document for transfusion-related iron overload. Semin Hematol 2001;38(Suppl 1):2–4.

Childhood Immune Thrombocytopenic Purpura: Diagnosis and Management

Victor Blanchette, FRCP[a],*, Paula Bolton-Maggs, DM, FRCP[b]

KEYWORDS

- Immune thrombocytopenic purpura • Immunoglobulin G
- Intravenous anti-D • Combined cytopenias • Splenectomy

Immune thrombocytopenic purpura (ITP) is an autoimmune disorder characterized by a low circulating platelet count caused by destruction of antibody-sensitized platelets in the reticuloendothelial system.[1] ITP can be classified based on patient age (childhood versus adult), duration of illness (acute versus chronic), and presence of an underlying disorder (primary versus secondary). Persistence of thrombocytopenia, generally defined as a platelet count of less than $150 \times 10^9/L$ for longer than 6 months, defines the chronic form of the disorder. Secondary causes of ITP include collagen vascular disorders, such as systemic lupus erythematosus (SLE); immune deficiencies, such as common variable immunodeficiency (CVID); and some chronic infections (eg, HIV and hepatitis C).

This article focuses on the diagnosis and management of children (under 18 years of age) who have acute and chronic ITP. Emphasis is placed on areas of controversy and new therapies.

PATHOPHYSIOLOGY

The pathophysiology of ITP increasingly is understood better (reviewed by Cines and Blanchette.[1]) Not surprisingly, it is complex with involvement of many players in the human immune orchestra, including antibodies, cytokines, antigen-presenting cells, costimulatory molecules, and T and B lymphocytes (including T-helper, T-cytotoxic, and T-regulatory lymphocytes). Current knowledge is summarized later.

A version of this article was previously published in the *Pediatric Clinics of North America*, 55:2.
[a] Division of Hematology/Oncology, The Hospital for Sick Children, Department of Pediatrics, University of Toronto, 555 University Avenue, Toronto, Ontario M5G 1X8, Canada
[b] University Department of Haematology, Manchester Royal Infirmary, Oxford Road, Manchester M13 9WL, United Kingdom
* Corresponding author.
E-mail address: victor.blanchette@sickkids.ca (V. Blanchette).

Hematol Oncol Clin N Am 24 (2010) 249–273
doi:10.1016/j.hoc.2009.11.004
0889-8588/10/$ – see front matter © 2010 Elsevier Inc. All rights reserved.

A key element in the pathophysiology of ITP is loss of self tolerance leading to the production of autoantibodies directed against platelet antigens. Evidence for an "anti-platelet factor" in the plasma of subjects who have ITP was provided in a seminal report from Harrington and coworkers[2] in 1951. The investigators demonstrated that the infusion of plasma from subjects who had ITP into volunteers induced a rapid fall in platelet count and a clinical picture that mimics ITP. The "antiplatelet factor" subsequently was confirmed as an immunoglobulin.[3] Now it is known that the auto-antibodies in patients who have ITP mostly are of the IgG class with specificity against platelet-specific antigens, in particular, glycoproteins IIb/IIIa and Ib/IX. Unfortunately, accurate detection of platelet autoantibodies is difficult and not available routinely in most clinical hematology laboratories; clinicians should be aware that indirect platelet autoantibody tests (tests that detect free autoantibodies in the plasma) are inferior to direct tests (tests that detect platelet-bound autoantibodies) and that even with the best direct tests performed in expert immunohematology laboratories, the positivity rate in patients who have well-characterized ITP does not exceed 80%.[4] A negative platelet antibody test, therefore, does not exclude a diagnosis of ITP. For this reason, platelet antibody testing is not recommended as part of the routine diagnostic strategy.[5]

It is increasingly clear that cellular immune mechanisms play a pivotal role in ITP.[1] The production of antiplatelet antibodies by B cells requires antigen-specific, CD4-postive, T-cell help (**Fig. 1**). It also is possible that in some ITP cases, cytotoxic T cells play a role in the destruction of platelets. A possible sequence of events in ITP is as follows. A trigger, possibly an infection or toxin, leads to the formation of anti-bodies/immune complexes that attach to platelets. Antibody-coated platelets then bind to antigen-presenting cells (macrophages or dendritic cells) through low-affinity Fcγ receptors (Fcγ RIIA/Fcγ RIIIA) and are internalized and degraded. Activated antigen-presenting cells then expose novel peptides on the cell surface and with costimulatory help facilitate the proliferation of platelet antigen-specific, CD4-positive, T-cell clones. These T-cell clones drive autoantibody production by platelet antigen-specific B-cell clones. As part of the platelet destructive process in ITP, cryptic epitopes from platelet antigens are exposed, leading to the formation of secondary platelet antigen-specific T-cell clones, with stimulation of new platelet antigen-specific B-cell clones and broadening of the immune response. The autoan-tibody profile of individual patients who have ITP reflects activity of polyclonal autoreactive B-cell clones derived by antigen-driven affinity selection and somatic mutation.

Although increased platelet destruction clearly plays a key role in the pathogenesis of ITP, it is now recognized that impaired platelet production also is important in many cases. In adults, as many as 40% of ITP cases may have reduced platelet turnover, reflecting the inhibitory effect of platelet autoantibodies on megakaryopoiesis.[6] Studies of platelet kinetics in children who have ITP are limited but it is possible that a similar situation exists. There also is evidence that platelet autoantibodies may induce thrombocytopenia by inhibiting proplatelet formation.[7] Circulating thrombo-poietin (TPO) levels in patients who have ITP typically are normal or increased only slightly, reflecting the normal or only slightly reduced TPO receptor mass in this acquired platelet disorder. In contrast, TPO levels are high in inherited platelet produc-tion disorders, such as thrombocytopenia-absent radii or congenital amegakaryocytic thrombocytopenia.[8] TPO testing generally is not available, but these observations have led to the question of whether or not TPO or molecules mimicking TPO may increase platelet production and be a new treatment strategy in ITP. Several such agents currently are in clinical trials.

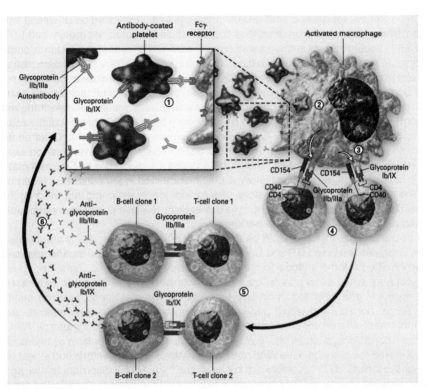

Fig. 1. Pathogenesis of epitope spread in ITP. The factors that initiate autoantibody production are unknown. Most patients have antibodies against several platelet-surface glycoproteins at the time the disease becomes clinically evident. Here, glycoprotein IIb/IIIa is recognized by autoantibody (*orange,* inset), whereas antibodies that recognize the glycoprotein Ib/IX complex have not been generated at this stage (1). Antibody-coated platelets bind to antigen-presenting cells (macrophages or dendritic cells) through Fcγ receptors and then are internalized and degraded (2). Antigen-presenting cells not only degrade glycoprotein IIb/IIIa (*light blue* oval), thereby amplifying the initial immune response, but also may generate cryptic epitopes from other platelet glycoproteins (*light blue* cylinder) (3). Activated antigen-presenting cells (4) express these novel peptides on the cell surface along with costimulatory help (represented in part by the interaction between CD154 and CD40) and the relevant cytokines that facilitate the proliferation of the initiating CD4-positive T-cell clones (T-cell clone 1) and those with additional specificities (T-cell clone 2) (5). B-cell immunoglobulin receptors that recognize additional platelet antigens (B-cell clone 2) thereby also are induced to proliferate and synthesize antiglycoprotein Ib/IX antibodies (*green*) in addition to amplifying the production of anti-glycoprotein IIb/IIIa antibodies (*orange*) by B-cell clone 1 (6). (*From* Cines DB, Blanchette VS. Immune thrombocytopenic purpura. N Engl J Med 2002;346:995–1008; with permission. Copyright © 2002, Massachusetts Medical Society. All rights reserved.)

DIFFERENTIAL DIAGNOSIS

Primary ITP is a diagnosis of exclusion. The question, "When does a low platelet count not mean ITP?" is important, especially for atypical cases. When an unexpected low platelet count in a child is obtained, artifact or laboratory error should be considered first and excluded. Pseudothrombocytopenia is an example of spurious thrombocytopenia that is caused by platelet aggregation and clumping in the presence of ethylenediamine tetraacetic acid (EDTA) anticoagulant.[9] Examination of well-stained blood smears prepared from a venous blood sample collected separately into EDTA and 3.8% sodium citrate anticoagulant usually confirms or excludes pseudothrombocytopenia. A smear prepared from the collection tube with EDTA should demonstrate platelet clumping, whereas a smear prepared from the tube with sodium citrate should not. Some patients, however, have platelets that also clump in citrate anticoagulant.

A detailed history, careful physical examination, and results of selected tests confirm or eliminate common causes of secondary thrombocytopenia, such as SLE. A positive antinuclear antibody is common in children who have ITP and, as an isolated finding, does not confirm or exclude SLE;[10] more specific tests, such as an anti–double-stranded DNA test, should be ordered if a diagnosis of SLE-associated ITP is suspected. A transfusion history should be obtained in all cases and, depending on the age of the child, the history should include questioning about drug use (prescription and nonprescription) and sexual activity. If relevant, testing for antibodies to hepatitis C and HIV should be performed.

A detailed family history should be obtained in all cases. Especially in children who have apparent "chronic" ITP and isolated moderate thrombocytopenia, the possibility of an inherited thrombocytopenia should be considered. The topic, "inherited thrombocytopenia: when a low platelet count does not mean ITP," is the focus of an excellent review.[11] The inherited thrombocytopenias can be classified based on platelet size (large, normal, and small) and gene mutations. They include conditions, such as the MYH9-related macrothrombocytopenias, Wiskott-Aldrich syndrome (WAS), and rare conditions, such as gray platelet syndrome (**Box 1**). The pattern of inheritance (eg, X-linked in boys who have WAS) and abnormalities on peripheral blood smear (eg, Döhle-like inclusions in neutrophils of patients who have MYH9 disorders or pale agranular platelets in gray platelet syndrome) may provide important clues to the underlying disorder. Failure of patients who have apparent "chronic ITP" and moderate thrombocytopenia to respond to front-line platelet-enhancing therapies, such as high-dose intravenous (IV) immunoglobulin G (IVIG) or IV anti-D, should prompt consideration of an alternate diagnosis. Additional investigation in such cases should include screening for type 2B von Willebrand disease, pseudo–von Willebrand disease, and Bernard-Soulier syndrome. In males who have small platelets, WAS or X-linked thrombocytopenia should be considered. These latter conditions can be confirmed by screening for mutations in the WASP gene. Boys who have WASP gene mutations may have significant immunologic abnormalities.

CHILDHOOD ACUTE IMMUNE THROMBOCYTOPENIC PURPURA
Clinical and Laboratory Features

Thrombocytopenia for less than 6 months defines the entity acute ITP. Typically, children who have acute ITP are young, of previous good health, and present with sudden onset of bruising or a petechial rash. In a series of 2031 children who had newly diagnosed ITP, reported by Kühne and colleagues[12] in 2001 for the Intercontinental Childhood ITP Study Group (ICIS), the mean age at presentation was 5.7 years. Approximately 70% of the cohort were children ages 1 to 10 years with 10% of the cohort infants (older than 3 and less than 12 months old) and the remainder 20% older children (ages 10 to 16 years).[13] Male and female children were affected approximately equally with the caveat that boys outnumbered girls in young children, especially those less than 1 year of age (**Fig. 2**).[12] The predominance of boys who had ITP in children under 10 years of age is reported in several other studies.[14–16] In approximately two thirds of cases, the onset of acute ITP is preceded by an infectious

> **Box 1**
> **Inherited thrombocytopenias classified by platelet size**
>
> *Small platelets [MPV < 7 fL]*
>
> WAS
>
> X-linked thrombocytopenia
>
> *Normal-sized platelets [MPV 7–11 fL]*
>
> Thrombocytopenia-absent radii
>
> Congenital amegakaryocytic thrombocytopenia
>
> Radioulnar synostosis and amegakaryocytic thrombocytopenia
>
> Familial platelet disorder with associated myeloid malignancy
>
> *Large/giant platelets [MPV > 11 fL]*
>
> MYH9[a] syndromes
>
> - May-Hegglin anomaly
> - Fechtner syndrome
> - Epstein syndrome
> - Sebastian syndrome
>
> Mediterranean thrombocytopenia
>
> Bernard-Soulier syndrome
>
> Velocardiofacial/DiGeorge syndrome
>
> Paris-Trousseau thrombocytopenia/Jacobsen syndrome
>
> Gray platelet syndrome
>
> *Abbreviation:* MPV, mean platelet volume.
> [a] MYH9 gene encodes for the nonmuscle myosin heavy-chain IIA.
> *Data from* Drachman JG. Inherited thrombocytopenia: when a low platelet count does not mean ITP. Blood 2004;103:390–8.

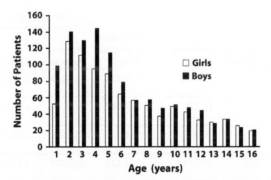

Fig. 2. Age (years) of children who had newly diagnosed ITP entered into the Intercontinental Childhood ITP Registry. (*From* Kühne T, Imbach P, Bolton-Maggs PHB, et al. Newly diagnosed idiopathic thrombocytopenic purpura in childhood: an observational study. Lancet 2001;358:2122–25; with permission.)

illness, most often an upper respiratory tract infection; in a minority of cases, ITP follows a specific viral illness (rubella, varicella, mumps, rubeola, or infectious mono-nucleosis) or immunization with a live virus vaccine.[17,18] The risk for ITP after mumps-measles-rubella vaccine is estimated at approximately 1 in 25,000 doses.[19] In children who have acute ITP, the interval between the preceding infection and the onset of purpura varies from a few days to several weeks, with the most frequent interval approximately 2 weeks.[20] Physical examination at presentation is remarkable only for the cutaneous manifestations of severe thrombocytopenia with bruising or a pete-chial rash present in almost all cases (**Table 1**). Clinically significant lymphadenopathy or marked hepatosplenomegaly are atypical features; however, shotty cervical adenopathy is common in young children and a spleen tip may be palpable in 5% to 10% of cases.[20,21] Epistaxis (often minor, sometimes severe) is a presenting symptom in approximately one quarter of affected children; hematuria occurs less frequently.[20]

The key laboratory finding in children who have acute ITP is isolated, and often severe, thrombocytopenia. In more than half of cases, platelet counts at presentation are less than 20×10^9/L (**Fig. 3**). Other hematologic abnormalities are consistent with a diagnosis of childhood acute ITP only if they can be explained easily (eg, anemia secondary to epistaxis/menorrhagia) or atypical lymphocytosis in cases of infectious mononucleosis. The one exception is mild eosinophilia, which is a common finding.[21] The blood smear shows a marked decrease in platelets with some platelets that are large (megathrombocytes) (**Fig. 4**). A bone marrow aspirate, if performed, typically shows normal to increased numbers of megakaryocytes, many of which are immature (see **Fig. 4**). An increase in the number of bone marrow eosinophil precursors is present in some cases.

Natural History of Childhood Acute Immune Thrombocytopenic Purpura

The natural history of childhood acute ITP is well documented (reviewed by Blanchette and Carcao[22]). Complete remission, defined as a platelet count greater than 150×10^9/L within 6 months of initial diagnosis and without the need for ongoing platelet-enhancing therapy, occurs in at least two thirds of cases. This excellent outcome

Table 1
Presenting features in children who have acute immune thrombocytopenic purpura

Investigator	Number of Cases	Male:Female Ratio	Preceding Infectious Illness	Hemorrhagic Manifestations		
				Purpura/ Petechiae	Epistaxis	Hematuria
Choi (1950–1964)[a,20]	239	117:122	119/239	235/239	76/239	20/239
Lusher (1956–1964)[21]	152	69:83	122/146	—	46/152	8/152
Blanchette (1974–1982)[22]	80	37:43	58/80	75/80	20/80	3/80
Bolton-Maggs (1995–1996)[14]	427	213:214	245/427	310/427	85/427	6/427
Total	898	436:462	544/892 (60.9%)	620/746 (83.1%)	227/898 (25.3%)	37/898 (4.1%)

[a] Years in parenthesis represent the period of observation.

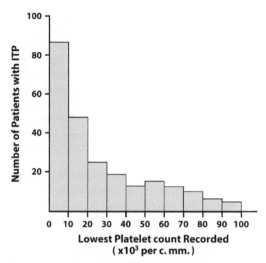

Fig. 3. Lowest platelet count observed in children who had ITP. (*From* Choi SI, McClure PD. Idiopathic thrombocytopenic purpura in childhood. Can Med Assoc J 1967;97:562–8; with permission. Copyright © 1967, Canadian Medical Association.)

seems independent of any management strategy. As an example, in the prospective study reported by Kühne and colleagues,[12] complete remission rates of 68%, 73%, and 66% were reported in children who received no treatment, IVIG, or corticosteroids, respectively. These data are similar to the 76% complete remission rate reported by George and colleagues[5] on the basis of a review of 12 case series involving 1597 cases. A recent study of children from five Nordic studies described a simple clinical score that predicts early remission.[23] If confirmed, this could identify those children who might be left without active therapy for low platelet counts. Predictors of early remission were abrupt onset of illness, preceding infection, male gender, age under 10 years, wet purpura, and a platelet count less than 5×10^9/L.

The outcome for children who have acute ITP who continue to manifest thrombocytopenia beyond 6 months from initial presentation generally is good. Published reports

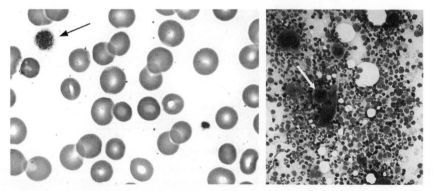

Fig. 4. Blood smear and bone marrow aspirate from a child who had ITP showing large platelets (blood smear [*left*]) and increased numbers of megakaryocytes, many of which appear immature (bone marrow aspirate [*right*]).

suggest that as many as one third of such children have spontaneous remission of their illness from a few months to several years after initial diagnosis.[5,24] In one study, 61% was predicted at 15 years of follow-up.[25] Most spontaneous remissions occur early, and the number of children who have severe thrombocytopenia (platelet counts $<20 \times 10^9/L$) and who are symptomatic with bleeding symptoms and, therefore, are therapy dependent more than 1 year after initial diagnosis is small. In a Swiss-Canadian retrospective analysis of 554 children who had newly diagnosed ITP and platelet counts less than $20 \times 10^9/L$, the percentages of children who had platelet counts less than $20 \times 10^9/L$ at 6, 12, 18, and 24 months after diagnosis were 9%, 6%, 4%, and 3%, respectively (**Fig. 5**).[26] This is the small subgroup of children for whom splenectomy ultimately may need to be considered.

The case for treatment of children who have acute ITP relates to those who have significant bleeding and consideration of the very small, but finite, risk for intracranial hemorrhage (ICH). The risk of this feared complication was 0.9% in a series of 1693 children reviewed by George and colleagues.[5] This figure, however, probably is an overestimate reflecting that reports in the literature mainly are from academic centers that likely are referred the most severe cases. Based on data in the United Kingdom, Lilleyman has estimated an incidence of 0.2% of ICH in children who have newly diagnosed ITP,[27] a figure consistent with the 0.17% incidence rate (3 of 1742 children who had newly diagnosed acute ITP) reported by Kühne and colleagues[13] on behalf of the ICIS.

Whatever the true incidence of ICH in children who have acute ITP, there is no doubt that this event is a devastating and sometimes fatal complication in this generally benign childhood disorder. The percent of cases of ICH occurring within 4 weeks of initial diagnosis varied from 19% to 50% in different reports;[5,27,28] in one retrospective review, 10% (7/69) of cases of ICH occurred within 3 days of diagnosis of ITP.[29] Trauma to the head and use of antiplatelet drugs, such as aspirin, were identified as risk factors for ICH in children who had ITP and very low platelet counts.[30]

Unfortunately, a prospective randomized controlled trial to determine definitively whether or not therapeutic intervention can decrease the incidence of ICH significantly

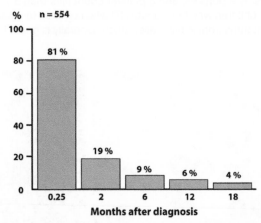

Fig. 5. Percentage of children (n = 554) who had ITP and platelet counts below $20 \times 10^9/L$ at 1 week, 2, 6, 12, and 18 months after diagnosis of acute ITP. Swiss-Canadian retrospective analysis. (*From* Imbach P, Akatsuka J, Blanchette V, et al. Immunthrombocytopenic purpura as a model for pathogenesis and treatment of autoimmunity. Eur J Pediatr 1995;154 (Suppl 3):S60–4; with permission.)

in children who have newly diagnosed ITP and platelet counts below 20×10^9/L is not feasible, because of the large numbers of cases required to ensure a statistically significant outcome. Physicians who care for children who have acute ITP, therefore, must act in the best interest of each child without the benefit of definitive data. Because of the significant morbidity and mortality associated with ICH and the availability of highly effective platelet-enhancing therapies, some recommend that families of young children who have newly diagnosed acute ITP at risk for ICH (who have platelet counts $<10 \times 10^9$/L) be offered the option of treatment using the minimum therapy necessary to increase the platelet count rapidly to a safe, hemostatic level. There is no current evidence, however, that such a management strategy significantly reduces the incidence of ICH in children who have ITP, although intuitively this seems probable.

In addition, there is evidence to suggest that the rate of platelet response to frontline therapies (corticosteroids or IVIG) in the subset of children who have ITP and clinically significant hemorrhage is suboptimal.[31] Discussion with parents and children, if of appropriate age, should include consideration of best available evidence with regard to the three key issues: (1) to treat or not to treat (2) to perform a bone marrow aspirate or not and (3) to hospitalize or not.

TO TREAT OR NOT TO TREAT
Observation

The case for observation of children who have acute ITP rests with the knowledge that acute ITP is, for the majority of affected children, a benign self-limiting disorder, usually with mild clinical symptoms and has a low risk for serious bleeding (approximately 3% with ICH being rare) and the fact that there are no prospective studies that clearly indicate a decrease in the incidence of ICH associated with treatment.[32] Several children who had ITP-associated ICH were receiving platelet-enhancing therapy at the time of the hemorrhage.[28] In addition, all treatments suffer from the disadvantage of side effects, which can be severe.

Guidelines for initial management of children who have acute ITP have been published and reflect the ongoing debate, "to treat or not to treat".[5,33–36] Recommendations from the Working Party of the British Committee for Standards in Haematology General Haematology Task Force state that treatment of children who have acute ITP should be decided on the basis of clinical symptoms in addition to cutaneous signs, not the platelet count alone.[36] The Working Party considered it appropriate to manage children who have acute ITP and mild clinical disease expectantly, with supportive advice, and a 24-hour contact point irrespective of the platelet count. Based on these guidelines, intervention is reserved for the few children who have overt hemorrhage and platelet counts below 20×10^9/L or those who have organ- or life-threatening bleeding irrespective of the circulating platelet count.[34,36] Many clinicians in Europe manage children who have ITP expectantly (ie, without medication to increase the platelet count) because of the rapid remissions in most cases, the low risk for bleeding, and toxicities of currently available medical therapies. Data are reported from the United Kingdom and Germany promoting the use of advice and support to children and their families during the usually short duration of the illness.[15,32,37]

Corticosteroids

The corticosteroid treatment regimen used to treat children who have newly diagnosed ITP in most reported studies, and worldwide, is oral prednisone at a dose of 1 to 2 mg/kg per day given in divided doses and continued for a few weeks. Two randomized studies support the benefit of corticosteroid therapy in children who have ITP. In the first study, conducted by Sartorius[38] and reported in 1984, 73 children ages 10 months to 14 years who had newly diagnosed ITP were randomized to receive oral prednisolone (60 mg/m^2 per day for 21 days) or a placebo. Platelet responses were significantly faster in the corticosteroid-treated group, with 90% of children achieving a platelet count of 30 × 10^9/L within the first 10 days of treatment compared with 45% of children in the placebo no-treatment group. The Rumpel-Leede test, which measures capillary resistance (blood vessel integrity), became negative sooner in the corticosteroid-treated group. In the second study, reported by Buchanan and Holtkamp[39] in 1984, 27 children who had acute ITP were randomized to receive oral prednisone (2 mg/kg per day for 14 days, with tapering and discontinuation of cortico-steroids by day 21) or placebo. Although there was a definite trend in favor of cortico-steroids, only on day 7 of therapy did the prednisone-treated patients have significantly higher platelet counts, lower bleeding scores, and shorter bleeding times than children receiving placebo. Taken together, these two studies suggest limited early benefit from conventional dose oral corticosteroid therapy in children who have acute ITP.

The risks and benefits of high-dose corticosteroid therapy administered orally or IV to children who have acute ITP merit discussion. In a study of 20 children random-ized to receive oral megadose methylprednisolone (30 mg/kg for 3 days followed by 20 mg/kg for 4 days) or IVIG (0.4 g/kg × 5 days), Özsoylu and colleagues[40] reported that 80% of children in both groups had platelet counts greater than 50 × 10^9/L by 72 hours after the start of treatment. Corticosteroids were given before 9:00 AM and adverse effects were not observed. In contrast, Suarez and colleagues[41] reported that hyperactivity and behavioral problems occurred in 5 of 9 children who had acute ITP given 6 to 8 mg/kg per day of oral prednisone for 3 days or until platelet counts had increased to 20 × 10^9/L. Immediate platelet responses with this regimen were impressive: the mean time to achieve a platelet count of 20 × 10^9/L was 1.9 ± 0.6 days (range 1–3 days).

A commonly used high-dose corticosteroid regimen is that reported by van Hoff and Ritchey.[42] The investigators treated 21 consecutive children who had ITP using IV methylprednisolone (30 mg/kg, maximum dose 1 g) given daily for 3 days. The median time to achieving a platelet count greater than 20 × 10^9/L was 24 hours. Ten children (48%) had transient glycosuria but no cases of hyperglycemia were observed. Similar results were reported by Jayabose and colleagues,[43] who treated 20 children who had acute ITP with IV methylprednisolone (5 mg/kg per day in four divided doses). By 48 hours from start of treatment, 90% of children had platelet counts greater than 20 × 10^9/L, and all children achieved this hemostatic threshold by 72 hours from the start of treatment. No patients developed symptomatic hyperglycemia or hyper-tension; the investigators did not comment about weight gain or mood/behavioral changes. The authors' experience with short-course oral prednisone (4 mg/kg per day × 4 days without tapering) is complementary. Eighty-three percent of children who had acute ITP and platelet counts less than 20 × 10^9/L achieved a platelet count above 20 × 10^9/L within 48 hours of starting corticosteroid therapy (**Fig. 6**).[44]

On the basis of these studies, it can be concluded that a clinically significant incre-ment in platelet count can be achieved rapidly in the majority of children who have acute ITP after the administration of high-doses of corticosteroids (approximately 4 mg/kg per day of prednisone or an equivalent corticosteroid preparation) adminis-tered orally or parenterally. The frequency and severity of corticosteroid toxicity relates to dose and duration of therapy and merits further study. If a decision is made to use corticosteroid therapy for children who have acute ITP, it seems wise

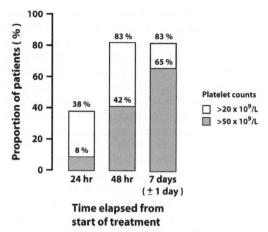

Fig. 6. Platelet response to short-course oral prednisone (4 mg kg^{-1} d^{-1} for 4 d) among 25 children who had acute ITP. (*From* Carcao MD, Zipursky A, Butchart S, et al. Short-course oral prednisone therapy in children presenting with acute immune thrombocytopenic purpura (ITP). Acta Paediatr Suppl 1998;424:71–4; with permission.)

to use high-dose corticosteroid regimens for as short a period of time as is necessary to achieve a clinically meaningful endpoint (eg, cessation of bleeding or achievement of a platelet count >20 × 10^9/L). This approach minimizes the predictable, and sometimes serious, adverse effects of long-term corticosteroid therapy (reviewed by Beck and colleagues[45]). A fall in platelet count often occurs during the period of tapering corticosteroids but not usually to clinically significant levels.

Intravenous Immunoglobulin G

Imbach and colleagues[46] first reported that IV infusion of a pooled, largely monomeric IgG preparation produced a rapid reversal of thrombocytopenia in children who had acute and chronic ITP. This landmark observation was confirmed subsequently by several investigators (reviewed by Blanchette and Carcao[22]). Transient blockade of Fc receptors on macrophages in the reticuloendothelial system, especially the spleen, is believed to play a major role in the immediate, and often dramatic, platelet responses observed after treatment of children who have ITP using a high dose of IVIG (1–2 g/kg). Two Canadian prospective randomized clinical trials are instructive in the context of IVIG treatment of children who have acute ITP. In the first study, reported by Blanchette and colleagues[47] in 1993, 53 children who had acute ITP and platelet counts less than 20 × 10^9/L were randomized to receive IVIG (1 g/kg on 2 consecutive days), oral prednisone (4 mg/kg per day × 7 days with tapering and discontinuation by day 21), or expectant management (no treatment). The rate of platelet response was significantly faster in children who received treatment compared with those managed expectantly; for the endpoint of time (days) taken to achieve a platelet count greater than or equal to 20 × 10^9/L, IVIG and corticosteroids were equivalent, whereas IVIG was superior to oral corticosteroid therapy for the endpoint of time (days) taken to achieve a platelet count greater than 50 × 10^9/L. Bleeding symptoms were not recorded in this study, however; the platelet count alone was used as a surrogate marker for response. The follow-up Canadian randomized trial compared two IVIG treatment regimens (1 g/kg on 2 consecutive days and 0.8 g/kg once), oral prednisone (4 mg/kg per day for 7 days with tapering and discontinuation by day 21), and for the subset of children who were blood group rhesus (D) positive, IV anti-D (25 μg/kg on 2 consecutive days).[48] The key findings from this second randomized trial in children who had newly diagnosed ITP and platelet counts less than 20×10^9/L were (1) a single dose of IVIG (0.8 g/kg) was as effective as the larger dose of IVIG 1 g/kg for 2 days in raising the platelet count and (2) both IVIG regimens were superior to IV anti-D administered as 25 μg/kg for 2 days for the clinically important endpoint of time (number of days) to achieve a platelet count greater than or equal to 20×10^9/L. Bleeding symptoms were not recorded in the study. The choice of the 0.8 g/kg dose as a single infusion reflected the early observation by Imbach and colleagues[49] that in children who had acute ITP treated with 0.4 g/kg of IVIG daily for 5 consecutive days, platelet responses often were observed after the first two infusions. These studies show that treatment with corticosteroids or IVIG can produce a rapid rise in the platelet count of children who have ITP with the caveat that the effect on bleeding symptoms was not assessed. As a result of these observations, the authors recommend that if a decision is made to treat children who have newly diagnosed ITP with IVIG, the initial dose should be 0.8 to 1.0 g/kg administered as a single infusion with subsequent IVIG doses given based on the clinical situation and follow-up platelet counts. Reflex administration of a second dose of IVIG (ie, a total dose of 2 g/kg) generally is not necessary and for the majority of children only leads to an increased frequency of adverse side effects (eg, headache, nausea, or vomiting) and higher costs.

It generally is accepted that IVIG therapy in children who have ITP, although expensive, is safe. High doses (2 g/kg), however, frequently are associated with side effects, principally fever and headache.[47] Other uncommon but clinically significant treatment-associated adverse effects include neutropenia and hemolytic anemia caused by alloantibodies in the IVIG preparations and self-limiting aseptic meningitis that generally occurs a few days after IVIG therapy. This latter complication is characterized by severe headache and, for the subset of children who still are significantly thrombocytopenic, often prompts investigation with a CT scan to rule out an ICH. On a reassuring note, although IVIG is a human plasma–derived product, current commercially available IVIG preparations are treated with highly effective measures to inactivate lipid-coated viruses, such as HIV and hepatitis C.

Intravenous Anti-D

In 1983, Salama and colleagues[50] reported that the IV infusion of anti-D resulted in the reversal of thrombocytopenia in patients who had ITP and were rhesus (D) positive. The investigators speculated that the beneficial effect of anti-D was due to the competitive inhibition of reticuloendothelial function by preferential sequestration of immunoglobulin-coated autologous red blood cells (RBCs). These observations subsequently were confirmed by several investigators. In a report that detailed experience with IV anti-D treatment in 272 subjects who had ITP, Scaradavou and colleagues[51] documented several important findings, including (1) anti-D at conventional doses is ineffective in splenectomized subjects; (2) platelet responses are significantly better in children compared with adults; and (3) responders to IV anti-D generally respond on retreatment. There was a trend toward a higher platelet count after therapy in patients who received 40 to 60 μg/kg of IV anti-D compared with those who received less than or equal to 40 μg/kg. The dose response to IV anti-D is of importance. A recent report by Tarantino and colleagues,[52] describing the results of a prospective randomized clinical trial of IV anti-D (50 μg/kg and 75 μg/kg) and IVIG (0.8 g/kg) in 101 children who had acute ITP and platelet counts less than 20×10^9/L, clearly established that IV anti-D (75 μg/kg) is superior to IV anti-D (50 μg/kg) and equivalent to IVIG (0.8 g/kg) with respect to the numbers of cases with platelet counts greater than 20×10^9/L at 24 hours after therapy.

Short-term adverse effects, such as fever, chills, and nausea/vomiting, are more frequent with a 75-µg/kg than a 50-µg/kg dose and are likely related to release of pro-inflammatory cytokines/chemokines after IV anti-D.[53] These side effects can be ameliorated/prevented by premedication of patients with acetaminophen/corticosteroids. The most predictable adverse effect of anti-D therapy in subjects who are rhesus (D) positive is a fall in hemoglobin level due to RBC destruction by infused RBC alloantibodies. The fall in hemoglobin occurs within 1 week of the anti-D therapy with recovery generally evident by day 21. In the Scaradavou study, the mean hemoglobin decrease was 0.8 g/dL at 7 days post IV anti-D treatment, and only 16% of cases had a hemoglobin decrease greater than 2.1 g/dL.[51] In occasional cases, abrupt severe intravascular hemolysis is reported after therapy; the majority of these cases were in adults, some of whom had comorbid diseases.[54] This complication also is reported in rare cases after IVIG therapy. Physicians who treat children who have ITP using anti-D should be aware of this complication and advise parents and children to report symptoms and signs, such as excessive tiredness or pallor or passage of dark (tea-colored) urine, promptly. No clinically significant increase in treatment-related hemolysis has been reported with 75 versus 50 µg/kg of IV anti-D, and a single dose of 75 µg/kg of anti-D now can be recommended as standard dosing for the treatment of children who have acute ITP and are rhesus (D) positive.

TO PERFORM A BONE MARROW ASPIRATE OR NOT

There is consensus that bone marrow aspiration is not necessary for children who have newly diagnosed typical acute ITP if management involves observation or plasma based therapies, such as IVIG or anti-D. The contentious issue is whether or not a bone marrow aspirate should be performed in children who have typical acute ITP before starting corticosteroids to avoid missing, and therefore treating inappropriately, an underlying leukemia. The results of a retrospective study of bone marrow aspirates performed in children who have suspected acute ITP are instructive in this regard.[55] No children who had typical laboratory features, defined as a normal hemoglobin level and total white blood cell and neutrophil count for age, had underlying leukemia; cases of leukemia, however, were observed in children who had atypical laboratory features. A bone marrow examination, therefore, should be considered mandatory in atypical cases of childhood acute ITP, defined as those who have lassitude, protracted fever, bone or joint pain, and unexplained anemia, neutropenia, or macrocytosis. The diagnosis should be questioned, particularly in those children who fail to remit. The most common diagnosis to emerge after isolated thrombocytopenia in a well child is aplastic anemia.

TO HOSPITALIZE OR NOT

The majority of children who have newly diagnosed acute ITP and platelet counts less than 20×10^9/L are hospitalized. The figure was 83% in the first United Kingdom National Survey[14] and 78% of 1995 children who had newly diagnosed ITP reported by Kühne and colleagues[12] on behalf of the ICIS. This high hospitalization rate is driven by the decision to treat and the perceived need for a bone marrow aspirate before starting corticosteroid therapy. If a conservative management approach is used, with bone marrow aspiration and treatment reserved for selected cases only (eg, those with atypical features or clinically significant bleeding), a low rate of hospitalization can be achieved.[37] Outpatient infusion of IVIG or anti-D also is an option in selected cases.

CHRONIC IMMUNE THROMBOCYTOPENIC PURPURA

Conventionally, chronic ITP is defined as thrombocytopenia (platelet count less than $150 \times 10^9/L$) persisting for longer than 6 months from the onset of illness. Using this definition, approximately 20% to 25% of children manifest chronic ITP at 6 months after the initial diagnosis of ITP. Many children who have platelet counts in the range of 30 to $150 \times 10^9/L$, however, require no platelet-enhancing therapy and some enter a spontaneous complete remission in the 6 to 24 months after initial presentation.[24] The clinically important subgroup of children is those who have platelet counts less than or equal to $20 \times 10^9/L$ at 6 months from initial diagnosis and who require ongoing platelet-enhancing therapy because of bleeding symptoms. This is the small group of children for whom second-line therapies (eg, rituximab) or splenectomy may need to be considered, approximately 5% of children who have acute ITP at the time point of 18 months after initial presentation.[26]

MANAGEMENT
Presplenectomy Management

Medical management is preferred over splenectomy for children who have chronic ITP for less than 12 months. Treatment options include oral corticosteroids (including pulse oral dexamethasone), IVIG, and IV anti-D (reviewed by Blanchette and Price[56]). Avoidance of medications known to affect platelet function adversely, especially aspirin, should be stressed and high-risk competitive or contact activities should be avoided during periods of severe thrombocytopenia. The goal should be to maintain a hemostatically "safe" platelet count while avoiding the potential toxicities and cost of overtreatment, in particular the well-known adverse effects of protracted corticosteroid therapy. If treatment is recommended, the authors' preference is to use short courses of relatively high-dose oral prednisone (4 mg/kg per day for 4 days, maximum daily dose 180 mg), IVIG (0.8 to 1.0 g/kg once), or, for children who are rhesus (D) positive, IV anti-D (75 μg/kg once), with all treatments given intermittently based on clinical need. Treatment is, in the main, outpatient based and parents and children (if of an appropriate age) should be informed about the risk, benefits, and alternatives to treatment, including the remote risk for transfusion-transmitted infections with virus-inactivated plasma-based therapies, such as IVIG and IV anti-D. The advantage of anti-D over IVIG in this clinical setting relates to the ease of administration (anti-D can be infused over 5–10 minutes compared with several hours for IVIG), significantly lower cost in some countries, and a comparable platelet-enhancing effect.

Splenectomy

Guidelines for splenectomy in children who have ITP are conservative, reflecting the significant spontaneous remissions that occur in children who have early chronic ITP and the small but finite risk of overwhelming postsplenectomy sepsis, a complication especially worrisome in children under 6 years of age. A group of United Kingdom pediatric hematologists recommended in 1992 that in children who have ITP, "splenectomy should not be considered before at least six months and preferably 12 months from the time of diagnosis, unless there are very major problems".[33] New guidelines published in 2003 state that splenectomy rarely is indicated in children who have ITP but comment that "severe lifestyle restrictions, crippling menorrhagia and life-threatening hemorrhage may give good reason for the procedure".[36] Practice guidelines developed for the American Society of Hematology (ASH) advocate that elective splenectomy be considered in children who have persistence of ITP for at least 12 months and who manifest bleeding symptoms and a platelet count below 10×10^9/L (children ages 3 to 12) or 10 to 30×10^9/L (children ages 8 to 12 years).[5] Only a few scenarios were considered, however. The efficacy and relative safety of splenectomy led Mantadakis and Buchanan[57] to recommend splenectomy for children older than 5 years who have had symptomatic ITP longer than 6 months' duration and whose quality of life is affected adversely by hemorrhagic manifestations, constant fear of bleeding, or complication of medical therapies. In contrast, the Israeli ITP Study Group recommends early splenectomy in children not responding rapidly to corticosteroid therapy.[58] This seems premature as many children likely remit spontaneously given time.

If elective splenectomy is performed, the laparoscopic technique is preferred; accessory spleens often are present and should be removed at the time of surgical intervention. Preoperative treatment with corticosteroids, IVIG, or anti-D is considered appropriate for children who have platelet counts less than 30×10^9/L. The outcome after splenectomy in children who have primary ITP is good, and a complete remission rate of approximately 70% can be expected after the procedure (**Table 2**). Some of the children reported in these series, however, may have entered a spontaneous remission over time without splenectomy. In adults, potential predictors of success after splenectomy include imaging studies to document the sites of platelet destruction and the historical response to medical therapies, such as IVIG and IV anti-D.[63–65] The results of imaging studies are insufficiently specific, however, and reports of the predictive value of prior responses to medical therapies too conflicting to recommend that this information be used to determine reliably whether or not a splenectomy should be performed in children who have chronic ITP.

PROTECTION AGAINST OVERWHELMING POSTSPLENECTOMY INFECTION

Before elective splenectomy, children who have ITP should be immunized with the hemophilus influenza type b and pneumococcal vaccines; depending on their age and immunization history, meningococcal vaccine also is recommended.[66] Because the protection provided after immunization is incomplete (not all pneumococcal serotypes are included in the currently available vaccines), daily prophylaxis with penicillin, or an equivalent antibiotic if the child is allergic to penicillin, is recommended for children up to 5 years of age and for at least 1 year after splenectomy to prevent pneumococcal sepsis, in particular. Some physicians recommend continuing antibiotic prophylaxis into adulthood. All febrile episodes should be assessed carefully and the use of

Table 2
Complete remission rates after splenectomy in children who had immune thrombocytopenic purpura

	Number of Cases	Complete Remission (%)
ASH review[5]	271	72
Blanchette (1992)[59]	21	81
Ben Yehuda (1994)[58]	27	67
Mantadakis (2000)[57]	38	76
Aronis (2004)[60]	33	79
Kühne (2006)[61]	134	67
Wang (2006)[62]	65	89
	589	74

parenteral antibiotics considered because overwhelming postsplenectomy infection can occur despite immunization and use of antibiotic prophylaxis. Children should wear a medical alert bracelet indicating that they have had a splenectomy and when traveling abroad should carry an explanatory letter and a supply of antibiotics to be started in the event of a febrile episode while arranging for medical assessment. In the United Kingdom, patients are issued with a card stating that they are asplenic.

EMERGENCY TREATMENT

On rare occasions, children who have acute ITP and severe thrombocytopenia may manifest symptoms or signs suggestive of organ- or life-threatening hemorrhage (eg, ICH). Management of such cases is challenging and should involve measures that have the potential to increase the circulating platelet count rapidly. An approach commonly used involves the immediate IV administration of methylprednisolone (30 mg/kg, maximum dose 1 g) over 20 to 30 minutes plus a larger than usual (two- to threefold) infusion of donor platelets in an attempt to boost the circulating platelet count temporarily. After administration of IV methylprednisolone and platelets, an infusion of IVIG (1 g/kg) should be started with IVIG and methylprednisolone repeated daily as indicated clinically, generally for at least 1 to 2 days. Survival of transfused donor platelets may be improved after IVIG therapy.[67] Depending on the specific clinical circumstances, an emergency splenectomy may need to be considered. Continuous infusion of platelets may be beneficial in selected cases. Experience with recombinant factor VIIa is limited but this hemostatic agent can be administered rapidly and should be considered in critical situations.[68]

COMBINED CYTOPENIAS

The combination of ITP and clinically significant autoimmune hemolytic anemia (Evans's syndrome) or autoimmune neutropenia occurs in a minority of cases.[69–73] Affected children often are older than those who present with typical acute ITP. The clinical course is variable and often prolonged with significant morbidity and mortality reported in retrospective series (**Table 3**). Response to single-agent therapy or splenectomy often is poor;[74] combination immunosuppressive therapy may yield improved results.[74–77] Underlying causes for the combined cytopenias include SLE, CVID, and the autoimmune lymphoproliperative syndrome (ALPS). Malignancies (eg, Hodgkin's disease and lymphomas) and chronic infections (eg, HIV and hepatitis C) also need to be considered. The possibility of these conditions should be kept in

Table 3 Retrospective reviews of patients who had Evans's syndrome					
Investigator	Number of Cases	Median Age at Onset (y)	Male:Female Ratio	Associated Neutropenia	Number of Deaths
Wang (1988)[69]	10	7.5	6:4	50%	3/10
Savaşan (1997)[70]	11	5.5	10:1	55%	4/11
Matthew (1997)[71]	42	7.7	22:20	38%	3/42
Blouin (2005)[72]	36	4.0	20:16	27%	3/36
	99		58:41	37%	13/99 (13.1%)

mind in children who have combined immune cytopenias and appropriate investigations performed.

Features of CVID include recurrent bacterial infections (especially sinopulmonary), gastrointestinal disturbances similar to those seen in children who have inflammatory bowel disease, and granulomatous disease, especially affecting the lungs.[78–82] Laboratory features include low serum IgG levels and in some cases low serum IgA and IgM levels, absent or impaired specific antibody responses to infection or vaccination, and variable abnormalities of the immune system (eg, decreased numbers or function of T and B cells). Approximately 10% to 20% of subjects who have CVID manifest autoimmune cytopenias.[79] Treatment consists of regular IVIG replacement therapy.[82] Caution should be exercised about performing splenectomy in cases of CVID-associated ITP because of the risk for overwhelming postsplenectomy infection.

ALPS is a rare but important disorder because of defects in programmed cell death of lymphocytes.[83–87] Mutations in the Fas receptor, Fas ligand, and caspase genes are identified in approximately 70% of cases. Clinical features of the disorder include massive lymphadenopathy, most often in the cervical and axillary areas, and hepatosplenomegaly. The laboratory hallmark of ALPS is an increased number of double-negative (CD4-negative and CD8-negative) T cells that express the α/β T-cell receptor. Defective in vitro antigen-induced apoptosis in cultured lymphocytes can be demonstrated in affected cases. For accurate diagnosis of ALPS, these tests should be performed by laboratories familiar with the test methods and in which local normal values are established.[88] The best frontline treatment of patients who have ALPS is with mycophenolate mofetil (MMF); in the largest series of ALPS reported to date of treatment with this immunosuppressive agent, a response rate of 92% was observed.[89] Splenectomy should be avoided in ALPS cases because of the high risk for overwhelming postsplenectomy sepsis.

NEW THERAPIES

First-line therapies in children include corticosteroids, high-dose IVIG, and, for children who are rhesus positive, IV anti-D. Splenectomy is the traditional second-line treatment of those children who have well-established, symptomatic chronic ITP who have failed or are intolerant of first-line therapies. An array of third-line therapies is available for children in whom splenectomy is refused or contraindicated. Agents include azathioprine, cyclophosphamide, danazol, vinca alkaloids, dapsone, cyclosporine, MMF, or combination therapy. As with adults, current evidence supporting effectiveness and safety of these therapies in children who have severe chronic refractory ITP is minimal.[5,90] The decision to choose one of these agents or combinations usually is based on physician preferences and experience. A major difficulty with many of these third-line therapies is modest response rates and frequently a slow onset of action. In addition, bone marrow suppression and an increased incidence of infection complicate treatment with many of the immunosuppressive agents. Before physicians can confidently know the best management for their patients, these treatments, and perhaps combinations of agents and new approaches to treatment, must be evaluated for effectiveness and safety in prospective cohort studies of consecutive patients or randomized controlled trials. Such trials should include measurement of relevant clinical outcomes (eg, bleeding manifestations and quality of life) other than the platelet count alone.[90]

Rituximab is a human murine (chimeric) monoclonal antibody directed against the CD20 antigen expressed on pre-B and mature B lymphocytes. Rituximab eliminates most circulating B cells with recovery of B-cell counts 6 to 12 months after therapy.

Rituximab currently is indicated for the treatment of lymphoma in adults. Because of its ability to deplete autoantibody-producing lymphocytes, it is used off-label to treat patients who have a variety of autoimmune diseases. Experience with rituximab therapy for patients who have ITP is greatest for adults. In a recent systematic review that involved 313 patients from 19 studies, Arnold and colleagues[91] reported a complete response rate, defined as a platelet count greater than 150×10^9/L, in 43.6% of cases (95% CI, 29.5% to 57.7%); 62.5% of cases (95% CI, 52.6% to 72.5%) achieved platelet counts greater than 50×10^9/L. The treatment regimen used most frequently was 375 mg/m^2 administered weekly for 4 weeks. The median time to response was 5.5 weeks and the median response duration 10.5 months. Durable responses were more frequent in patients who achieved complete remission. The largest pediatric series reported data including 36 patients, ages 2.6 to 18.3 years, six of whom had Evans's syndrome.[92] Responses, defined as a platelet count greater than 50×10^9/L during 4 consecutive weeks starting in weeks 9 to 12 after 4 weekly doses of rituximab (375 mg/m^2 per dose), were observed in 31% of cases (CI, 16% to 48%). In adults who had chronic ITP, durable responses lasting longer than 1 year were more likely in complete responders, and these patients also were more likely to respond to retreatment after relapse.[93,94] Although these results are promising, there is an urgent need for randomized control trials to define the role of rituximab as a splenectomy-sparing strategy or as treatment of patients who fail splenectomy and who have severe, symptomatic ITP. Clinically severe, short- and medium-term adverse effects after rituximab therapy for patients who have ITP fortunately are rare. They include therapy-associated serum sickness, immediate and delayed neutropenia, and reactivation of coexisting chronic infections (eg, hepatitis B).[95,96] The recent report of two patients who had SLE who developed progressive multifocal leukoencephalopathy after rituximab therapy prompted an alert from the Food and Drug Administration's MedWatch Program.[96] Although changes in circulating immunoglobulin levels are observed in some children after rituximab therapy, it seems that IVIG replacement therapy for otherwise healthy pediatric patients who have ITP and who do not have underlying immunodeficiency treated with rituximab is unnecessary.[92]

TPO is the primary growth factor in regulation of platelet production.[97] Megakaryopoiesis is controlled by signaling through the c-Mpl receptor present on megakaryocytes and platelets. On the basis that platelet production is impaired in some patients who have ITP, studies evaluated the use of a pegylated, truncated form of human TPO (PEG-megakaryocyte growth and development factor [MGDF]) with encouraging results. PEG-MGDF was immunogenic and induced production of neutralizing anti-TPO antibodies in some recipients, resulting in thrombocytopenia.[98] It was withdrawn, therefore, from further clinical investigation. Recently, nonimmunogenic thrombopoietic peptides (AMG 531) and small nonpeptide molecules (eltrombopag and AKR-501) have been developed[99] (reviewed by Kuter[100]). AMG 531 consists of a peptide-binding domain, which stimulates megakaryopoiesis in the same way as TPO, and a carrier Fc domain. AMG 531 activates c-Mpl receptors to stimulate the growth and maturation of megakaryocytes and this effect ultimately results in increased production of platelets. Preliminary studies with AMG 531 in adults who have ITP are encouraging.[101,102] A prospective pediatric study is underway. Eltrombopag and AKR-501 are small-molecule thrombopoietic receptor agonists administered orally.[99] Early results with eltrombopag in adults who have ITP also are encouraging.[103] Apart from reversible marrow fibrosis in some adult patients treated with AMG 531, these novel platelet-enhancing therapies seem remarkably nontoxic. Their true place in the management of children who have ITP remains to be determined through prospective clinical trials. It should be borne in mind that, based on experience in adults, recurrence of thrombocytopenia in cases of chronic, refractory ITP is likely in most cases once these novel thrombopoiesis-stimulating agents are discontinued.

FUTURE DIRECTIONS

Although much has been learned about the pathogenesis and treatment of ITP over the past 3 decades, many questions remain unanswered. Optimal management of children who have newly diagnosed acute ITP and platelet counts less than 20 × 10^9/L remains the subject of debate and there is an urgent need for a well-designed large trial to address the issues of to treat or not, to perform a bone marrow aspirate or not, and whether or not to hospitalize such children. Experience from the United Kingdom suggests that promotion of conservative guidelines for management of childhood acute ITP can result in a decrease in the frequency of treatment and invasive procedures, such as bone marrow aspirates.[104] The role of new therapies, such as rituximab and thrombopoietic agents, remains to be defined by well-designed, prospective clinical trials. All future clinical trials for childhood ITP should include outcome measures more than the platelet count alone (eg, bleeding scores, health-related quality-of-life assessments, and economic analyses).[105–111] Finally, exchange of information between adult and pediatric hematologists who care for patients who have ITP must be encouraged, especially with regard to guidelines for investigation and management.[112]

REFERENCES

1. Cines DB, Blanchette VS. Immune thrombocytopenic purpura. N Engl J Med 2002;346:995–1008.
2. Harrington WJ, Minnich V, Hollingsworth JW, et al. Demonstration of a thrombocytopenic factor in the blood of patients with thrombocytopenic purpura. J Lab Clin Med 1951;38:1–10.
3. Shulman NR, Marder VJ, Weinrach RS. Similarities between known antiplatelet antibodies and the factor responsible for thrombocytopenia in idiopathic purpura. Physiologic, serologic and isotopic studies. Ann N Y Acad Sci 1965; 124:499–542.
4. Berchtold P, Muller D, Beardsley D, et al. International study to compare antigen-specific methods used for the measurement of antiplatelet autoantibodies. Br J Haematol 1997;96:477–83.
5. George JN, Woolf SH, Raskob GE, et al. Idiopathic thrombocytopenic purpura: a practice guideline developed by explicit methods for the American Society of Hematology. Blood 1996;88:3–40.
6. Louwes H, Lathori OAZ, Vellenga E, et al. Platelet kinetic studies in patients with idiopathic thrombocytopenic purpura. Am J Med 1999;106:430–4.
7. Takahashi R, Sekine N, Nakatake T. Influence of monoclonal antiplatelet glycoprotein antibodies on in vitro human megakaryocyte colony formation and proplatelet formation. Blood 1999;93:1951–8.
8. Cremer M, Schulze H, Linthorst G, et al. Serum levels of thrombopoietin, IL-11, and IL-6 in pediatric thrombocytopenias. Ann Hematol 1999;78:401–7.
9. Payne BA, Pierre RV. Pseudothrombocytopenia: a laboratory artifact with potentially serious consequences. Mayo Clin Proc 1984;59:123–5.
10. Lowe EJ, Buchanan GR. Idiopathic thrombocytopenic purpura diagnosed during the second decade of life. J Pediatr 2002;141:253–8.

11. Drachman JG. Inherited thrombocytopenia: when a low platelet count does not mean ITP. Blood 2004;103:390–8.
12. Kühne T, Imbach P, Bolton-Maggs PHB, et al. Newly diagnosed idiopathic thrombocytopenic purpura in childhood: an observational study. Lancet 2001; 358:2122–5.
13. Kühne T, Buchanan GR, Zimmerman S, et al. A prospective comparative study of 2540 infants and children with newly diagnosed idiopathic thrombocytopenic purpura (ITP) from the Intercontinental Childhood ITP Study Group. J Pediatr 2003;143:605–8.
14. Bolton-Maggs PHB, Moon I. Assessment of UK practice for management of acute childhood idiopathic thrombocytopenia purpura against published guidelines. Lancet 1997;350:620–3.
15. Sutor AH, Harms A, Kaufmehl K. Acute immune thrombocytopenia (ITP) in childhood: retrospective and prospective survey in Germany. Semin Thromb Hemost 2001;27:253–67.
16. Rosthoj S, Hedlund-Treutiger I, Rajantie J, et al. Duration and morbidity of newly diagnosed idiopathic thrombocytopenic purpura in children. A prospective Nordic study of an unselected cohort. J Pediatr 2003;143:302–7.
17. Oski FA, Naiman JL. Effect of live measles vaccine on the platelet count. N Engl J Med 1966;275:352–6.
18. Miller E, Waight P, Farrington CP, et al. Idiopathic thrombocytopaenic purpura and MMR vaccine. Arch Dis Child 2001;84:227–9.
19. Black C, Kaye JA, Jick H. MMR vaccine and idiopathic thrombocytopenic purpura. Br J Clin Pharmacol 2003;55:107–11.
20. Choi SI, McClure PD. Idiopathic thrombocytopenic purpura in childhood. Can Med Assoc J 1967;97:562–8.
21. Lusher JM, Zuelzer WW. Idiopathic thrombocytopenic purpura in childhood. J Pediatr 1966;68:971–9.
22. Blanchette VS, Carcao M. Childhood acute immune thrombocytopenic purpura: 20 years later. Semin Thromb Hemost 2003;29:605–17.
23. Edslev PW, Rosthøj S, Treutiger I, et al. A clinical score predicting a brief and uneventful course of newly diagnosed idiopathic thrombocytopenic purpura in children. Br J Haematol 2007;138:513–6.
24. Imbach P, Kühne T, Müller D, et al. Childhood ITP: 12 months follow-up data from the prospective Registry I of the Intercontinental Childhood ITP Study Group (ICIS). Pediatr Blood Cancer 2006;46:351–6.
25. Reid MM. Chronic idiopathic thrombocytopenic purpura: incidence, treatment and outcome. Arch Dis Child 1995;72:125–8.
26. Imbach P, Akatsuka J, Blanchette V, et al. Immunthrombocytopenic purpura as a model for pathogenesis and treatment of autoimmunity. Eur J Pediatr 1995; 154(Suppl 3):S60–4.
27. Lilleyman JS. On behalf of the Paediatric Haematology Forum of the British Society of Haematology. Intracranial haemorrhage in idiopathic thrombocytopenic purpura. Arch Dis Child 1994;71:251–3.
28. Lee MS, Kim WC. Intracranial hemorrhage associated with idiopathic thrombocytopenic purpura: report of seven patients and a meta-analysis. Neurology 1998;50:1160–3.
29. Butros LJ, Bussel JB. Intracranial hemorrhage in immune thrombocytopenic purpura: a retrospective analysis. J Pediatr Hematol Oncol 2003;25:660–4.
30. Woerner SJ, Abildgaard CF, French BN. Intracranial hemorrhage in children with idiopathic thrombocytopenic purpura. Pediatrics 1981;67:453–60.

31. Medeiros D, Buchanan GR. Major hemorrhage in children with idiopathic thrombocytopenic purpura: immediate response to therapy and long-term outcome. J Pediatr 1998;133:334–9.
32. Bolton-Maggs PHB, Dickerhoff R, Vora AJ. The non-treatment of childhood ITP (or "The art of medicine consists of amusing the patient until nature cures the disease"). Semin Thromb Hemost 2001;27:269–75.
33. Eden OB, Lilleyman JS. On behalf of the British Paediatric Haematology Group. Guidelines for management of idiopathic thrombocytopenic purpura. Arch Dis Child 1992;67:1056–8.
34. Lilleyman JS. Management of childhood idiopathic thrombocytopenic purpura. Br J Haematol 1999;105:871–5.
35. De Mattia D, Del Principe D, Del Vecchio GC, et al. Acute childhood idiopathic thrombocytopenic purpura: AIEOP concensus guidelines for diagnosis and treatment. Haematologica 2000;85:420–4.
36. Provan D, Newland A, Norfolk D, et al. Working Party of the British Committee for Standards in Haematology General Haematology Task Force. Guidelines for the investigation and management of idiopathic thrombocytopenic purpura in adults, children and in pregnancy. Br J Haematol 2003;120:574–96.
37. Dickerhoff R, von Ruecker A. The clinical course of immune thrombocytopenic purpura in children who did not receive intravenous immunoglobulins or sustained prednisone treatment. J Pediatr 2000;137:629–32.
38. Sartorius JA. Steroid treatment of idiopathic thrombocytopenic purpura in children. Preliminary results of a randomized cooperative study. Am J Pediatr Hematol Oncol 1984;6:165–9.
39. Buchanan GR, Holtkamp CA. Prednisone therapy for children with newly diagnosed idiopathic thrombocytopenic purpura. A randomized clinical trial. Am J Pediatr Hematol Oncol 1984;6:355–61.
40. Özsoylu S, Sayli TR, Öztürk G. Oral megadose methylprednisolone versus intravenous immunoglobulin for acute childhood idiopathic thrombocytopenic purpura. Pediatr Hematol Oncol 1993;10:317–21.
41. Suarez CR, Rademaker D, Hasson A, et al. High-dose steroids in childhood acute idiopathic thrombocytopenia purpura. Am J Pediatr Hematol Oncol 1986;8:111–5.
42. van Hoff J, Ritchey AK. Pulse methylprednisolone therapy for acute childhood idiopathic thrombocytopenic purpura. J Pediatr 1988;113:563–6.
43. Jayabose S, Patel P, Inamdar S, et al. Use of intravenous methylprednisolone in acute idiopathic thrombocytopenic purpura. Am J Pediatr Hematol Oncol 1987;9:133–5.
44. Carcao MD, Zipursky A, Butchart S, et al. Short-course oral prednisone therapy in children presenting with acute immune thrombocytopenic purpura (ITP). Acta Paediatr Suppl 1998;424:71–4.
45. Beck CE, Nathan PC, Parkin PC, et al. Corticosteroids versus intravenous immune globulin for the treatment of acute immune thrombocytopenic purpura in children: a systematic review and meta-analysis of randomized controlled trials. J Pediatr 2005;147:521–7.
46. Imbach P, Barandun S, d'Apuzzo V, et al. High-dose intravenous gammaglobulin for idiopathic thrombocytopenic purpura in childhood. Lancet 1981;1228–31.
47. Blanchette VS, Luke B, Andrew M, et al. A prospective, randomized trial of high-dose intravenous immune globulin G therapy, oral prednisone therapy, and no therapy in childhood acute immune thrombocytopenic purpura. J Pediatr 1993;123:989–95.

48. Blanchette V, Imbach P, Andrew M, et al. Randomised trial of intravenous immunoglobulin G, intravenous anti-D and oral prednisone in childhood acute immune thrombocytopenic purpura. Lancet 1994;344:703–7.

49. Imbach P, Wagner HP, Berchtold W, et al. Intravenous immunoglobulin versus oral corticosteroids in acute immune thrombocytopenic purpura in childhood. Lancet 1985;464–8.

50. Salama A, Mueller-Eckhardt C, Kiefel V. Effect of intravenous immunoglobulin in immune thrombocytopenia. Competitive inhibition of reticuloendothelial system function by sequestration of autologous red blood cells? Lancet 1983;193–5.

51. Scaradavou A, Woo B, Woloski BMR, et al. Intravenous anti-D treatment of immune thrombocytopenic purpura: experience in 272 patients. Blood 1997; 89:2689–700.

52. Tarantino MD, Young G, Bertolone SJ, et al. Single dose of anti-D immune globulin at 75 µg/kg is as effective as intravenous immune globulin at rapidly raising the platelet count in newly diagnosed immune thrombocytopenic purpura in children. J Pediatr 2006;148:489–94.

53. Newman GC, Novoa MV, Fodero EM, et al. A dose of 75 µg/kg/d of i.v. anti-D increases the platelet count more rapidly and for a longer period of time than 50 µg/kg/d in adults with immune thrombocytopenic purpura. Br J Haematol 2001;112:1076–8.

54. Gaines AR. Disseminated intravascular coagulation associated with acute hemoglobinemia or hemoglobinuria following $Rh_o(D)$ immune globulin intravenous administration for immune thrombocytopenic purpura. Blood 2005;106: 1532–7.

55. Calpin C, Dick P, Poon A, et al. Is bone marrow aspiration needed in acute childhood idiopathic thrombocytopenic purpura to rule out leukemia? Arch Pediatr Adolesc Med 1998;152:345–7.

56. Blanchette VS, Price V. Childhood chronic immune thrombocytopenic purpura: unresolved issues. J Pediatr Hematol Oncol 2003;25:S28–33.

57. Mantadakis E, Buchanan GR. Elective splenectomy in children with idiopathic thrombocytopenic purpura. J Pediatr Hematol Oncol 2000;22:148–53.

58. Ben-Yehuda D, Gillis S, Eldor A, et al. Clinical and therapeutic experience in 712 Israeli patients with idiopathic thrombocytopenic purpura. Acta Haematol 1994; 91:1–6.

59. Blanchette VS, Kirby MA, Turner C. Role of intravenous immunoglobulin G in autoimmune hematologic disorders. Semin Hematol 1992;29:72–82.

60. Aronis S, Platokouki H, Avgeri M, et al. Retrospective evaluation of long-term efficacy and safety of splenectomy in chronic idiopathic thrombocytopenic purpura in children. Acta Paediatr 2004;93:638–42.

61. Kühne T, Blanchette V, Buchanan GR, et al. Splenectomy in children with idiopathic thrombocytopenic purpura: a prospective study of 134 children from the Intercontinental Childhood ITP Study Group. Pediatr Blood Cancer 2007; 49:829–34.

62. Wang T, Xu M, Ji L, et al. Splenectomy for chronic idiopathic thrombocytopenic purpura in children: a single centre study in China. Acta Haematol 2006;115: 39–45.

63. Najean Y, Rain J-D, Billotey C. The site of destruction of autologous [111] In-labelled platelets and the efficiency of splenectomy in children and adults with idiopathic thrombocytopenic purpura: a study of 578 patients with 268 splenectomies. Br J Haematol 1997;97:547–50.

64. Holt D, Brown J, Terrill K, et al. Response to intravenous immunoglobulin predicts splenectomy response in children with immune thrombocytopenic purpura. Pediatrics 2003;111:87–90.
65. Bussel JB, Kaufmann CP, Ware RE, et al. Do the acute platelet responses of patients with immune thrombocytopenic purpura (ITP) to IV anti-D and to IV gammaglobulin predict response to subsequent splenectomy? Am J Hematol 2001;67:27–33.
66. Price VE, Dutta S, Blanchette VS, et al. The prevention and treatment of bacterial infections in children with asplenia or hyposplenia: practice considerations at the Hospital for Sick Children, Toronto. Pediatr Blood Cancer 2006;46:597–603.
67. Baumann MA, Menitove JE, Aster RH, et al. Urgent treatment of idiopathic thrombocytopenic purpura with single-dose gammaglobulin infusion followed by platelet transfusion. Ann Intern Med 1986;104:808–9.
68. Barnes C, Blanchette V, Canning P, et al. Recombinant FVIIa in the management of intracerebral haemorrhage in severe thrombocytopenia unresponsive to platelet-enhancing treatment. Transfus Med 2005;15:145–50.
69. Wang WC. Evans syndrome in childhood: pathophysiology, clinical course, and treatment. Am J Pediatr Hematol Oncol 1988;10:330–8.
70. Savaşan S, Warrier I, Ravindranath Y. The spectrum of Evans' syndrome. Arch Dis Child 1997;77:245–8.
71. Mathew P, Chen G, Wang W. Evans syndrome: results of a national survey. J Pediatr Hematol Oncol 1997;19:433–7.
72. Blouin P, Auvrignon A, Pagnier A, et al. [Evans' syndrome: a retrospective study from the ship (french society of pediatric hematology and immunology) (36 cases)]. Arch Pediatr 2005;12:1600–7 [in French].
73. Calderwood S, Blanchette V, Doyle J, et al. Idiopathic thrombocytopenia and neutropenia in childhood. Am J Pediatr Hematol Oncol 1994;16:95–101.
74. Norton A, Roberts I. Management of Evans syndrome. Br J Haematol 2005;132: 125–37.
75. Scaradavou A, Bussel J. Evans syndrome: results of a pilot study utilizing a multi-agent treatment protocol. J Pediatr Hematol Oncol 1995;17:290–5.
76. Uçar B, Akgün N, Aydoğdu SD, et al. Treatment of refractory Evans' syndrome with cyclosporine and prednisone. Pediatr Int 1999;41:104–7.
77. Williams JA, Boxer LA. Combination therapy for refractory idiopathic thrombocytopenic purpura in adolescents. J Pediatr Hematol Oncol 2003;25:232–5.
78. Cunningham-Rundles C. Hematologic complications of primary immune deficiencies. Blood Rev 2002;16:61–4.
79. Michel M, Chanet V, Galicier L, et al. Autoimmune thrombocytopenic purpura and common variable immunodeficiency. Analysis of 21 cases and review of the literature. Medicine 2004;83:254–63.
80. Knight AK, Cunningham-Rundles C. Inflammatory and autoimmune complications of common variable immune deficiency. Autoimmun Rev 2006;5:156–9.
81. Brandt D, Gershwin ME. Common variable immune deficiency and autoimmunity. Autoimmun Rev 2006;5:465–70.
82. Wang J, Cunningham-Rundles C. Treatment and outcome of autoimmune hematologic disease in common variable immunodeficiency (CVID). J Autoimmun 2005;25:57–62.
83. Sneller MC, Dale JK, Straus SE. Autoimmune lymphoproliferative syndrome. Curr Opin Rheumatol 2003;15:417–21.
84. Oliveira JB, Fleischer T. Autoimmune lymphoproliferative syndrome. Curr Opin Allergy Clin Immunol 2004;4:497–503.

85. Rao VK, Straus SE. Causes and consequences of the autoimmune lymphoproliferative syndrome. Hematology 2006;11:15–23.
86. Worth A, Thrasher AJ, Gaspar HB. Autoimmune lymphoproliferative syndrome: molecular basis of disease and clinical phenotype. Br J Haematol 2006;133:124–40.
87. Savaşan S, Warrier I, Buck S, et al. Increased lymphocyte Fas expression and high incidence of common variable immunodeficiency disorder in childhood Evans' syndrome. Clin Immunol 2007;125:224–9.
88. Teachey DT, Manno CS, Axsom KM, et al. Unmasking Evans syndrome: T-cell phenotype and apoptotic response reveal autoimmune lymphoproliferative syndrome (ALPS). Blood 2005;105:2443–8.
89. Rao VK, Dugan F, Dale JK, et al. Use of mycophenolate mofetil for chronic, refractory immune cytopenias in children with autoimmune lymphoproliferative syndrome. Br J Haematol 2005;129:534–8.
90. Vesely SK, Perdue JJ, Rizvi MA, et al. Management of adult patients with persistent idiopathic thrombocytopenic purpura following splenectomy. A systematic review. Ann Intern Med 2004;140:112–20.
91. Arnold DM, Dentali F, Crowther MA, et al. Systematic review: efficacy and safety of rituximab for adults with idiopathic thrombocytopenic purpura. Ann Intern Med 2007;146:25–33.
92. Bennett CM, Rogers ZR, Kinnamon DD, et al. Prospective phase 1/2 study of rituximab in childhood and adolescent chronic immune thrombocytopenic purpura. Blood 2006;107:2639–42.
93. Cooper N, Stasi R, Cunningham-Rundles S, et al. The efficacy and safety of B-cell depletion with anti-CD20 monoclonal antibody in adults with chronic immune thrombocytopenic purpura. Br J Haematol 2004;125:232–9.
94. Perrotta AL. Re-treatment of chronic idiopathic thrombocytopenic purpura with Rituximab: literature review. Clin Appl Thromb Hemost 2006;12:97–100.
95. Larrar S, Guitton C, Willems M, et al. Severe hematological side effects following Rituximab therapy in children. Haematologica 2006;91:101–2.
96. Anonymous. Rituxan warning. FDA Consum 2007;41:2.
97. Kaushansky K. Thrombopoietin. N Engl J Med 1998;339:746–54.
98. Li J, Yang C, Xia Y, et al. Thrombocytopenia caused by the development of antibodies to thrombopoietin. Blood 2001;98:3241–8.
99. Erickson-Miller CL, DeLorme E, Tian SS, et al. Discovery and characterization of a selective, nonpeptidyl thrombopoietin receptor agonist. Exp Hematol 2005;33:85–93.
100. Kuter DJ. New thrombopoietic growth factors. Blood 2007;109:4607–16.
101. Newland A, Caulier MT, Kappers-Klunne M, et al. An open-label, unit dose-finding study of AMG 531, a novel thrombopoiesis-stimulating peptibody, in patients with immune thrombocytopenic purpura. Br J Haematol 2006;135:547–53.
102. Bussel JB, Kuter DJ, George JN, et al. AMG 531, a thrombopoiesis-stimulating protein, for chronic ITP. N Engl J Med 2006;355:1672–81.
103. Bussel JB, Cheng G, Saleh MN, et al. Eltrombopag for the treatment of chronic idiopathic thrombocytopenic purpura. N Engl J Med 2007;357:2237–47.
104. Bolton-Maggs PHB. Management of immune thrombocytopenic purpura. Paediatr Child Health 2007;17:305–10.
105. Buchanan GR, Adix L. Outcome measures and treatment endpoints other than platelet count in childhood idiopathic thrombocytopenic purpura. Semin Thromb Hemost 2001;27:277–85.

106. Barnard D, Woloski M, Feeny D, et al. Development of disease-specific health-related quality of life instruments for children with immune thrombocytopenic purpura and their parents. J Pediatr Hematol Oncol 2003;25:56–62.
107. von Mackensen S, Nilsson C, Jankovic M, et al. Development of a disease-specific quality of life questionnaire for children and adolescents with idiopathic thrombocytopenic purpura (ITP-QoL). Pediatr Blood Cancer 2006;47:688–91.
108. Klaassen RJ, Blanchette VS, Barnard D, et al. Validity, reliability and responsiveness of a new measure of health-related quality of life in children with immune thrombocytopenic purpura: the Kids' ITP Tools. J Pediatr 2007;150:510–5.
109. Buchanan GR, Adix L. Grading of hemorrhage in children with idiopathic thrombocytopenic purpura. J Pediatr 2002;141:683–8.
110. Page KL, Psaila B, Provan D, et al. The immune thrombocytopenic purpura (ITP) bleeding score: assessment of bleeding in patients with ITP. Br J Haematol 2007;138:245–8.
111. O'Brien SH, Ritchey AK, Smith KJ. A cost-utility analysis of treatment for acute childhood idiopathic thrombocytopenic purpura (ITP). Pediatr Blood Cancer 2007;48:173–80.
112. Cines DB, Bussel JB. How I treat idiopathic thrombocytopenic purpura (ITP). Blood 2005;106:2244–51.

Index

Note: Page numbers of article titles are in **boldface** type.

A

Hematol Oncol Clin N Am 24 (2010) 275–286
doi:10.1016/S0889-8588(10)00009-2
0889-8588/10/$ – see front matter © 2010 Elsevier Inc. All rights reserved.

hemonc.theclinics.com

Moving?

Make sure your subscription moves with you!

To notify us of your new address, find your **Clinics Account Number** (located on your mailing label above your name), and contact customer service at:

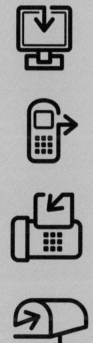

Email: journalscustomerservice-usa@elsevier.com

800-654-2452 (subscribers in the U.S. & Canada)
314-447-8871 (subscribers outside of the U.S. & Canada)

Fax number: 314-447-8029

Elsevier Health Sciences Division
Subscription Customer Service
3251 Riverport Lane
Maryland Heights, MO 63043

*To ensure uninterrupted delivery of your subscription, please notify us at least 4 weeks in advance of move.

Printed and bound by CPI Group (UK) Ltd, Croydon, CR0 4YY

03/10/2024

01040449-0008